Corrective Osteotomies of the Lower Extremity after Trauma

Edited by G. Hierholzer and K. H. Müller

With 214 Figures

Springer-Verlag Berlin Heidelberg New York Tokyo

G. Hierholzer, Professor Dr. med.
Ärztlicher Direktor der
Berufsgenossenschaftlichen
Unfallklinik Duisburg-Bucholz
Großenbaumer Allee 250
D-4100 Duisburg

K. H. Müller, Priv.-Doz. Dr. med.
Erster Oberarzt der
Berufsgenossenschaftlichen
Krankenanstalten „Bergmannsheil Bochum"
Universitätsklinik und Poliklinik
Hunscheidtstraße 1
D-4630 Bochum

Translated from the German by Terry C. Telger

ISBN-13:978-3-642-70776-6 e-ISBN-13:978-3-642-70774-2
DOI: 10.1007/978-3-642-70774-2

Library of Congress Cataloging in Cataloging in Publication Data. Korrekturosteotomien nach Traumen an der unteren Extremität. Corrective osteotomies of the lower extremity after trauma. Translation of: Korrekturosteotomien nach Traumen an der unteren Extremität.
Includes index.
1. Extremities, Lower-Surgery. 2. Osteotomy.
3. Extremities, Lower Wounds and injuries-Complications and sequelae. I. Hierholzer, G. (Günther), 1933.
II. Müller, K. H., 1944. III. Title.
RD779.K67 1985 617'.58099 85-25103

Softcover reprint of the hardcover 1st edition 1985

Typesetting: With a system of the Springer Produktions-Gesellschaft.

2124/3020-543210

List of Contributors

Ahlers, J., Dr. med.
Unfallchirugische Abteilung der Chirurgischen Universitätsklinik, Langenbeckstr. 1, D-6500 Mainz 1

Baur, W., Dr. med.
Orthopädische Klinik Wichernhaus, D-8501 Rummelsberg/Nürnberg

Betz, A., Dr. med.
Chirurgische Klinik der Universität –Innenstadt– Nußbaumstraße 20, D-8000 München 2

Burri, C., Prof. Dr. med.
Direktor der Abteilung für Unfallchirurgie, Hand-, Plastische und Wiederherstellungschirurgie der Universität Ulm, Steinhövelstraße 9, D-7900 Ulm

Conradi, H. W., Dr. med.
Chirurgische Universitätsklinik, Berufsgenossenschaftliche Krankenanstalten „Bergmannsheil", Hunscheidtstraße 1, D-4630 Bochum

Decker, S., Prof. Dr. med.
Leitender Arzt der Unfallabteilung des Friederikenstiftes, Humboldtstraße 5, D-3000 Hannover 1

Friedebold, G., Prof. Dr. med.
Direktor der Orthopädischen Klinik und Poliklinik der Freien Universität im Oskar-Helene-Heim, Clayallee 229, D-1000 Berlin 33

Gotzen, L., Prof. Dr. med.
Direktor der Unfallchirurgischen Klinik der Universitätsklinik, Baldinger Straße, D-3550 Marburg

Gras, U., Dr. med.
Berufsgenossenschaftliche Unfallklinik, Großenbaumer Allee 250, D-4100 Duisburg 28

Hanke, J., Dr. med.
Abteilung Unfallchirurgie am Universitätsklinikum der Gesamthochschule, Hufelandstraße 55, D-4300 Essen

Hierholzer, G., Prof. Dr. med.
Ärztlicher Direktor der Berufsgenossenschaftlichen Unfallklinik, Großenbaumer Allee 250, D-4100 Duisburg 28

Hölter, H. W., Dr. med.
Abteilung Unfallchirurgie am Universitätsklinikum der Gesamthochschule, Hufelandstraße 55, D-4300 Essen

Hörster, G., Priv.-Doz. Dr. med.
Oberarzt der Berufsgenossenschaftlichen Unfallklinik, Großenbaumer Allee 250, D-4100 Duisburg 28

Holz, U., Priv.-Doz. Dr. med.
Leitender Arzt der Abteilung für Unfallchirurgie, Katharinenhospital, Kriegsbergstraße 60, D-7000 Stuttgart 1

Illgner, A., Dr. med.
Unfallchirurgische Klinik der Med. Hochschule, Karl-Wiechert-Allee 9, D-3000 Hannover 61

Jungbluth, K. H., Prof. Dr. med.
Direktor der Abteilung für Unfallchirurgie der Chirurgischen Universitätsklinik Hamburg-Eppendorf, Martinistraße 62, D-2000 Hamburg 20

Kleining, R., Priv.-Doz. Dr. med.
Oberarzt der Berufsgenossenschaftliche Unfallklinik, Großenbaumer Allee 250, D-4100 Duisburg 28

Kuner, E. H., Prof. Dr. med.
Ärztlicher Direktor der Abteilung für Unfallchirurgie der Chirurgischen Universitätsklinik, Hugstetterstraße 55, D-7800 Freiburg

Lies, A., Dr. med.
Oberarzt der Chirurgischen Universitätsklinik, Berufsgenossenschaftliche Krankenanstalten „Bergmannsheil", Hunscheidtstraße 1, D-4630 Bochum

Ludolph, E., Dr. med.
Oberarzt der Berufsgenossenschaftlichen Unfallklinik, Großenbaumer Allee 250, D-4100 Duisburg 28

Morscher, E., Prof. Dr. med.
Vorsteher der Orthopädischen Universitätsklinik, Kantonspital, CH-4055 Basel

Müller, K. H., Priv.-Doz. Dr. med.
Erster Oberarzt der Chirurgischen Universitätsklinik, Berufsgenossenschaftliche Krankenanstalten „Bergmannsheil", Hunscheidtstraße 1, D-4630 Bochum

Müller, M. E., Prof. Dr. med.
Stiftung Maurice E. Müller für Fortbildung und Forschung in orthopädischer Chirurgie, Murtenstraße 35, CH-3008 Bern

Müller-Färber, J., Priv.-Doz. Dr. med.
Chefarzt der Abteilung für Unfall- und Wiederherstellungschirurgie, Kreiskrankenhaus Heidenheim, Schloßhausstraße 100, D-7920 Heidenheim

Muhr, G., Prof. Dr. med.
Direktor der Abteilung für Unfallchirurgie der Chirurgischen Universitätsklinik im Landeskrankenhaus, D-6650 Homburg/Saar

Oest, O., Prof. Dr. med.
Chefarzt der Orthopädischen Klinik, Rosenstraße 2, D-4030 Ratingen

Perren, S. M., Prof. Dr. med.
Leiter des Laboratoriums für experimentelle Chirurgie, Schweizerisches Forschungsinstitut, CH-7270 Davos/Murtenstraße 35, CH-3008 Bern

Peternek, E., Dr. med.
Oberarzt der Chirurgischen Universitätsklinik, Berufsgenossenschaftliche Krankenanstalten „Bergmannsheil", Hunscheidtstraße 1, D-4630 Bochum

Pfeiffer, U., Dr. med.
Orthopädische Klinik Wichernhaus, D-8501 Rummelsberg/Nürnberg

Pfister, U., Priv.-Doz. Dr. med.
Direktor der Abteilung für Unfallchirurgie, Städtisches Klinikum, Moltkestraße 14, D-7500 Karlsruhe 1

Probst, J., Prof. Dr. med.
Ärztlicher Direktor der Berufsgenossenschaftlichen Unfallklinik, Prof.-Küntscher-Straße 8, D-8110 Murnau

Rogmans, D., Dr. med.
Orthopädische Klinik und Poliklinik der Freien Universität im Oskar-Helene-Heim, Clayallee 229, D-1000 Berlin 33

Ritter, G., Prof. Dr. med.
Direktor der Unfallchirurgischen Abteilung der Chirurgischen Universitätsklinik, Langenbeckstraße 1, D-6500 Mainz 1

Skuginna, A., Dr. med.
Oberarzt der Berufsgenossenschaftlichen Unfallklinik, Großenbaumer Allee 250, D-4100 Duisburg 28

Schadewaldt, H., Prof. Dr. med.
Direktor des Institutes für Geschichte der Medizin, Medizinische Einrichtungen der Universität Düsseldorf, Moorenstraße 5, D-4000 Düsseldorf 1

Scheuer, I., Dr. med.
Oberarzt der Chirurgischen Universitätsklinik, Berufsgenossenschaftliche Krankenanstalten „Bergmannsheil", Hunscheidtstraße 1, D-4630 Bochum

Schlickewei, W., Dr. med.
Abteilung für Unfallchirurgie der Chirurgischen Universitätsklinik, Hugstetterstraße 55, D-7800 Freiburg

Schmit-Neuerburg, K. P., Prof. Dr. med.
Direktor der Abteilung Unfallchirurgie am Universitätsklinikum der Gesamthochschule, Hufelandstraße 55, D-4300 Essen

Schneider, R., Prof. Dr. med.
Spez.-Arzt für Chirurgie F.M.H., Klinik Linde, CH-2502 Biel

Schneppendahl, G., Dr. med.
Berufsgenossenschaftliche Unfallkilinik, Großenbaumer Allee 250, D-4100 Duisburg

Schweiberer, L., Prof. Dr. med.
Direktor der Chirurgischen Klinik der Universität —Innenstadt—, Nußbaumstraße 20, D-8000 München 2

Störmer, B., Dr. med.
Oberarzt der Berufsgenossenschaftlichen Unfallklinik, Großenbaumer Alle 250, D-4100 Duisburg 28

Strigl, M. P., Dr. med.
Berufsgenossenschaftliche Unfallklinik, Großenbaumer Allee 250, D-4100 Duisburg 28

Strosche, H., Dr. med.
Chirurgische Universitätsklinik, Berufsgenossenschaftliche Krankenanstalten „Bergmannsheil", Hunscheidtstraße 1, D-4630 Bochum

Tscherne, H., Prof. Dr. med.
Direktor der Unfallchirurgischen Klinik der Med. Hochschule, Karl-Wiechert-Allee 9, D-3000 Hannover 61

Wagner, H., Prof. Dr. med.
Chefarzt der Orthopädischen Klinik Wichernhaus, D-8501 Rummelsberg/Nürnberg

Walter, E., Dr. med.
Abteilung für Unfallchirurgie, Katharinenhospital, Kriegsbergstraße 60, D-7000 Stuttgart 1

Weigand, H., Prof. Dr. med.
Oberarzt der Unfallchirurgischen Abteilung der Chirurgischen Universitätsklinik, Langenbeckstr. 1, D-6500 Mainz 1

Weller, S., Prof. Dr. med.
Ärztlicher Direktor der Berufsgenossenschaftlcihen Unfallklinik, Rosenauer Weg 95, D-7400 Tübingen

Wentzensen, A., Dr. med.
Oberarzt der Berufsgenossenschaftlichen Unfallklinik, Rosenauer Weg 95, D-7400 Tübingen

Willenegger, H., Prof. Dr. med.
AO-International, Murtenstraße 35, CH-3008 Bern

Witt, A. N., Prof. Dr. med., Dr. med. h.c.
em. Direktor der Orthopädischen Universitätsklinik, Harlachingerstraße 51, D-8000 München 80

Wolff, R., Dr. med.
Oberarzt der Orthopädischen Klinik und Poliklinik der Freien Universität Berlin im Oskar-Helene-Heim, Clayallee 229, D-1000 Berlin 33

Wolf, J.-D., Dr. med.
Oberarzt der Chirurgischen Universitätsklinik, Berufsgenossenschaftliche Krankenanstalten „Bergmannsheil", Hunscheidtstraße 1, D-4630 Bochum

Wörsdörfer, O., Priv.-Doz. Dr. med.
Oberarzt der Abteilung für Unfallchirurgie, Hand-, Plastische und Wiederherstellungschirurgie der Universität Ulm, Steinhövelstr. 9, D-7900 Ulm

Zeiler, G., Dr. med.
Oberarzt der Orthopädischen Klinik Wichernhaus, D-8501 Rummelsberg/Nürnberg

Zilch, H., Priv.-Doz. Dr. med.
Oberarzt der Orthopädischen Klinik und Poliklinik der Freien Universität Berlin im Oskar-Helene-Heim, Clayallee 229, D-1000 Berlin 33

Preface

The reconstructive surgery of posttraumatic deformities has made significant advances in recent years. Reports on technical progress and clinical results are encouraging, even though they have often raised patient expectations to an unrealistic level. The operative methods available to us today enable corrective osteotomies to be performed with a high degree of accuracy and success. Precisely because the sequelae of trauma are so difficult to schematize, every case must be evaluated individually based on a critical assessment of subjective complaints, diagnosis and prognosis before a decision can be made. The planning and execution of corrective procedures are carried out with the same meticulous care as for idiopathic limb deformities. However, the occurrence of a traumatizing event with its immediate and long-term complications calls for special insight in the setting of therapeutic goals. It is essential that the patient be appraised of the results that can reasonably be expected and of the risks that are involved. Success in therapeutic procedures requires detailed theoretical knowledge, thorough operative training, and a strong commitment on the part of the surgeon. It is these aspects of the corrective surgery of posttraumatic deformities with which the editors are principally concerned.

Corrective osteotomies for posttraumatic deformities of the lower extremity formed the topic of a recent symposium held to commemorate the 65th birthday of Dr. Jörg Rehn, to whom the publication of this book is gratefully dedicated. The symposium offered convincing proof of the ability and willingness of surgeons and orthopedists to work together. The editors express thanks to all the authors for their contributions and for enriching the discussion. We also gratefully acknowledge the support of Springer-Verlag in bringing the book to press.

September 1984

G. Hierholzer, Duisburg
K. H. Müller, Bochum

Contents

Jörg Rehn

Jörg Rehn was born in Hamburg, Germany, on March 15, 1918. He studied medicine in Freiburg and Marburg and became a licenced physician in 1944. Following World War II and captivity as a prisoner of war, he began his medical practice with Professor F. Büchner at the Pathological Institute and continued it with Professor Heilmayer at the Medical Clinic of the University of Freiburg in the elementary disciplines of medicine. In April of 1948 he began specialized training at the Surgical Clinic of the University of Freiburg, which at that time was headed by his father, professor Eduard Rehn.

In 1952, when the directorship of the clinic passed to Professor Hermann Krauss, a pupil of Sauerbruchs, Prof. Dr. Jörg Rehn received recognition as a specialist in surgery. Even while working with Professors Buchner and Heilmayer, Dr. Rehn conducted experimental and clinical research in addition to his work as a practicing physician. In 1956 he wrote the thesis *Studies in Experimental Animals on the Pathogenesis of Burn Diseases* to qualify as a lecturer in surgery. In 1957 he became a staff physician at the Surgical Clinic of Freiburg University and was appointed extracurricular professor in 1961. From September, 1962, to March, 1983, he was Chief of Staff of the Surgical Clinic of the Bergmannsheil Medical Facility in Bochum. Professor Rehn was instrumental in setting up the Medical Department of Ruhr University along the lines of the "Bochum model."

Besides his outstanding contributions to basic medicosurgical research and general surgery, his main field of activity, true to the Lexer-Rehn school, has been in trauma and reconstructive surgery and its complications. Professor Rehn has headed the Bergmannsheil Surgical Clinic with great enthusiasm and sacrifice. In the process, he has not only enhanced the reputation of this venerable trauma clinic, but has helped it to become one of the leading trauma centers in the German-speaking world. Jörg Rehn has been fortunate in that both his father and his grandfathers were successful, respected, self-assured yet modest surgeons whose examples helped to guide his professional career. With this tradition behind him, and with his spirited commitment to clinical practice and scientific research, Professor Rehn has become one of our foremost representatives of trauma surgery. He has served as President of the German Society of Traumatology (1971) and President of the German Society of Plastic and Reconstructive Surgery (1972). Today Professor Rehn is an honorary member of the German Society of Traumatology and of the Swiss Society of Trauma Medicine and Occupational Diseases. His surgical, scientific and creative activity as well as his sense of duty as a physician and a human being serve as a spendid model for his students. Professor Rehn creates for them a climate of freedom in which both cooperation and independence and flourish. His authority and personality are a source of inspiration and support for all his colleagues.

K. H. Müller

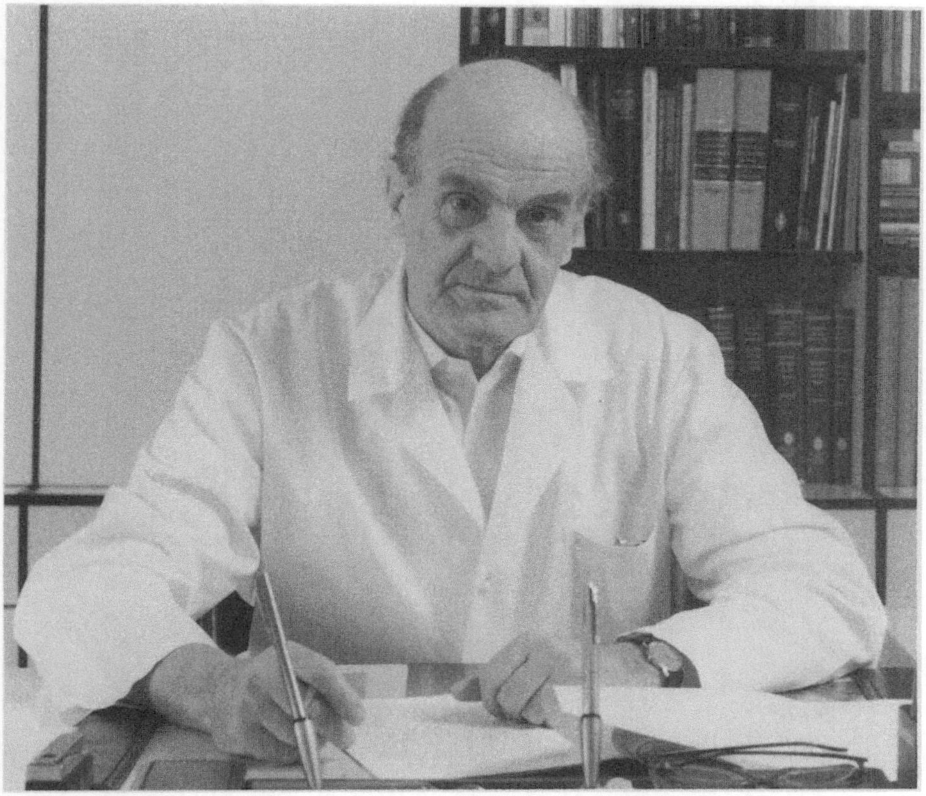

Jörg Rehn

A Tribute to Jörg Rehn

G. Hierholzer

This symposium commemorating the 65th birthday of Professor Jörg Rehn is an occasion for congratulations and for appreciation of his many years of surgical and scientific endeavor and, for many of us, a welcome opportunity to express our thanks. It is no small task to deliver this tribute, for I realize that I am speaking for many who wish also to express their esteem and their affection. Nevertheless, I feel that my admiration, respect and friendship for Jörg Rehn entitle me to place my own interpretation on how best to express this tribute. I believe that if it is appropriate for a junior to express thoughts concerning his relationship to his senior, it should not be to pass judgment or even to mete out praise, but rather to highlight aspects of his personality, attitudes and career and attempt to interpret his philosophies and goals in the hope that others will profit fron them. Jörg Rehn is anchored in tradition. It is important to emphasize this point, because often it is no longer fasionable to see value in it. He affirms the German heritage, respects family history, and builds upon it through an exemplary commitment to his profession. He has demonstrated that there is both a justification and a need for pride in the achievements of our ancestors, and that this pride need not prevent one from starting humbly and advancing through hard work. Jörg Rehn has earned our admiration through his work and accomplishments. The concept of depending on the state is as foreign to him as the notion of refusing to serve society.

His life after graduating medical school was disrupted by the approach of World War II, enforced Labor Service, military duties during the war, and the trying postwar years. I believe it is important to recall the stresses to which this generation was subjected during their training and during a significant portion of their careers. In the future, it is likely that such trials will be repeated, because subsequent generations tend to forget the past and thus remove one of the most important barriers to the repetition of past mistakes.

Jörg Rehn had outstanding teachers. Through them, he was guided toward clinical work and stimulated to conduct scientific research. But his recollections from that period also show how much his encounters and experiences sharpened his innate talent for critical observation. The relevance of this fact to questions of today may be expressed as follows: Despite the ability to think critically and to exercise criticism, Jörg Rehn has never given cause to doubt his willingness to make sacrifices, his readiness to cooperate, and his strong sense of duty. Perhaps we sould spend more time teaching and learning the value of combining these virtues. He has shown that progress which preserves continuity with the past is more fruitful than the practice of invalidating the past. His regard for progress is illustrated by the special professional structures which he instituted in the mid-1960's at the Bergmannsheil Surgical Clinic, and which since have become standard at other clinics.

Jörg Rehn has always recognized the fundamental relevance of scientific research to clinical practice and has served the advancement of surgery through his own contributions and by stimulating and guiding his colleagues. It would be futile to try to list his scientific achievements, and he probably would not wish me to do so. But we must not neglect his attitude toward changes in the approach to scientific study. If this attitude were to be expressed fully and with the sharpness that is his custom, many would feel compelled to lower their heads like churchgoers after a harsh sermon.

The main question he asks us is how far we still pursue science for its own sake. Certainly, the clinician must incorporate the field of applied research into his scientific mission. But even he hust continually examine the relationship of means to goals in order to determine whether the boundary of scientific claim as once defined by Bacon has been crossed. In conversation, Jörg Rehn is not hesitant to state misgivings about any manuscript or lecture that disregards the principles of the scientific method. His criticism is particularly sharp when it is apparent that egotism is the main motivation for a publication or even for the recording of observations. He urgently warns against a trend that discourages the reading of original works and encourages the posting of scientific data without allowing for their discussion.

Even as a clinician, he manifests a profound awareness of the scientific foundations of medicine. I have never seen Jörg Rehn perform surgery derived purely from empiricism. To him, empirical observation is mainly valuable as a stimulus for objective inquiry. The observation itself is only a guide, and he is reluctant to elevate it to the status of proof. His sense of responsibility toward his patients has not diminished his critical outlook. In his world there is no place for the hasty implementation of procedures that lack an adequate foundation. The notion of celebrating case numbers or displaying pride in a clinical success is foreign to him, although such occasions have been known to impart a softer and sometimes even boyish cast to his features. For Jörg Rehn, grappling with surgical indications is far more rewarding than the drive for technical perfection. He is particularly interested in helping young colleagues find the necessary approach to the conduct of high-risk procedures and training them in the avoidance, recognition and treatment of complications.

As a matter of personal concern, it seems appropriate to comment briefly on the debate that appears to persist in public circles with regard to medical issues. It is very apparent that neither the media nor various groups and committees can even approach the mentality and professional conduct that are the hallmark of the competent physician. It is dangerous from the patient's standpoint and oppressive from ours how, with blatently ideological intent and through the generalization of isolated incidents, increasing aspersions are being cast on the vocation of medicine.

Jörg Rehn is a surgeon, and as such he expects an assigned task to be carried out in a concise and timely fashion. In bringing this tribute to a conclusion, I return to the theme of gratitude with which I began. We know, however, that it is better to express thanks with actions than with words. With this in mind, I believe that our task in the future is to join our honored guest in seeing to it that his his guiding principles are upheld. We must retain the freedom necessary to organize and create and, in the spirit of Dahlmann, vehemently resist external influences on theory, research and clinical practice. We must encourage individual initiative and champion the performance principle, which are essential to the rational and successful evolution of medicine. Finally, we must preserve the traditional concepts of medical ethics that urge a liberal attitude and the willingness to help even in high-risk situations. May the fear of forensic complications never diminish the courage for medical and above all surgical action.

Dear Jörg, allow me to close with a very personal word to you. I am aware of how greatly your personality has influenced my life for more than two decades. I thank you for your guiding presence and am not hesitant to express my sincere feelings on this occasion.

I. Basic Principles

Pathophysiology of Posttraumatic Deformities of the Lower Extremity

E. Morscher

The speciality of orthopedics owes its name to Nicolas Andry (1658 – 1741), who was concerned with the prevention and correction of angular deformities of the spine and extremities. "Orthos" means "straight" as well as "correct," implying that that which is straight is also correct.

As we examine the normal axial relationships of the lower extremities, their ranges of variation, and the effects of deviations, it must be remembered that the election of operative treatment is not just a matter of defining "normal limits" and deciding what is inside or outside a particular region of a bell-shaped curve. Rather, it is a matter of establishing the degree of axial deviation beyond which a deformity may be said to have an immediate or potential *pathologic significance*. A deformity derives this significance not only from its association with pain, disability, and the development of posttraumatic osteoarthritis, but also from asthetic considerations, which very often are the source of greatest concern to the patient, at least initially. An axial deformity acquires true pathological significance when compensatory mechanisms fail.

It is known, for example, that a valgus deformity of the tibia can usually be adequately compensated by supination in the subtalar joint. On the other hand, varus angulation of the tibia quickly leads to decompensation due to the limited range of pronation in the subtalar joint, resulting in pain or even a rigid pes planus deformity.

Especially during the growth period, axial deformities can trigger compensatory mechanisms that must be taken into account during the planning of corrective procedures (cf. Chapter VI).

The age of the child and the growth potential of the affected epiphyseal plate are basic considerations in this regard.

An alteration or correction of axial alignment can occur in either of two ways:

1. It can be accomplished by enchondral longitudinal growth, in which, according to Pauwels, the epiphyseal plate tends to become oriented at right angles to the resultant (vectorial sum) of the forces exerted on it. The closer the deformity is to the epiphysis, the more quickly and effectively the correction is achieved.

2. An axial deformity can be corrected to some extent by appositional growth in thickness on the concave side of the deformity and by resorptive processes on the convex side.

With traumatic disturbances of epiphyseal plate function, there are four basic ways in which vectors can be used to characterize the growth disturbance

Corrective Osteotomies of the Lower Extremity
Edited by G. Hierholzer, K. H. Müller

Table 1. Posttraumatic Growth Disturbances

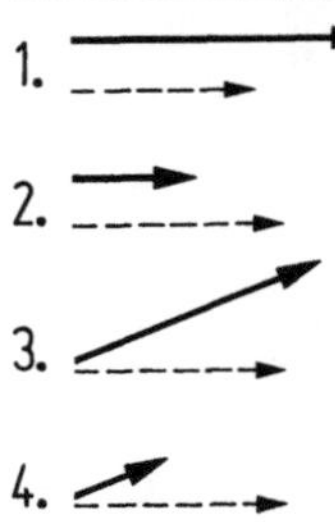

1.	V: + R: =	Lengthening
2.	V: + R: =	Shortening
3.	V: + R: =	Lengthening Deformity
4.	V: + R: =	Lengthening Shortening

qualitatively in terms of its direction and quantitatively in terms of its rate. These are illustrated in Table 1.

The approach to treatment in such cases will depend on whether the epiphyseal plates are still open or whether growth is concluded. An axial deformity should *never* be regarded as an isolated lesion, but should always be viewed within the general context of statics and dynamics. Thus, for example, excessive external torsion of the tibia can compensate for excessive anteversion of the femoral neck.

When bones of the lower extremity are affected with multiple deformities in the same direction, the effects of these deformities add together in a morphologic sense but are potentiated from the standpoint of degenerative change.

Determination of the *frontal leg axes* depends essentially on what is occurring in the horizontal plane, not only with regard to torsion of the bone but also in terms of rotation in the joints.

The extension of the knee joint is variable, and even a mild genu recurvatum will produce varus deviation of the knee. Accordingly, a distinction must be made at examination between extension in the "neutral position" and maximum extension, which generally corresponds to a recurvatum.

As the degree of recurvatum increases, there is an increasing tendency for the patellae and knees to rotate inward, causing the knees to separate and simulate a genu varum. The greater the initial internal rotation of the knees, the greater this effect. In all individuals there is a tendency for the knees to rotate inward when the feet are placed parallel, except in cases where there is retroversion of the femoral neck or marked external torsion of the tibia.

When we examine the leg axes with the feet parallel, we notice a difference between males and females, with about 60% of males showing a genu varum, as opposed to only 34% of females. The prevalence of genu valgum is 12% in males versus 22% in females [8]. But the angle that is critical with regard to the development of osteoarthritis depends basically on the position of the feet, and this varies greatly from one individual to the next.

Another factor to be considered when evaluating leg axes is that the femoral and tibial axes are not straight. The femur is convex on its anterolateral side, and the tibia is convex posterolaterally. When the leg is extended, this results in what the French call an *effect manivelle*, or crank effect. Thus, internal rotation of the leg at the hip straightens the femur while accentuating the varus curvature of the tibia. When establishing a norm, it is of course necessary to consider age and gender. But constitution is also important, as illustrated by the prevalence of genu valgum in asthenic types and of genu varum in pyknics.

The importance of *individual* peculiarities is well known from the treatment of fresh fractures. For example, it is standard practice at most centers to leave the healthy leg undraped during the fixation of a tibial fracture so that the torsion of the fractured bone can be matched to that of the unaffected limb.

The *normal axial relationships* of the lower extremities are familiar to every orthopedist and need not be discussed here. However, the three-dimensionality of the physical axes is a point that is frequently neglected and ought to be emphasized. While we are accustomed to thinking in terms of three cardinal anatomic planes, we must always bear in mind that forces act *dynamically in space* and do not confine themselves to the planes that we arbitrarily define.

One need only consider the complex biomechanics of the femoral neck, whose anteversion cannot be measured directly, but must be represented indirectly by a projected angle during the planning of surgery. Earlier we alluded to the highly complex interrelationship that exists between genu recurvatum and genu varum.

With regard to the development of osteoarthritis, it is essential to consider the effect of an axial deformity under the dynamic conditions of gait. Of course, this approach is far more difficult and complicated and often requires the use of a specially equipped *gait laboratory*.

The measurement of joint mobility and skeletal axes on the examining table and the evaluation of roentgenograms can be supplemented by measurements of movements and forces in all three planes during gait. Objective measurements of walking speed, step length and step frequency are easily obtained in the gait laboratory. Progressive changes in joint angles, intramuscular electromyograms, and energy expenditure during walking are more difficult to study in quantitative terms. The magnitude and direction of the reaction forces exerted by the ground against the foot during gait can be precisely measured, however. Piezoelectric transducers can be used to measure and graphically record vertical load, gravitational forces in the sagittal and frontal planes, and free rotational moment. Measurements of force transmission yield much information on the nature of the progression, the mechanisms that compensate for axial deviations, limitations of joint motion, ligamentous instabilities, and muscular actions.

Like Bragard [1] and many others, we are accustomed to referring to the line connecting the center of the hip joint and the center of the ankle joint as the *mechanical axis* of the lower extremity. This line is meaningful only under the static conditions of stance. In static tests an angular deviation of only 3° is sufficient to completely unload the lateral compartment of the knee under a varus load, and the medial compartment under a valgus load [5]. But the mechanical axis that is operative during gait and therefore relevant to the pathogenesis of osteoarthritis is the line connecting the center of gravity of the body and the weight-supporting surface, i.e., the sole of the foot. During walking, when the loads on the knee are greatest, this line always passes medial to the center of the knee joint, causing a physiologic varus stress to be exerted on the knee during gait [2]. Only in the Duchenne gait, in which the center of the gravity of the body is shifted over the hip joint of the supporting leg, do the static and dynamic mechanical axes coincide. This fact explains why genu varum is so much more common in the elderly, and especially in osteoporosis, than genu valgum.

We now return to the central question – that of the clinical relevance and *pathologic significance* of the various axial limb deformities and the necessity of their surgical correction. The greatest controversy in this regard relates to torsion of the femur. For many years it was incorrectly assumed that torsional deformities of the femur would not undergo spontaneous correction, even in children [6,7]. As in cases of marked idiopathic anteversion, this belief resulted in a large number of unnecessary derotation osteotomies. To date there is no convincing evidence that an isolated, excessive anteversion unassociated with deformities of the acetabulum or other structures about the hip has ever led to osteoarthritis of the hip, although this possibility cannot be entirely ruled out [3]. In any case, we know that the reduction of the anteversion, especially in puberty, occurs in a manner analogous to a very slowly progressive slipping of the capital femoral epiphysis [4,9,10].

A coxa vara deformity, which usually is combined with retroversion of the femoral neck, generally does not lead to osteoarthritis of the hip when joint congruity is good, although it invariably causes significant functional impairment of the hip with leg shortening, a Trendelenburg-Duchenne limp, and limitation of hip abduction. These problems may be sufficient in themselves to warrant corrective surgery.

In the knee joint, we find that genu recurvatum is most common in individuals with constitutional connective-tissue weakness or hyperlaxity. Genu recurvatum may well be a cause of chronic knee complaints, most notably the painful cartilage depression caused by repeated engagement of the femoral condyles on the anterior margin of the tibial plateau or on the anterior horns [11,12,13].

It is well known that operative procedures on the tibial apophysis for correction of recurrent platellar dislocation or other conditions are contraindicated during the growth period.

With flexion deformity of the knee, pressure across the femoropatellar joint is markedly increased. Practice teaches us time and again that the development of a flexion contracture in the setting of a latent knee osteoarthrotis acutely accelerates the vicious cycle, resulting in a rapid progression of degenerative disease.

As mentioned previously, a varus deformity of the tibia has much greater pathologic significance than a corresponding valgus deformity. As evidence of this, we note that five times as many valgus osteotomies are necessary in adult patients as varus osteotomies. Also, our review of 400 tibial osteotomies has shown that the best results in varus deformities were obtained by making a slight overcorrection of the physiologic valgus. By contrast, a pathologic genu valgum should never be corrected to straightness and certainly should not be overcorrected to varus. Even at a relatively young age, varus positions can lead to chronic complaints with a concentration of stresses on the medial meniscus and corresponding premature degenerative changes in the medial part of the joint. A meniscectomy is of only temporary benefit in these cases, and degenerative changes will progress all the more rapidly once the meniscus has been removed. Osteoarthritic patients who present for operative treatment after a prior meniscectomy typically do so 20–30 years after the primary operation. This raises the question of whether the medial osteoarthritis was purely a result of the meniscectomy or whether the meniscectomy was necessitated by a primary varus deformity with premature degeneration of the meniscus. In any case, we are very liberal in our election of valgus osteotomy for chronic medial complaints associated with even a minor varus deformity. This contrasts with our very restrictive policy toward the use of meniscectomy.

The degree to which axial deformities of the foot can affect loads on the knee joint is generally known. Thus, the simple measure of elevating the outer edge of the shoe is often sufficient to reduce excessive loads on the medial part of the knee and relieve associated complaints.

Recognizing that a varus deformity of the hindfoot not only predisposes to supination sprains of the foot but also facilitates their recurrence following ligament reconstruction, we recently recommended that such cases be treated by combining a lateral ligament reconstruction with osteotomy of the calcaneus using the Dwyer technique [14].

Certainly, gait analysis will continue to yield many important insights into the effect of axial deformities on articular function and the transmission of stresses through the joints.

Even at the level of the clinical examination, one should not view a deformity as an isolated lesion, but should give attention to the overall condition of the lower extremity and the patient. Only in this way can one appreciate the totality of the problem and select a therapy (e.g., shoe insert, corrective surgery) that will afford the greatest long-term benefit to the patient.

References

1. Bragard K (1932) Das genu valgum, 1. Teil. Z Orthop 57 [Suppl]
2. Debrunner A, Seewald K (1964) Die Belastung des Kniegelenkes in der Frontalebene. Z Orthop 98:508
3. Halpern AA, Tanner J, Rinsky L (1980) Does persistent fetal anteversion contribute to osteoarthritis? Clin Orthop 145:213
4. Jani L (1979) Idiopathic anteversion of the femoral neck. Int Orthop 2:283–292
5. Kostuik JP, Schmidt O, Harris WR, Woolridge C (1975) A study of weight transmission through the knee joint with applied varus and valgus loads. Clin Orthop 108:95–98
6. Laer L von (1977) Beinlängendifferenzen und Rotationsfehler nach Oberschenkelfrakturen im Kindesalter. Arch Orthop Unfallchir 89:121–137
7. Laer L von (1982) Die klinische Bedeutung des posttraumatischen Rotationsfehlers nach Oberschenkelschaftfrakturen im Wachstumsalter. Hefte Unfallheilkd 158:159–162
8. Lerat JL, Moyen B, Bochu M (1982) Examen clinique des axes chez l'adulte. Rev Chir Orthop 68:37–43

9. Morscher E (1961) Die mechanischen Verhältnisse des Hüftgelenkes und ihre Beziehungen zum Halsschaftwinkel und insbesondere zur Antetorsion des Schenkelhalses während der Entwicklungsjahre. Z Orthop 94:374–394
10. Morscher E (1967) Development and clinical significance of the anteversion of the femoral neck. Reconstr Surg Traumatol 9:107–125
11. Morscher E (1971) Cartilage-bone lesions of the knee joint following injury. Reconstr Surg Traumatol 12:2–26
12. Morscher E (1978) Posttraumatic cartilage impression of the femoral condyle. Prog Orthop Surg 3:105–111
13. Morscher E (1979) Traumatische Knorpelläsionen am Kniegelenk. Chirurg 50:599–604
14. Morscher E, Baumann JU, Hefti F (1981) Die Kalkaneus-Osteotomie nach Dwyer, kombiniert mit lateraler Bandplastik bei rezidivierender Distorsio pedis. Z Unfallmed Berufskr 74:85–90

Indications for Corrective Osteotomy after Malunited Fractures

G. Hierholzer and P. M. Hax

Introduction

The indications for corrective osteotomy after malunited fractures of the lower extremity are based on a combination of clinical findings and theoretical aspects. It does not result from mechanical considerations alone. Of course, the various factors must be determined individually, but then they should be evaluated comparatively so that a final clinical decision can be made as to the most appropriate therapy. The discussion of special indications presumes that the general condition of the patient has been ascertained and the surgical risk is known. A posttraumatic deformity not only alters anatomy but also affects function in accordance with its location and extent. The secondary effects of an abnormal load-bearing alignment must be taken into account. The condition of the affected bony tissue, the neighboring joints, and functionally important soft-tissue structures have to be considered. Primary or secondary lesions influence not only the indication for osteotomy but also the selection of the operative procedure. The age and cooperativeness of the patient, the nature and severity of subjective complaints, professional and private living habits, and cosmetic aspects all must be included in the surgeon's evaluation. In this chapter we shall examine the main factors influencing the selection of patients for corrective surgery, the variable importance of these factors, and the need to recognize priorities. The following factors are emphasized:

1. Unphysiologic mechanical loads on the joints.
2. The functional aspect.
3. Effects on capsuloligamentous structures of adjacent joints.
4. Morphologic condition of the bone, cartilage and soft tissues.
5. Subjective complaints.
6. Cosmetic effects.

The indication for a corrective osteotomy usually results from a combination of these factors, although a single factor may be predominant in a particular case.

Unphysiologic Mechanical Loads

In the upper extremity, the significance of a posttraumatic deformity is largely functional. With deformities of the lower extremity, the resulting alteration of load-bearing alignment can assume an importance equal to or greater than that of the functional derangement. This is because in the lower extremity, the

Corrective Osteotomies of the Lower Extremity
Edited by G. Hierholzer, K. H. Müller

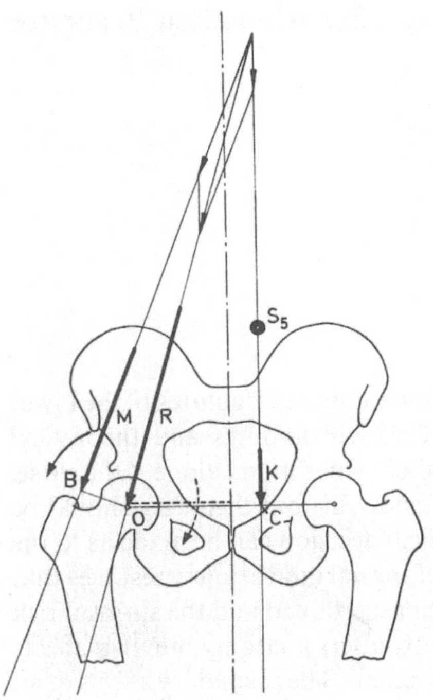

Fig. 1. Pressure load on the hip joint, represented as the resultant **R** of the muscular force **M** and gravity **S** [17]

vector of the pressure loads represents the sum (resultant) of muscular forces and body weight. Hence, the joints of the lower extremity are subjected to greater compressive loads than those of the upper extremity (Fig. 1). The resulting pressure across the hip joint can reach a level equal to 4.5 times the body weight [16,17]. The force vector acting on the head and neck of the femur accounts for the tendency of fractures in that region to displace and underscores the danger of a varus deformity. The surgical treatment of a fracture that has united with varus angulation consists of a valgus osteotomy to restore a normal neck-shaft angle, thereby correcting the abnormal mechnaical load and muscular insufficiency (Fig. 2). The technique is well standarized [5,13,14,19,21,24] and has a high rate of success.

Deformity in the opposite direction, posttraumatic coxa valga, concentrates stresses in the lateral part of the joint and may be the result of a treatment that was initially appropriate from a mechanical and biological standpoint (Fig. 3). In the treatment of a femoral neck fracture with a steep inclincation of the fracture line, main priority should be given to preserving or restoring the viability of the femoral head. With a steep fracture line a valgus osteotomy is the only means available for transforming disruptive shearing forces into interfragmental compression (Fig. 4) [14–16,28]. It is noteworthy that while this indication for primary valgus intertrochanteric osteotomy has been employed with increasing frequency, no long-term clinical studies are available on the sequelae of the operation. In our view, this procedure creates an unphysiologic stress pattern that justifies a secondary varus osteotomy as soon as subjective complaints or objective changes develop in the affected hip and knee.

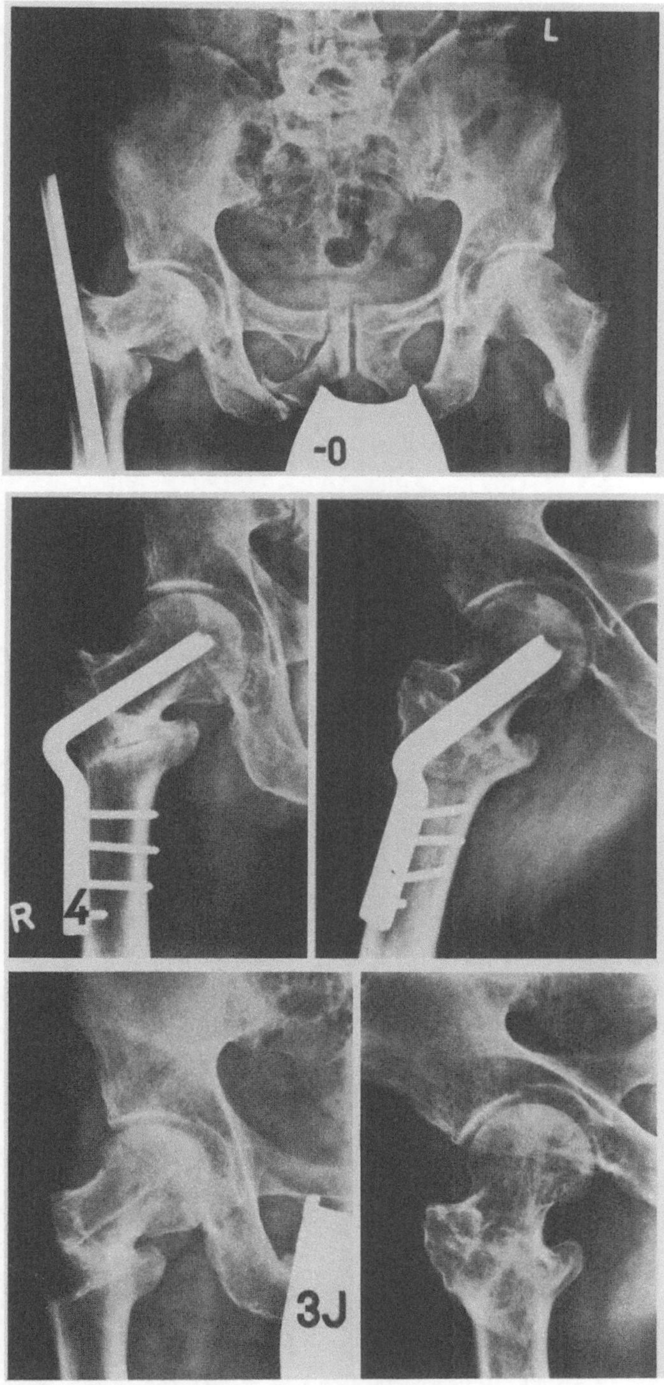

a

b

c

Fig. 2 a – c. A. L., 59 years of age. **a** Pertrochanteric fracture of the right femur that has united in varus. **b** Valgus osteotomy. **c** Three years after operation

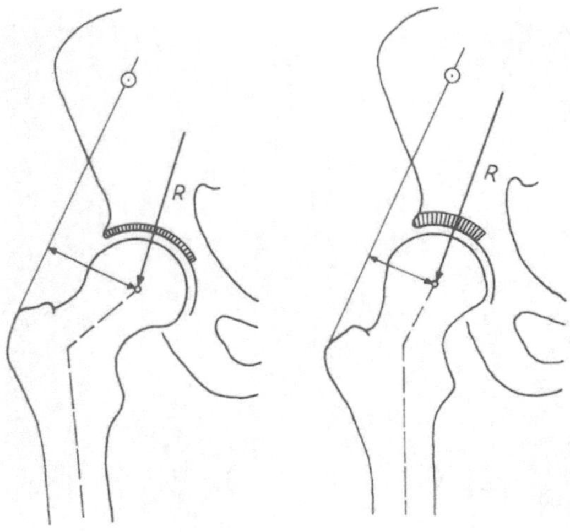

Fig. 3. Normal loading of the hip joint with a physilogic CCD angle (*left*). Valgus of the femoral neck (*right*) increases the resultant **R** and reduces the area of weight bearing

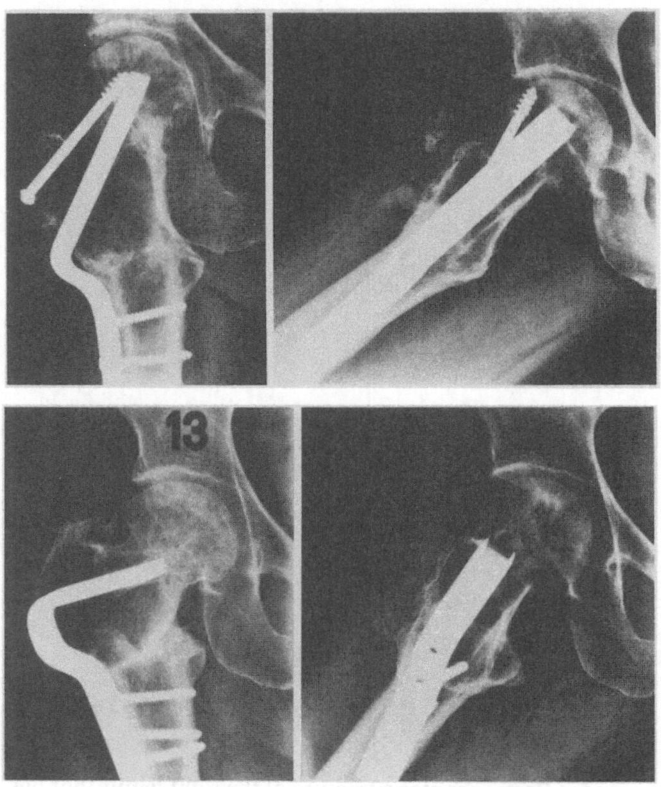

a

b

Fig. 4 a,b. C. K., 53 years of age. **a** Result of initial operation in which a subcapital fracture of the right femur was fixed with an angled blade plate, and a valgus osteotomy was done to eliminate shear forces in the fracture zone. **b** Restoration of a physiologic CCD angle by varus osteotomy after union of the fracture

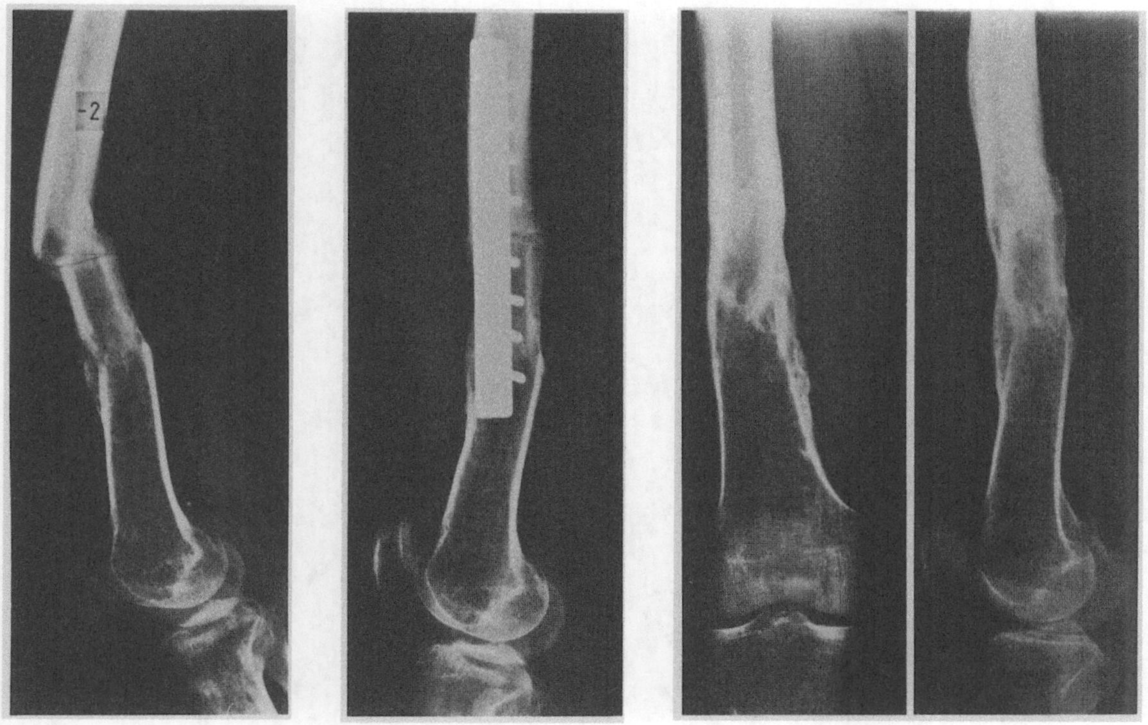

a **b** **c**

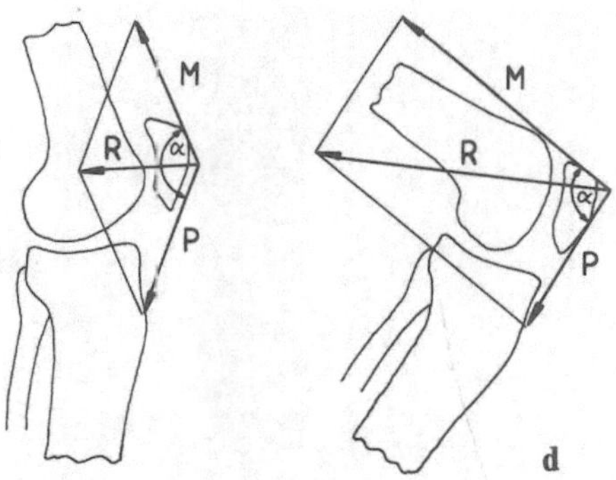

d

Fig. 5 a–d. E. B., 30 years of age. **a** Posttraumatic backward displacement of the femur. **b** Recurvatum osteotomy. **c** Four years after operation. **d** Diagrams indicate magnitude and direction of pressure load on the patellofemoral joint

In the tibia, increasing attention is being given to the treatment of axial deformities after fractures, especially when they are located in the frontal or sagittal planes [1,6,12,20,21,24,27]. The pathophysiology of tibial malunions is discussed by Hörster (see Chapter III, p. 127). Clinical observations indicate that the mechanical effects of a backward displacement of the femur on the knee joint are often underestimated. Powerful muscular structures bridge the knee joint anteriorly, and the increase in muscle tension associated with a backward displacement serves to keep the joint stable. This is accompanied by an increased pressure load across the knee, which is greatest in the femoropatellar region [2,8,10]. With passage of time, the functional compensation of the deformity with a sustained increase of compressive loading leads to osteoarthritic change (Fig. 5). In the tibia, a varus deformity exceeding 5°

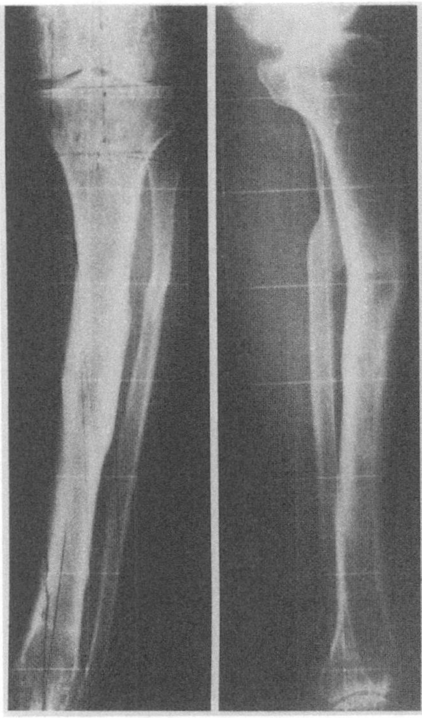

a

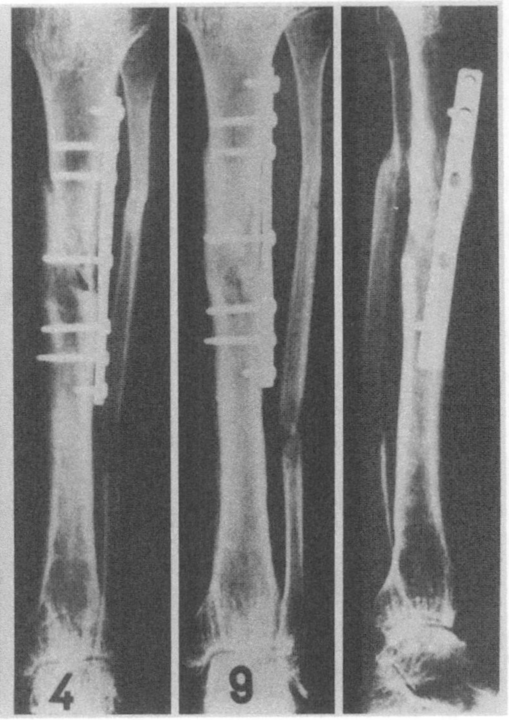

b

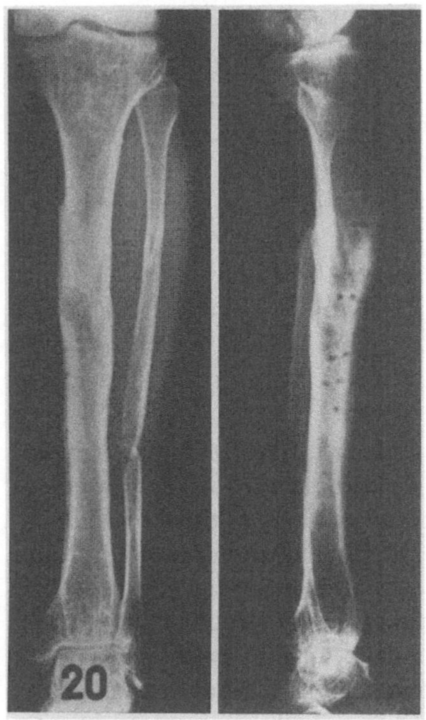

c

Fig. 6 a–c. H. H., 49 years of age. **a** Posttraumatic varus deformity of the left tibia. **b** Oblique tibial osteotomy (plated) and fibular osteotomy. **c** Appearance after union

leads to a concentration of stresses in the knee and ankle joints that necessitates correction (Fig. 6) – an instance where unphysiologic loads are the chief factor in the election of corrective osteotomy.

The Functional Aspect

An important clinical responsibility lies in recognizing the functional impact of a posttraumatic deformity and incorporating it into the indications for corrective osteotomy. The object of the corrective procedure is to improve or preserve joint mobility. On the other hand, the functional impact of a deformity associated with secondary changes may justify the sacrifice of joint mobility in deference to a higher functional priority, such as walking ability. The importance of function as a therapeutic goal is best illustrated by examples.

Rotational deformities of the femur apparently occur more frequently than they are diagnosed. Because the hip joint is spheroidal, these deformities do

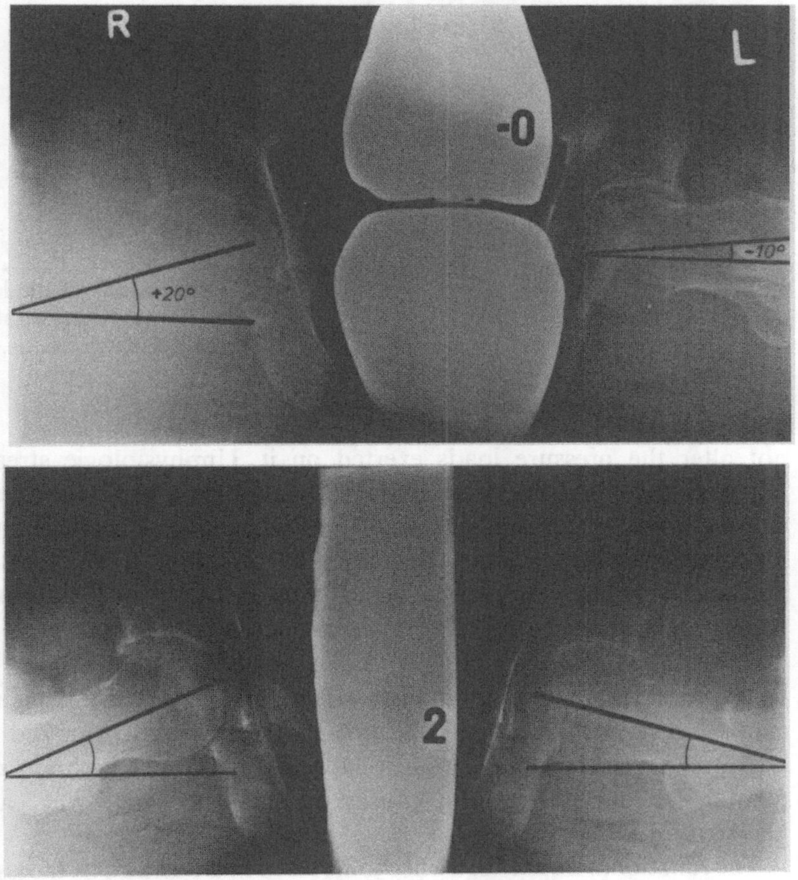

a

b

Fig. 7 a,b. R. V., 31 years of age. Rotational deformity of the left femur. **a** Anteversion film of the hips before and **b** after derotation osteotomy

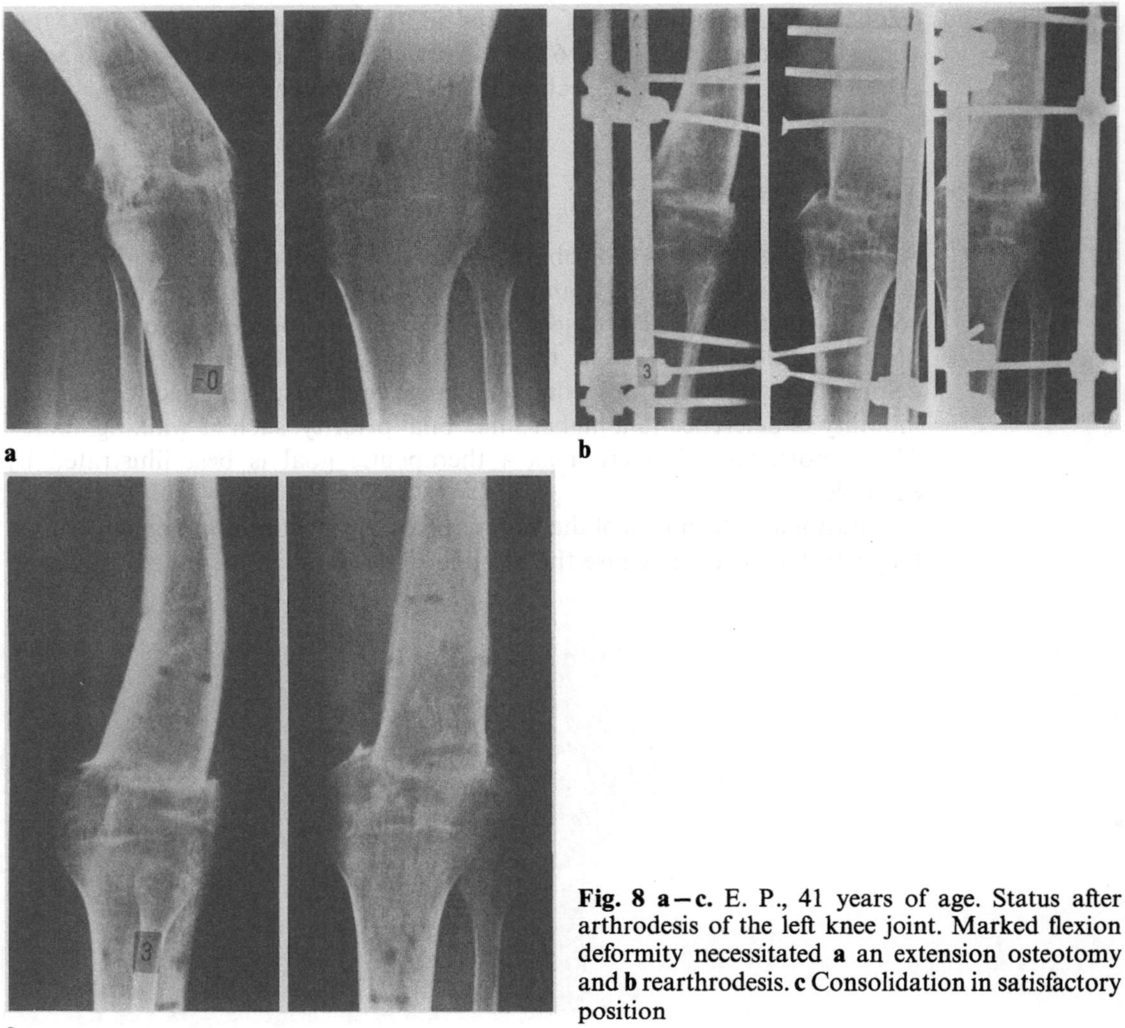

a b c

Fig. 8 a–c. E. P., 41 years of age. Status after arthrodesis of the left knee joint. Marked flexion deformity necessitated **a** an extension osteotomy and **b** rearthrodesis. **c** Consolidation in satisfactory position

not alter the pressure loads exerted on it. Unphysiologic stresses in the adjacent knee joint may remain subordinated for a prolonged period. If an external rotation deformity exists, it can be partially or entirely compensated for through muscular action. Sustained overexertion of the internal rotators and adductor muscles eventually leads to a functional disturbance of gait which, together with subjective complaints, becomes the principal indication for corrective osteotomy (Fig. 7). Even with a fracture near the hip that has healed in varus angulation and has altered the lever arm, muscular insufficiency with a positive Trendelenburg sign can lead to marked functional impairment. In the tibia, a rotational varus deformity hampers dorsal and plantar flexion of the foot, causes an unsteady gait, and can provide justification for surgery.

The functional impact of a knee joint fused in a position of excessive flexion is particularly noteworthy (Fig. 8). Flexion in excess of 15° seriously hampers gait and may render the patient incapable of walking. This profound

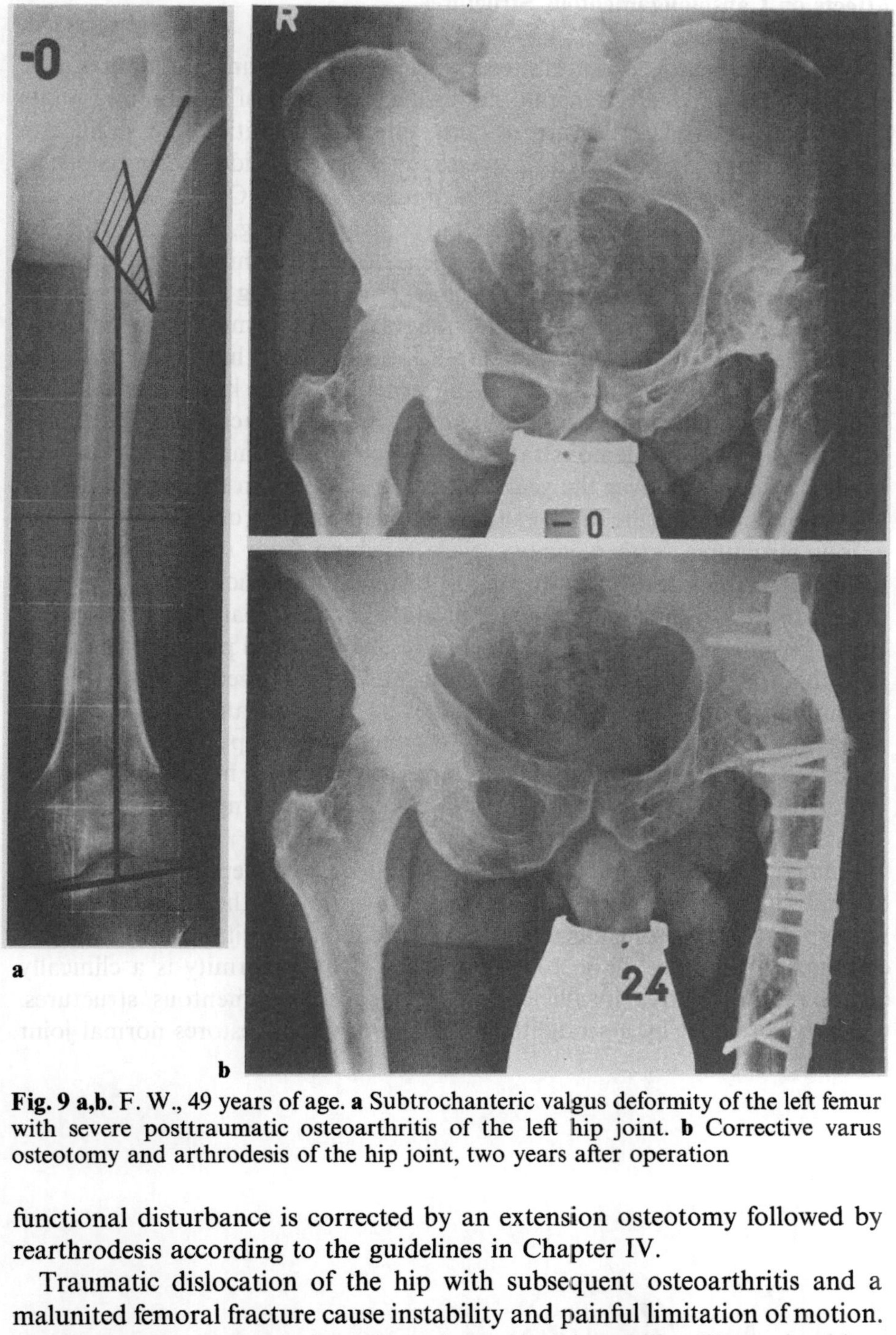

a

b

Fig. 9 a,b. F. W., 49 years of age. **a** Subtrochanteric valgus deformity of the left femur with severe posttraumatic osteoarthritis of the left hip joint. **b** Corrective varus osteotomy and arthrodesis of the hip joint, two years after operation

functional disturbance is corrected by an extension osteotomy followed by rearthrodesis according to the guidelines in Chapter IV.

Traumatic dislocation of the hip with subsequent osteoarthritis and a malunited femoral fracture cause instability and painful limitation of motion. The clinical picture is dominated by a loss of walking ability. The main object of corrective osteotomy in such cases is to restore ambulatory ability [9,18]. The complexity of the problem is illustrated by the case in Fig. 9. Restoration of walking ability in this patient required arthrodesis of the hip combined with osteotomy of the femoral shaft to normalize the loads on the knee.

Effects on Capsuloligamentous Structures

The nature and extent of deformities associated with malunited fractures have effects on the static and dynamic stabilizing structures of neighboring joints [3,4,7,10,11,15,16,23]. With varus and valgus deformities, the joints are subjected to unphysiologic tensile stresses on the convex side, causing capsular and ligamentous structures to become stretched and lax. On the concave side the structures may become atrophied and contracted (Fig. 10). The article by Kleining examines the efficacy of compensatory mechanisms for varus and valgus deformities of the knee and the danger of initiating a vicious cycle (cf. Chapter IV, p. 233). With an anterior angulation deformity, some compensation is assured by the dynamic stabilizing structures that bridge the knee joint. However, the posterior stabilizing structures of the knee are insufficient to maintain equilibrium in the face of a backward displacement. The clinical example (Fig. 11) demonstrates the effect of a genu recurvatum that gradually increased over the years following an injury in the growth period. This late condition is the result of a continuous stretching of the capsuloligamentous structures, with a vicious cycle resulting from malposition of the articular surfaces and the stretching of ligamentous structures.

Deformities of the foot frequently produce a state of painful irritation that may in turn lead to soft-tissue contractures. The clinical picture of impaired function and subjective complaints then must be analyzed in terms of both causative factors. The severity of changes in capsuloligamentous structures and especially the contracture of tendons may not be apparent until surgical exposure is obtained and may necessitate supplementary measures to correct the deformity, such as arthrolysis or Z-plastic lengthening of tendons (Fig. 12).

Finally, a malunited fracture that is associated with a depression of bone in the interligamentous region of the knee can produce the phenomenon of relative ligamentous insufficiency [3,5,10,11,23]. This situation is not uncommon in the knee (Fig. 10). One effect of the deformity is a clinically demonstrable relative insufficiency of the capsuloligamentous structures, which is corrected by a straightening osteotomy that restores normal joint relations (Fig. 13).

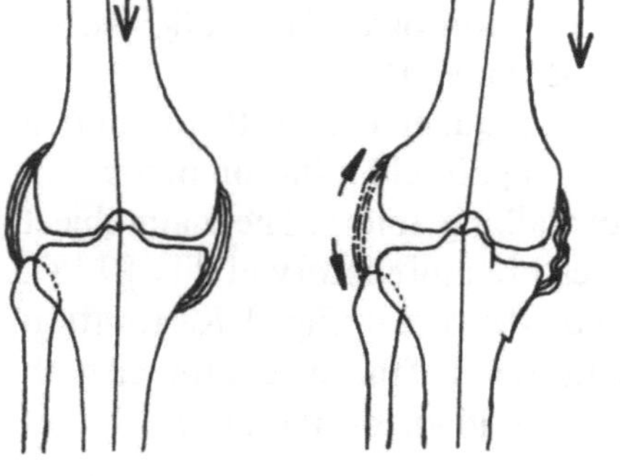

Fig. 10. *Left*: Normal loading of the knee joint. *Right*: Unphysiologic tension on the convex side of the axial deformity and relative laxness of the ligaments on the concave side due to depression of the medial tibial plateau after a fracture

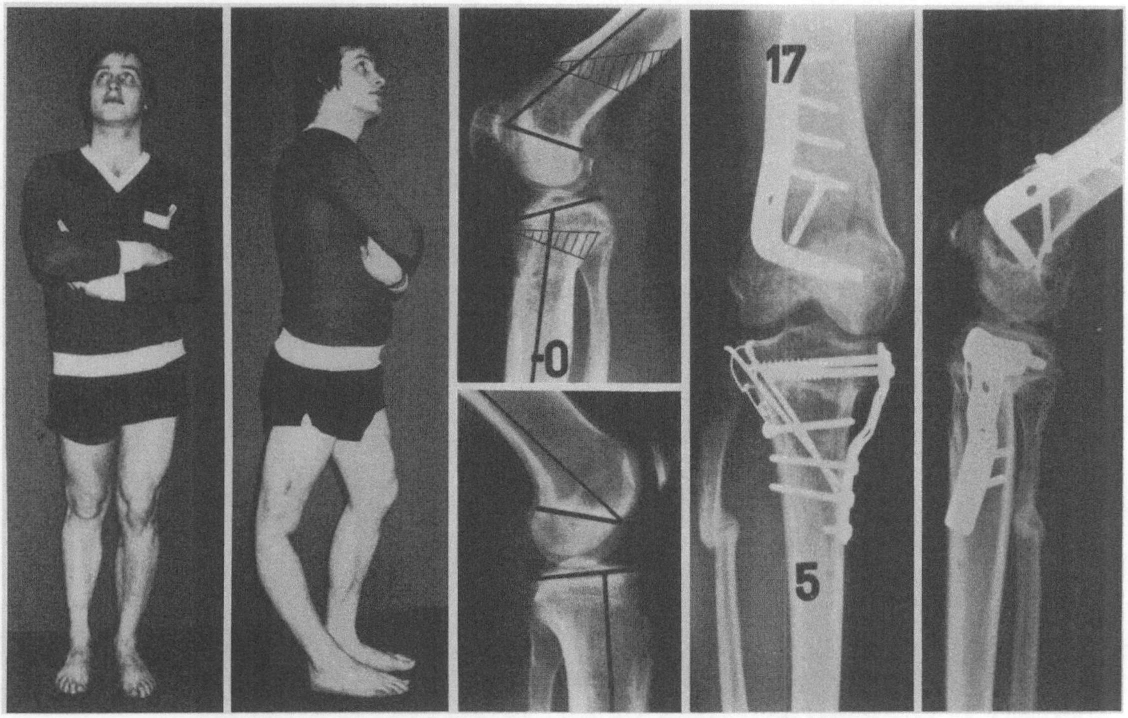

a b c

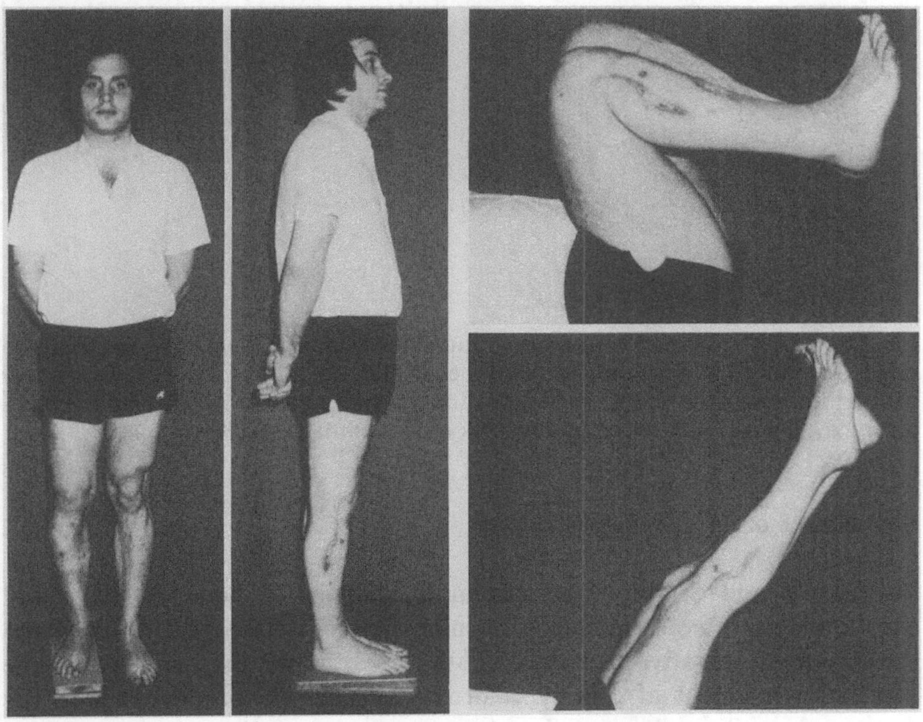

d

Fig. 11 a–d. D. W., 24 years of age. **a** Marked hyperextensibility of the right knee joint with forward displacement of the distal femur and proximal tibia in comparison to the left side (**b**). **c** Status after two-stage corrective osteotomy. **d** Clinical appearance and function at 18 months

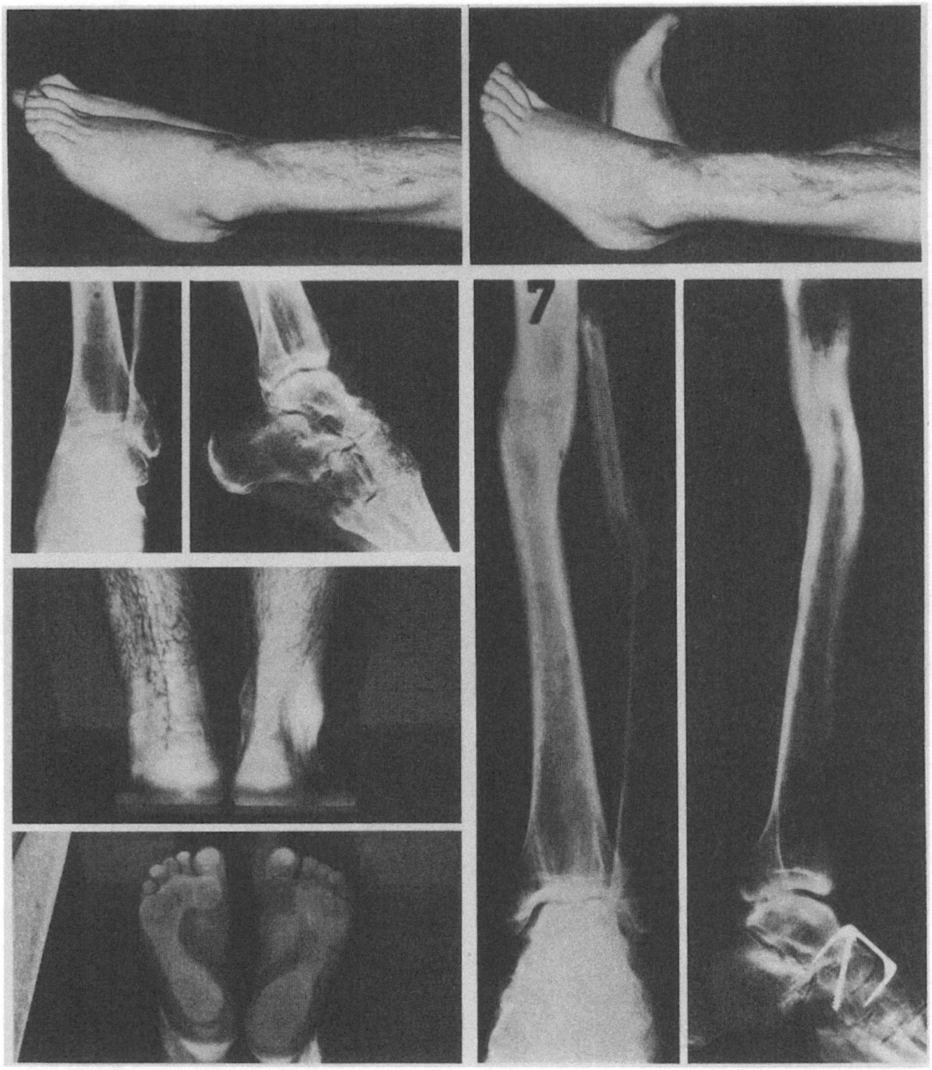

Fig. 12 a – d. H. S., 28 years of age. **a** Posttraumatic equinus of the left foot secondary to tarsal deformity (**b**) and shortening of the Achilles tendon. **c** Corrective osteotomy with arthrodesis of the talonavicular joint and lengthening of the Achilles tendon by Z-plasty. **d** Clinical result showing the areas of foot contact with the ground

Significance of Morphologic Damage

The nature and degree of posttraumatic damage to bone, cartilage and surrounding soft tissues influence the indication for corrective osteotomy and the choice of operative technique. Thus, for example, the prospect for the successful treatment of a bony deformity is inversely proportional to the degree of cartilage damage that has occurred in adjacent joints. If the degenerative process is advanced, it may present a contraindication to joint-preserving osteotomy. In this case arthrodesis is carried out as an adjunct to

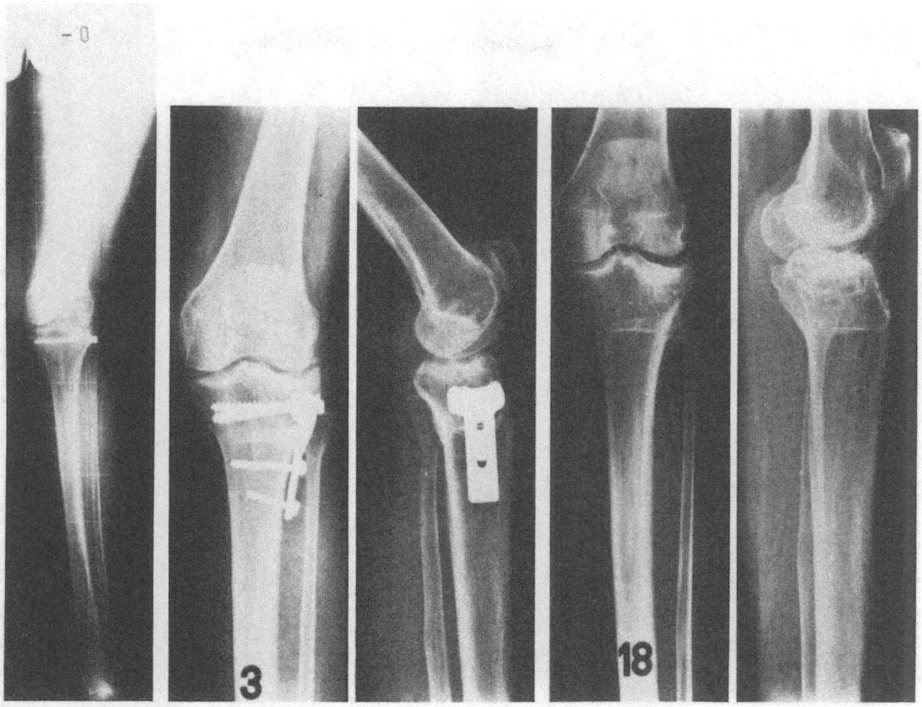

a b c

Fig. 13 a – c. M. D., 66 years of age. Fracture of the lateral tibial plateau. **a** Status after insufficient internal fixation. The fracture united with depression of the articular surface, relative laxness of the lateral collateral ligament, and valgus deformity. **b** Straightening osteotomy with interposition of bone graft. **c** Eighteen months after reoperation

the corrective osteotomy [9,18] (Fig. 14). On the other hand, if areas of healthy cartilage are still present in the joint next to the deformity, than planning of the corrective osteotomy can utilize these areas as load-bearing surfaces, even though this may require that a certain *unphysiologic* alignment be accepted. This approach is illustrated by the roentgenograms in Fig. 15, which show significant widening of the knee joint space following a varus osteotomy with slight overcorrection. Symptoms were greatly improved, and joint function was preserved.

When corrective surgery is indicated, a change in the bone tissue secondary to a previous infection or a sclerotic change due to other causes mainly affects the site at which the correction is performed. If the change is severe, the correction may not be done at the site of maximum deformity. If an infection is present and the nature and degree of the deformity indicate a need for osteotomy, this operation should be deferred until inflammation has subsided in accordance with pertinent guidelines. The residual tissue damage from the infection will mainly influence the selection of the stabilizing technique. Under these conditions we prefer external fixation with a joint-spanning frame, as this allows implants to be inserted outside the endangered area (Fig. 16). Damage to the skin and underlying soft-tissue layers in the form of extensive

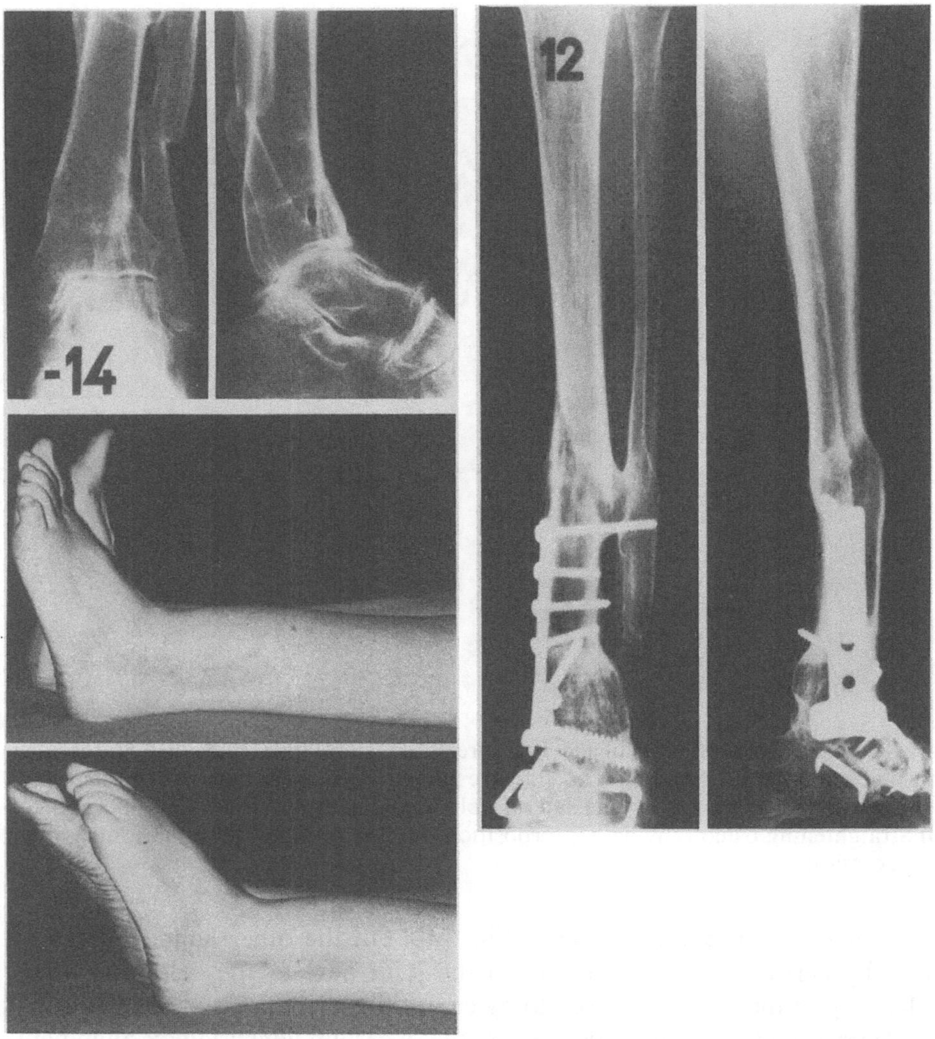

a b c

Fig. 14 a – c. E. D., 49 years of age. **a** Valgus and recurvatum deformity of the left distal tibia. **b** Corrective osteotomy combined with ankle and subtalar arthrodesis due to advanced osteoarthritis of neighboring joints. **c** Range of motion after operation

cicatrization, postthrombotic syndrome, or a significant arterial blood flow disturbance aggravate the risk of infection and call for atypical surgical approaches and atypical implantation techniques.

Significance of Subjective Complaints

The nature and severity of subjective complaints associated with posttraumatic deformity are by no means a secondary concern when weighing indications for corrective surgery [6,20,23,27]. In younger patients, the elasticity of the articular cartilage and conditioned state of the muscles provide a com-

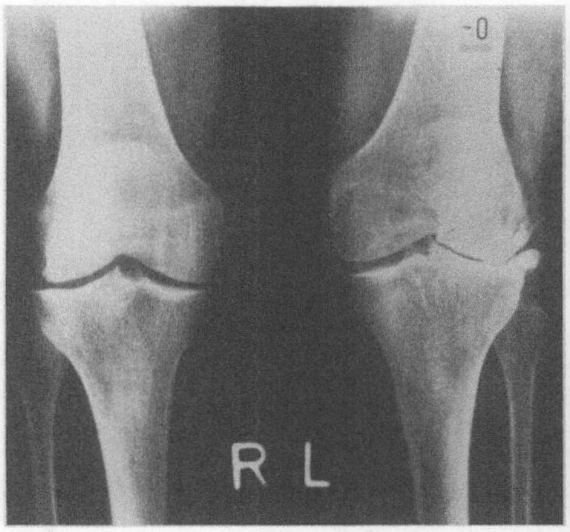

a

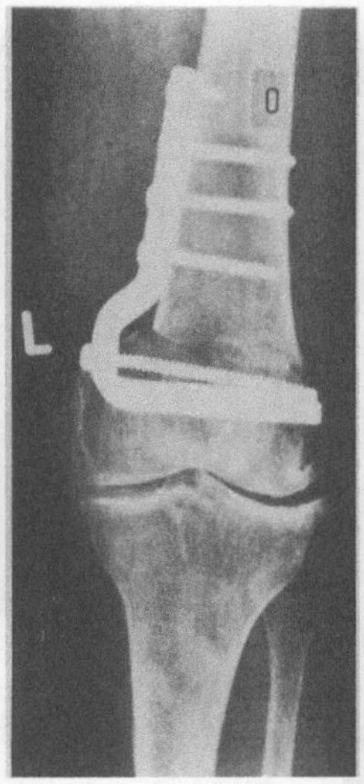

b

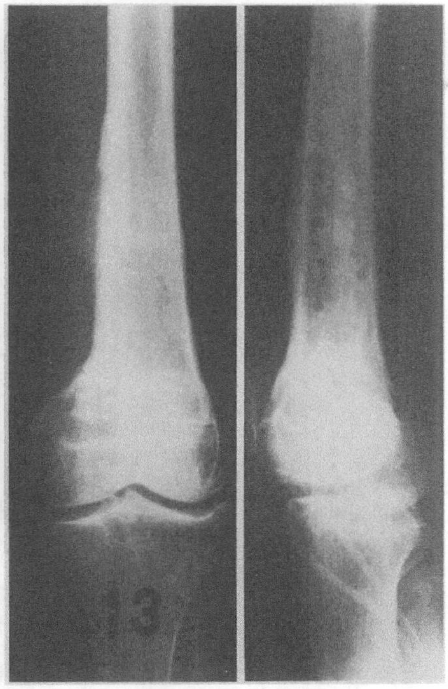

c

Fig. 15 a–c. G. J., 69 years of age. **a** Posttraumatic osteoarthritis of the knee with valgus deformity after condylar fracture of the left femur. **b** Varus osteotomy fixed with angled blade plate in a slightly overcorrected position to relieve stresses on the lateral part of the joint. **c** Roentgenograms at 13 months show marked improvement of joint spac

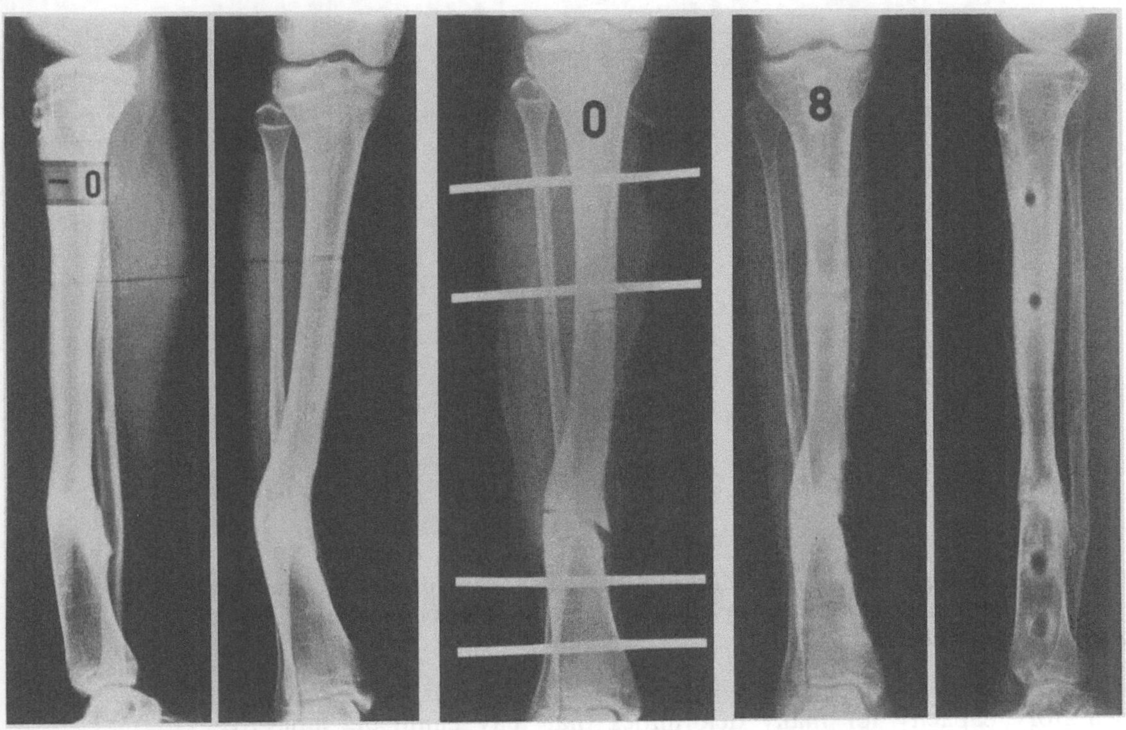

a b c

Fig. 16 a–c. S. S., 19 years of age. **a** Posttraumatic varus deformity of the right tibia. **b** Valgus osteotomy stabilized with external fixation due to a prlor history of infection and precarious soft tissues. **c** Eight months after operation

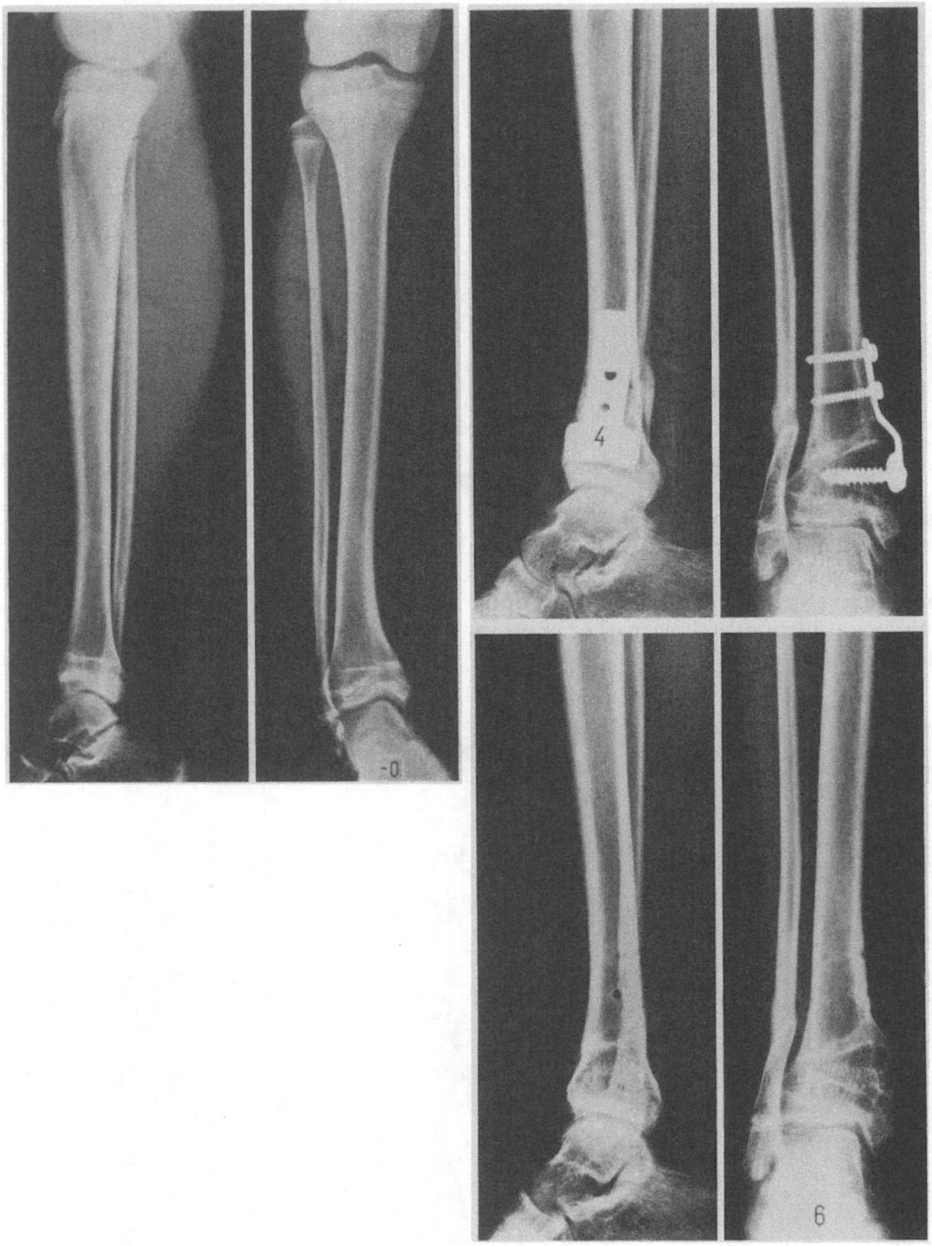

a b c

Fig. 17 a – c. M. A., 14 years of age. **a** Marked posttraumatic varus deformity of the right distal tibia with mild subjective complaints. **b** Corrective valgus osteotomy. **c** Result after removal of implants

pensatory capacity for many deformities that may eliminate subjective complaints as an early symptom. Thus, an absence of subjective complaints in young patients or the presence of minor complaints does not contraindicate an osteotomy that is indicated on the basis of impaired joint mechanics. This is illustrated by a patient with a marked varus deformity of the distal tibia that

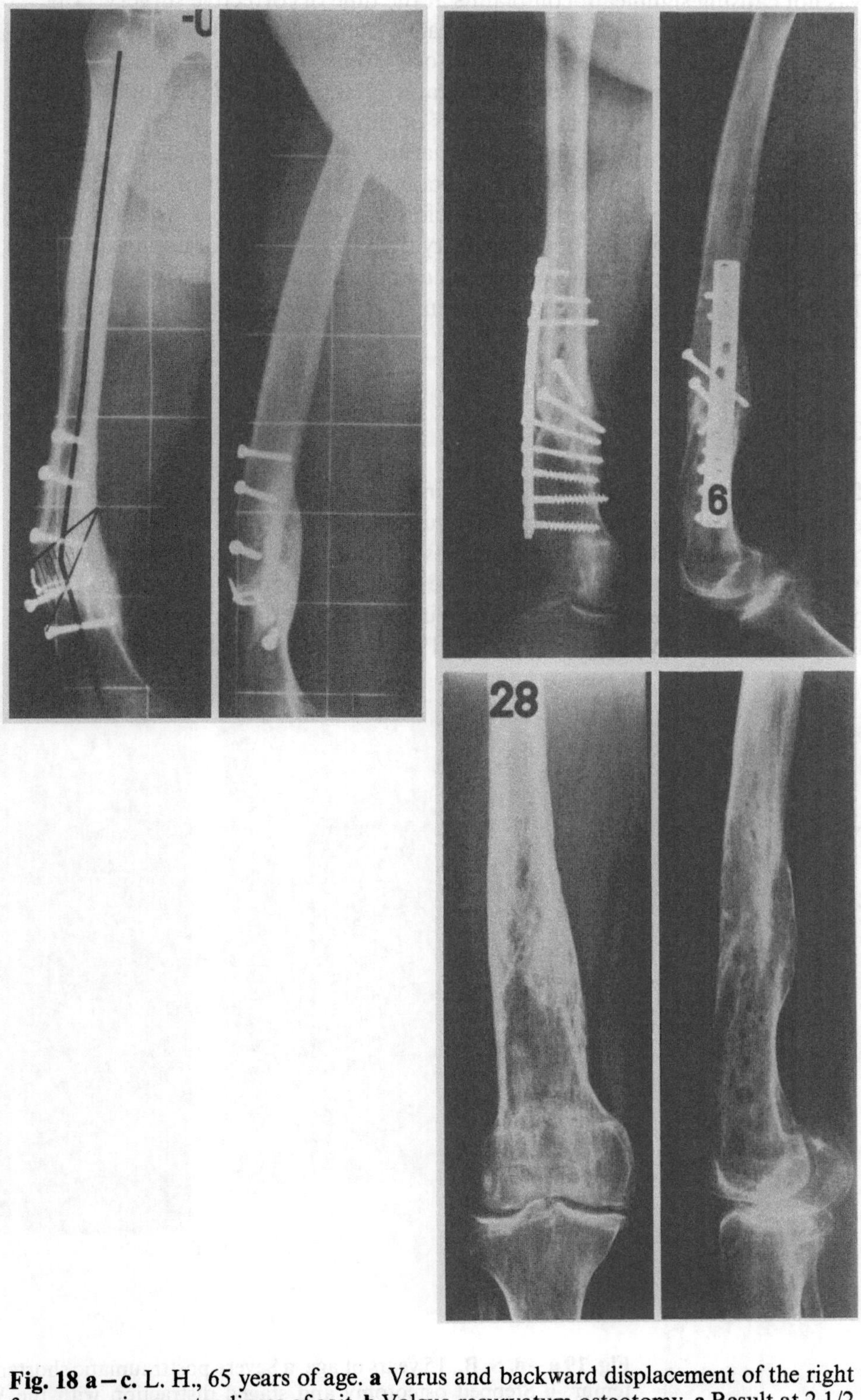

a b c

Fig. 18 a–c. L. H., 65 years of age. **a** Varus and backward displacement of the right femur, causing unsteadiness of gait. **b** Valgus-recurvatum osteotomy. **c** Result at 2 1/2 years

was not causing significant complaints at the time of corrective surgery (Fig. 17). In older patients, on the other hand, the presence of only moderate complaints may justify postponing an osteotomy that would appear to be indicated on the basis of roentgenograms. Neither would a prophylactic correction be appropriate in most cases of this type.

Attention should also be given to the nature of subjective complaints, which can assume decisive proportions. For example, the complaint of an unsteady gait in an elderly woman with a varus deformity secondary to a distal femoral fracture should be given a higher priority than the presence of unphysiologic mechanical loads and moderate general complaints (Fig. 18). This case also illustrates the overlap that exists between "functional sequelae" and "subjective complaints."

Cosmetic Effects

The consideration of cosmesis in selecting patients for corrective osteotomy after malunited fractures is not only justified but may be a predominant concern. We understand "cosmetic effects" to mean those effects that might be judged to require correction in the course of a critical medical evaluation. Two typical examples are presented, the first involving a significant posttraumatic shortening of the lower extremity (Fig. 19). Such deformities can be a source

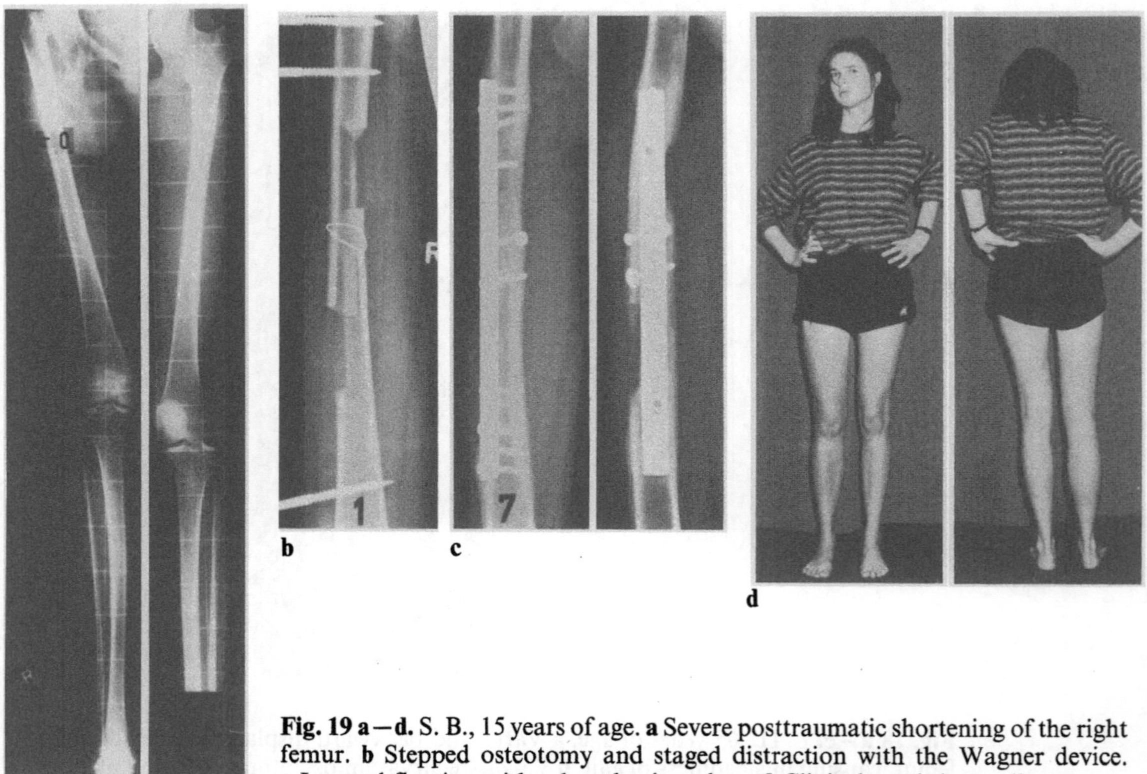

Fig. 19 a–d. S. B., 15 years of age. **a** Severe posttraumatic shortening of the right femur. **b** Stepped osteotomy and staged distraction with the Wagner device. **c** Internal fixation with a lengthening plate. **d** Clinical result is excellent

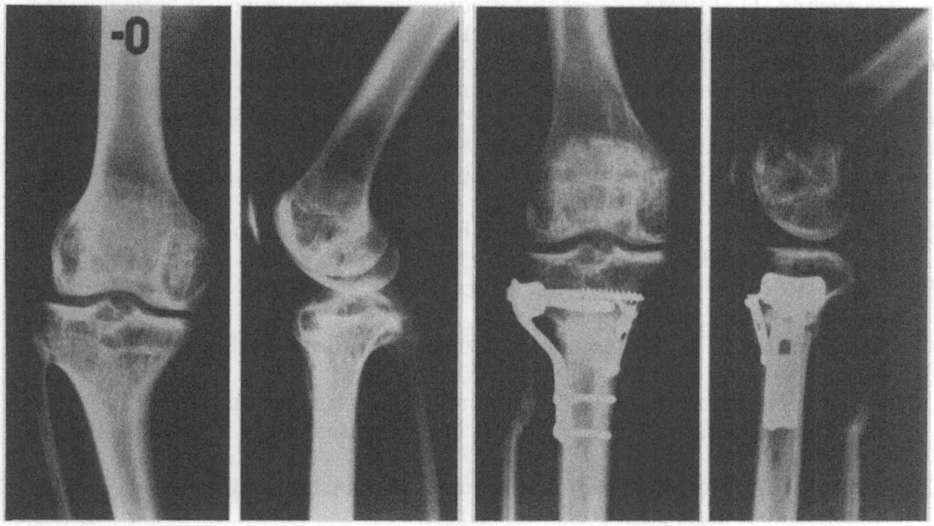

a **b**

Fig. 20 a,b. F. M., 25 years of age. **a** Varus deformity after right tibial condyle fracture in the growth period. **b** Corrected by valgus osteotomy

of serious psychological problems, especially in young people. When weighing the indication for a lengthening osteotomy, one should consider the guidelines presented by Scheuer and Lies (p. 151) as well as the therapeutic risks that are involved [22,25]. The significance of the cosmetic effects of a posttraumatic deformity is further illustrated by a patient at the end of the growth period in whom extensive burns precluded adequate primary stabilization of a tibial condylar fracture (Fig. 20). Besides the points noted above, the illustration demonstrates the importance of restoring anatomic form.

Summary

The indication for corrective osteotomy after malunited fractures of the lower extremity is based on clinical findings, the evaluation of joint mechanics, subjective complaints, and the cooperativeness of the patient. The significance of individual factors is variable, and these factors should be individually determined and comparatively evaluated when selecting patients for surgery. Discussions of these points are supplemented by clinical examples.

References

1. Endler F (1974) Biomechanische Probleme bei kombinierten Achsenfehlern der unteren Extremitäten. Orthop Praxis 7/X:423–430
2. Friedrich E, Schumpe G (1974) Der Patellaanpreßdruck bei Operation nach Bandi. Orthop Praxis 7/X:419–422
3. Greif E (1974) Korrektureingriffe nach Schienbeinkopfbrüchen. Vortrag 8. Unfallseminar Unfallchirurgische Klinik Medizinische Hochschule Hannover

4. Havemann D (1972) Korrekturosteotomien bei fehlgeheilten gelenknahen Frakturen der unteren Extremität. Aktuel Chir 7:361–368
5. Hierholzer G (1972) Operative Eingriffe zur Prophylaxe und Therapie der Arthrose bei Fehlstellungen nach Frakturen. Hefte Unfallheilkunde 110:155–161
6. Hippe P (1976) Die Indikation zur Korrektur diaphysärer Achsenfehler der unteren Extremitäten. Orthop Praxis 3/XII:299–303
7. Janssen G (1973) Die supramalleoläre Korrektur-Osteotomie nach Unterschenkelfraktur. Z Unfallmed Berufskr 66:191–195
8. Kehr H (1977) Korrekturosteotomien bei posttraumatischen Fehlstellungen am Femur. Arch Orthop Trauma Surg 87:325–331
9. Liechti R (1974) Die Arthrodese des Hüftgelenkes und ihre Problematik. Springer, Berlin Heidelberg New York.
10. Maquet PGJ (1976) Biomechanics of the knee. Springer, Berlin Heidelberg New York
11. Müller KH, Biebrach M (1977) Korrekturosteotomien und ihre Ergebnisse bei kniegelenknahen posttraumatischen Fehlstellungen. Unfallheilkunde 80:359–367
12. Müller ME, (Hrsg) (1967) Posttraumatische Achsenfehlstellungen an den unteren Extremitäten. Huber, Bern Stuttgart
13. Müller ME (1971) Die hüftnahen Femurosteotomien, 2. Aufl. Thieme, Stuttgart
14. Müller ME, Allgöwer M, Willenegger H (1977) AO-Manual, 2. Aufl. Springer, Berlin Heidelberg New York
15. Müller W (1976) Die Tibia-Osteotomie in der Therapie posttraumatischer Arthrosen am Kniegelenk. Vortrag 5. Reisensburger Workshop zur klinischen Unfallchirurgie. Hefte zur Unfallheilkunde 128:175–183
16. Pauwels F (1965) Gesammelte Abhandlungen zur funktionellen Anatomie des Bewegungsapparates. Springer, Berlin Heidelberg New York
17. Pauwels F (1973) Atlas zur Biomechanik der gesunden und kranken Hüfte. Springer, Berlin Heidelberg New York
18. Schneider R (1976) Die Arthrodese des Hüftgelenks mit Kreuzplatte und Beckenosteotomie. Huber, Bern Stuttgart Wien
19. Schneider R (1979) Die intertrochantere Osteotomie bei Coxarthrose. Springer, Berlin Heidelberg New York
20. Tönnis D (1977) Die Indikation zu Korrekturoperationen bei fehlerhafter Achsenstellung der Gliedmaßen. Aktuell Chir 12:13–24
21. Tscherne H, Gotzen L (1978) Posttraumatische Fehlstellungen. In: Chirurgie der Gegenwart IVa, 52:1–76. Urban & Schwarzenberg, München Berlin Wien
22. Wagner H (1971) Operative Beinverlängerung. Chirurg 42:260–266
23. Wagner H (1976) Indikation und Technik der Korrekturosteotomien der posttraumatischen Kniegelenkarthrose. Vortrag 5. Reisensburger Workshop zur klinischen Unfallchirurgie. Hefte zur Unfallheilkunde 128:155–174
24. Wagner H (1977) Prinzipien der Korrekturosteotomie am Bein. Orthopäde 6:145–177
25. Wagner H (1977) Surgical lengthening or shortening of femur and tibia. Technique and indications. In: Progress in Orthopaedic Surgery. Vol. 1: Leg Length Discrepancy/The Injured Knee Edited by D. S. Hungerford. Springer, Berlin, Heidelberg, New York
26. Weber BG, Cech O (1973) Pseudoarthrosen. Huber, Bern Stuttgart Wien
27. Zenker H (1972) Zur Indikation und Technik korrigierender Osteotomien im Schaftbereich langer Röhrenknochen. Arch Orthop Trauma Surg 74:205–223

Special Diagnosis and Preoperative Planning of Corrective Osteotomies

O. Oest

Introduction

With modern techniques of internal fixation [9], we are able to perform almost any corrective osteotomy of bone with a high degree of precision. But surgical correction of the axial alignment of a leg must be preceded by meticulous planning, because postoperative corrections are no longer possible after stable internal fixation has been applied. Preoperative planning of this type must be predicated on sound, reproducible morphologic data, i.e., on the actual morphology of the leg skeleton under conditions of functional loading. The external, clinical appearance of a leg can provide only a hint of the osseous deformities that exist and thus of the correction that is required. A thick soft-tissue envelope can be highly deceptive, and clinical measurements of angles or of intercondylar and intermalleolar distances often give an incomplete or misleading picture of actual limb alignment. A realistic image of the leg skeleton in the frontal plane (Fig. 1) can be obtained only by means of a long Weight-bearing roentgenogram [11–16,20].

Special Diagnosis – Whole-Leg Roentgenogram

The patient stands frontally on a step before a solid backrest such that the central beam of the x-ray tube is centered on the knee joint (Fig. 2). The next step is to frontalize the knee joint (Fig. 3) such that the femoral condyles are parallel to the film plane. This is done by having the patient flex the knee briefly so that the lower leg can be used as a directional guide [16]. When the lower leg is perpendicular to the film plane, the condylar axis will normally be parallel to the film plane. After final adjustments are made, the patient is instructed to bear most of his weight on the leg that is being filmed. In patients with a flexion contracture of the knee, frontalization of the knee joint is essential for obtaining a useful whole-leg film, because any external or internal rotation of the partially extended limb can mimic a valgus or varus deformity [2,16]. This can also occur in patients in whom leg rotation is restricted by osteoarthritis of the hip. With an external rotation contracture of the hip joint, frontalization can be accomplished only by rotating the patient in a medial direction. We find that similar considerations apply to the filming of hips with a slipped upper femoral epiphysis [8]. With combined axial deformities, especially those involving rotation of the femur, the concurrent determination of femoral neck anteversion is imperative [7].

Corrective Osteotomies of the Lower Extremity
Edited by G. Hierholzer, K. H. Müller

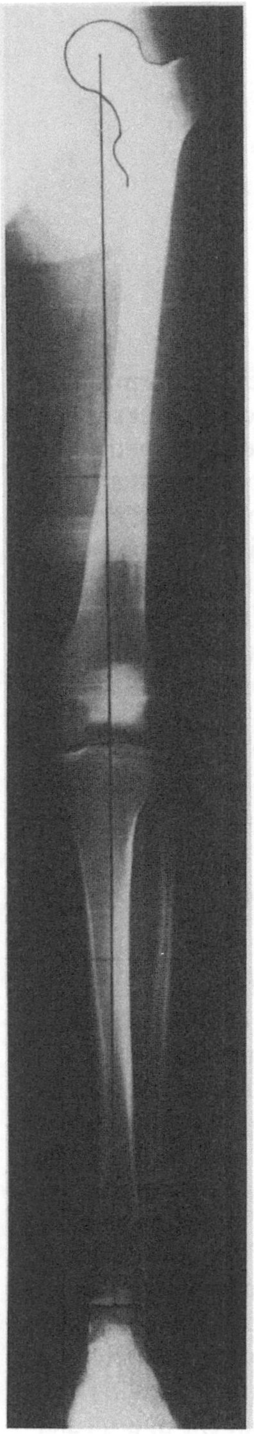

Fig. 1. Long roentgenogram of the lower extremity

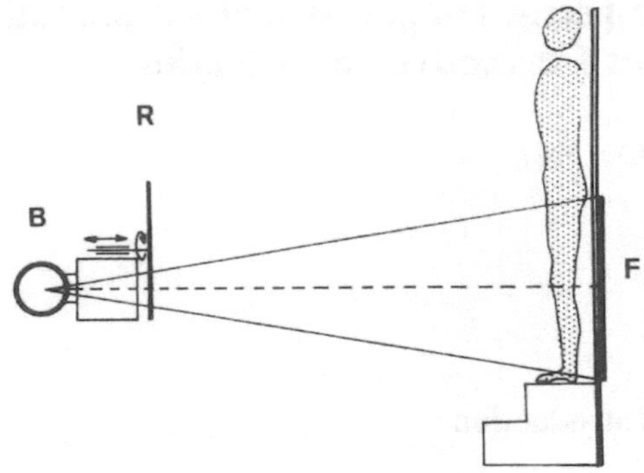

Fig. 2. The beam is centered on the knee joint at a distance of 3 m. **R** Rotating equalizing diaphragm, **B** x-ray tube, **F** film

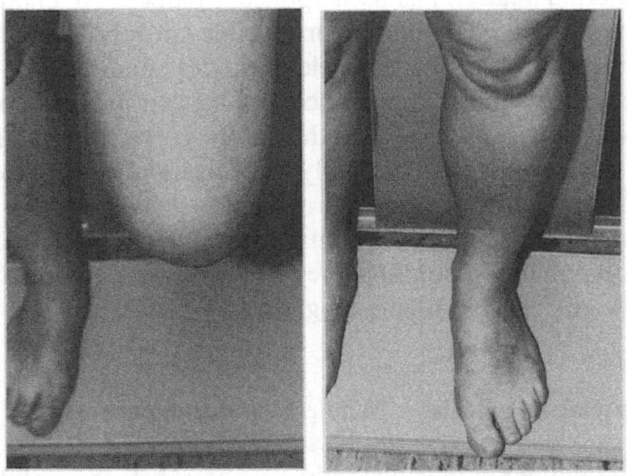

Fig. 3. Frontalization of the knee joint

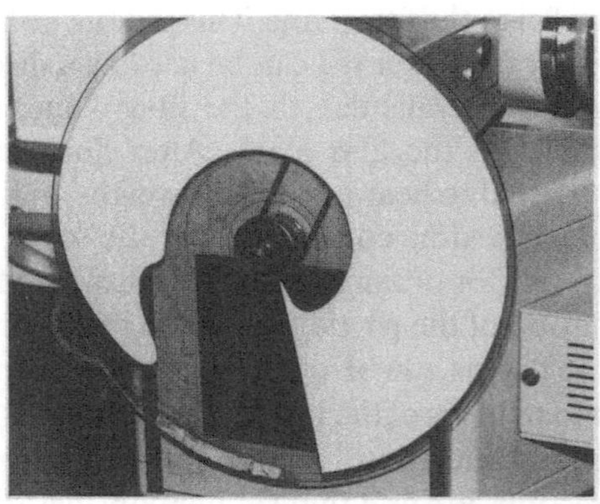

Fig. 4. Rotating equalizing diaphragm

Fig. 1. Long roentgenogram of the lower extremity

The x-ray tube is centered on the knee joint with a focus-film distance of 3 m [2,16]. Given the variations in the soft-tissue envelope of the leg, means must be used to equalize the exposure if a uniform image is to be obtained. For this purpose we use a rotating equalizing diaphragm [16], which is mounted in front of the beam restrictor of the x-ray tube (Fig. 4). The rotating diaphragm can be adjusted to individual leg length by varying its distance from the restrictor. This diaphragm changes the x-ray beam quantitatively but not qualitatively, i.e., it selectively modulates the exposure delivered to different segments of the limb, resulting in the generation of a relatively uniform image on the x-ray plate.

Evaluation of Films

The whole-leg roentgenogram is evaluated on a large, horizontal view box [2,16,20]. A 100-cm precision metal ruler, an adjustable protractor, the x-ray ischiometer of Müller [7], and a sharpened soft pencil are required. With simple axial deformities the evaluation can be done on the roentgenogram itself, but sometimes it is best to make a separate drawing on which the result of the correction can be shown. The individual steps are as follows:

1. *Locate the Center of the Femoral Head*
The center of the femoral head is determined using the x-ray ischiometer of Müller [7]. By laying the appropriate circle over the outline of the femoral head, the center usually can be easily located and marked. This may be difficult if the femoral head shows osteoarthritic deformity. If the contralateral head is intact, its center can be transferred to the image of the affected femur, or the outer portions of the upper femoral epiphysis and diaphyseal spine can be used as reference points according to the method of Hilgenreiner [4].

2. *Locate the Center of the Knee Joint*
First a horizontal line is drawn tangent to the femoral condyles to obtain the "knee baseline" (KB). The center of the knee joint is located by drawing lines vertical to the KB and tangent to the condyles of the femur and tibia that are closest to the intercondylar eminence (Fig. 5 a). The midpoint of the resulting line segment is the center of the knee joint [2].

3. *Locate the Center of the Ankle Joint*
A horizontal line is drawn tangent to the upper margin of the talus. The points where this line intersects the inner surfaces of the malleoli define the width of the ankle joint (Fig. 5 b). The midpoint of this line segment is found [2].

4. *Femoral and Tibial Shaft Axes*
The center of the femoral diaphysis is marked at two levels: at the junction of the proximal and middle thirds, and at the junction of the middle and distal thirds. The line connecting these points is the femoral shaft axis (FSA). The tibial shaft axis (TSA) is constructed in analogous fashion [2].

5. *Mechanical Axis*
The mechanical axis of the leg (MA) [5,6,18,19] extends from the center of the femoral head to the center of the ankle joint (Fig. 6).

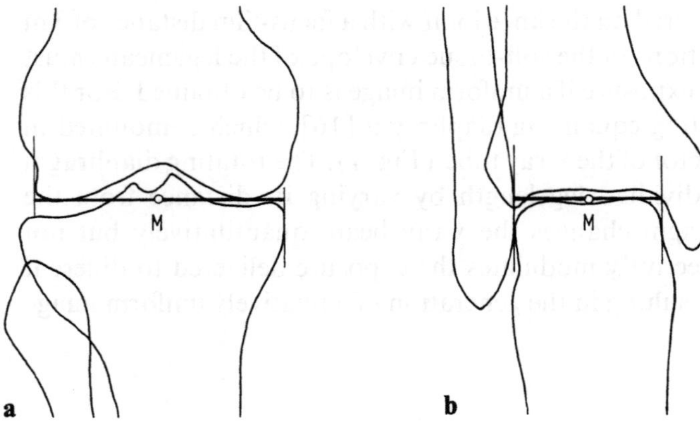

Fig. 5. a Locating the center of the knee joint (**M**); **b** locating the center of the ankle joint (**M**)

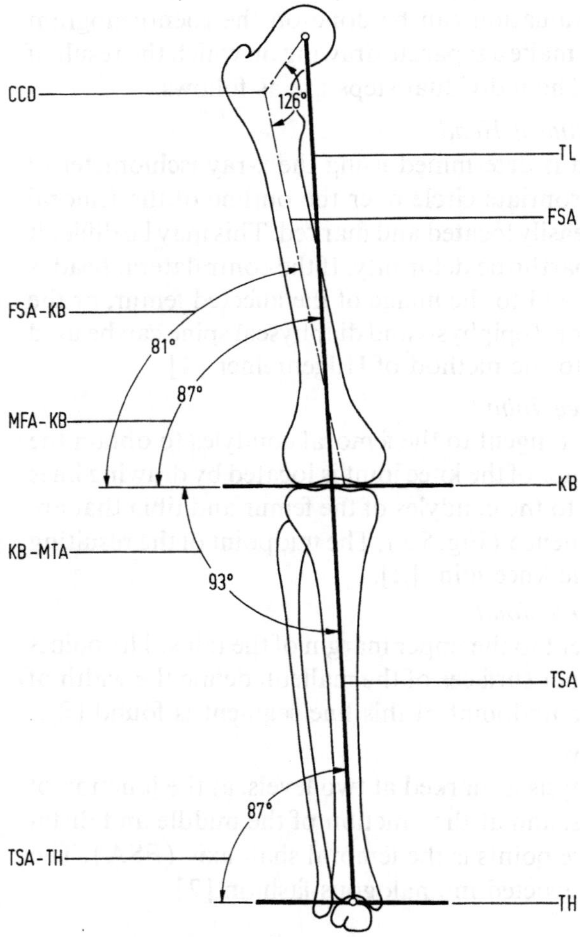

Fig. 6. Axes and angles relevant to the evaluation of a long roentgenogram of the lower extremity (abbreviations explained in text)

6. *Angle Measurements*

a) The angle of inclination of the femoral neck (CCD) is measured with the x-ray ischiometer of Müller [7]; 126° is normal.

b) Angle between the femoral shaft axis (FSA) and knee baseline (KB); 81–82° is normal.

c) Angle between the knee baseline (KB) and tibial shaft axis (TSA); 93° is normal.

d) Angle between the tibial shaft axis (TSA) and upper margin of the talus (TH); 87° is normal.

7. *Other Parameters*

a) Inclination of the knee baseline (in degrees).

b) Inclination of the upper margin of the talus (in degrees).

c) Inclination of the mechanical axis.

d) Medial or lateral deviation of the mechanical axis from the center of the knee joint.

e) Prominence of the lesser trochanter, the tibia-to-fibula distance, the width of the femoral condyles, and the position of the fibular head apex relative to the lateral border of the upper tibia for comparison of two long films with respect to the rotational position of the leg [2].

Planning the Osteotomy

1. *Extent of Genu Varum or Valgum*

The extent of the genu varum or valgum corresponds to the deviation of the mechanical axis of the leg from the center of the knee joint [3]. The greater this deviation, the stronger the indication for corrective osteotomy [12,15]. The classification of Gragard [1] recognizes three grades of severity of genu varum and genu valgum. This classification is itself a useful predictor of whether secondary osteoarthritis of the knee joint is likely to develop.

2. *Site of the Axial Deformity*

In most cases the site of a posttraumatic deformity is easily identified. It can be expressed indirectly in terms of the changes in the angles listed above. The presence of multiple axial changes can create a relatively complex situation that may require a special diagrammatic reconstruction of the leg skeleton to enable the planning of a multistage correction [10,17].

3. *Site of the Correction*

As a rule, the correction should be performed at the site of the previous fracture, unless this is contraindicated by biological concerns relating to the development of a nonunion or infection. The *angle of correction* corresponds to the angle of the axial deviation.

4. *Planning the Correction*

It must be decided whether a simple or combined axial deformity exists.

A simple axial deformity can usually be corrected by an osteotomy at the site of its occurrence. Osteotomies at sites distant from the deformity are exceptional. Combined axial deformities in the same direction add together, while deformities in opposite directions tend to cancel. The different changes may have either a varus effect or a valgus effect on the leg axis, as shown in Table 1. In terms of extent, an axial deformity near the knee joint will always have the most pronounced effect on the general limb axis. Spirig [20] recommends that preoperative drawings be made directly on the long roentgenogram. In our experience, however, it is sometimes advantageous to make a separate drawing on heavy paper, as this will allow a template to be made of the proposed osteotomy fragment so that the axial changes effected by the osteotomy can be simulated on the drawing.

Table 1. Varus or Valgus Effect of Various Factors on the Leg Axis

Varus effect	Valgus effect
1. Lengthening of the femoral neck	1. Shortening of the femoral neck
2. Reduction of the CCD angle	2. Increase in the CCD angle
3. Varus bowing of the femur	3. Valgus bowing of the femur
4. Increase in the FSA-KB angle	4. Reduction of the FSA-KB angle
5. Varus inclination of the KB	5. Valgus inclincation of the KB
6. Increase in the KB-TSA angle	6. Reduction of the KB-TSA angle
7. Varus bowing of the tibia	7. Valgus bowing of the tibia
8. Increase in the TSA-TH angle	8. Reduction of the TSA-TH angle

Below are several examples which illustrate the procedure for the planning of corrective osteotomies [2] (Fig. 7):

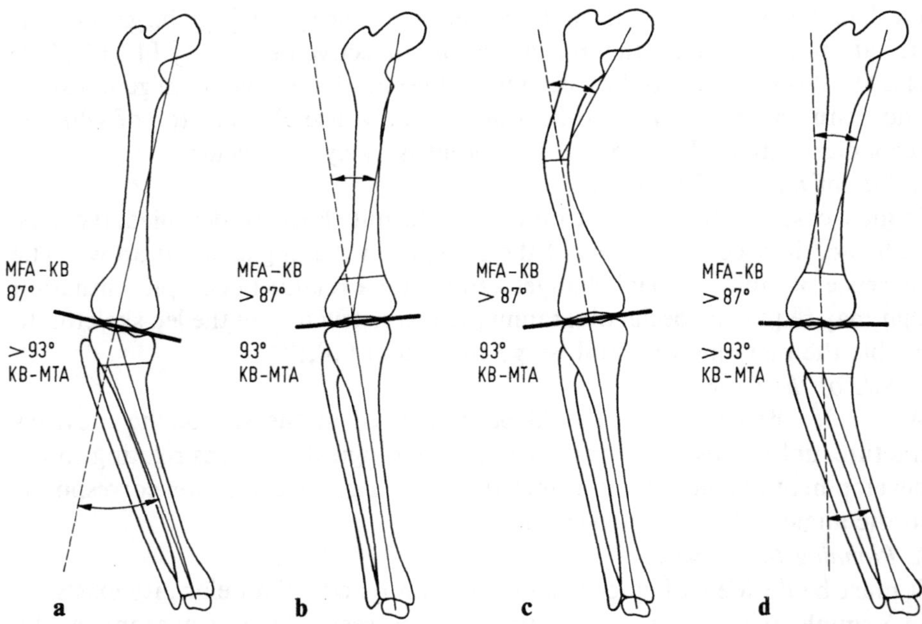

Fig. 7 a–d. Determining the angle of correction for a genu varum in which the axial deformity is located **a** in the upper tibia, **b** in the supracondylar region, **c** at the center of the femoral shaft, and **d** in the infra- and supracondylar regions (abbreviations explained in text)

a) Infracondylar osteotomy for genu varum with axial deformity of the upper tibia (Fig. 7 a). Proceed as follows:
- Extend the mechanical femoral axis (MFA) distally.
- Draw a horizontal line at the level of the proposed osteotomy.
- Find the intersection of this line with the extended mechanical femoral axis, and draw a line from that point to the center of the ankle joint.
- The angle formed by this line and the mechanical femoral axis equals the angle of correction.

b) Supracondylar osteotomy (Fig. 7 b) for genu varum with axial deformity of the distal femur:
- Extend the mechanical tibial axis (MTA) proximally.
- Draw a horizontal line at the level of the proposed osteotomy.
- Find the intersection of this line with the extended mechanical tibial axis, and draw a line from that point to the center of the femoral head.
- The angle formed by this line and the mechanical tibial axis equals the angle of correction.

c) With a deformity of the femoral shaft, the procedure is the same as that for the tibial shaft (Fig. 7 c):
For the same degree of deformity, osteotomies distant from the knee joint require a greater angular correction than osteotomies near the joint. To investigate this relationship, we determined the osteotomy angles on the whole-leg film of a genu valgum that would be needed at different levels of the tibia in order to correct axial alignment (Fig. 8). The plot of the measured values has the shape of an exponential function, i.e., the size of the correction angle increases not linearly but exponentially with

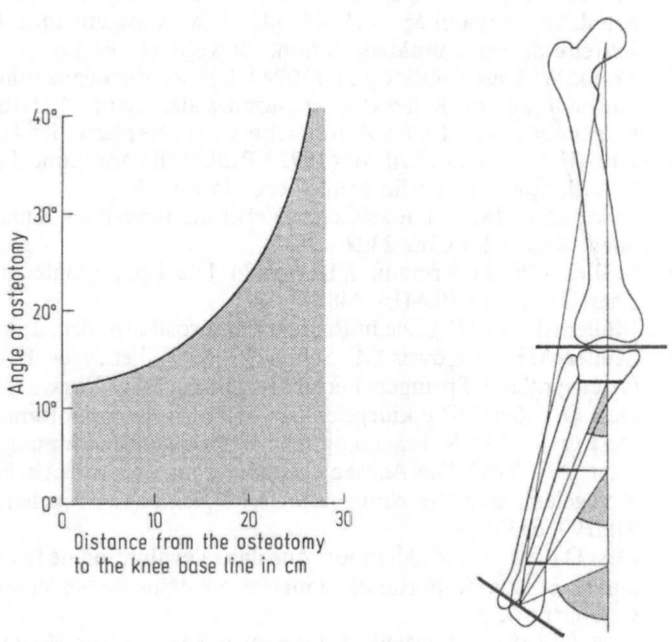

Fig. 8. Dependence of the correction angle on the level of the osteotomy

increasing distance from the knee baseline. This permits the following conclusions to be drawn:

- The size of the correction angle depends very strongly on the level of the osteotomy. The planning procedure described makes due allowance for this fact.
- A faulty osteotomy angle has a much greater impact on the mechanical limb axis close to the joint than at a distance from it.

d) If axial deformities are present at two levels and cause marked alteration of the MFA-KB and KB-MTA angles, corrections at two levels are necessary to restore alignment. A horizontal knee baseline is obtained by correcting the MFA-KB angle to 87° and the KB-MTA angle to 93° (Fig. 7 d). Comparison with the opposite extremity is always advised.

Summary

To perform an acurate corrective osteotomy for posttraumatic lower limb deformity, it is necessary to make preoperative drawings based on a long weight-bearing roentgenogram of the leg. The meticulous transferral of the planned correction from paper to the operated limb ensures an optimum therapeutic outcome. Only in this way can one avoid the disappointments that result from significant under- and overcorrections.

References

1. Bragard K (1932) Das Genu valgum. Z Orthop Chir [Suppl] 57
2. Frank W, Quadflieg KH (1974) Die Röntgenganzaufnahme der unteren Extremität. Inauguraldissertation, Universität Gießen
3. Frank W, Oest O, Rettig H (1974) Die Röntgenganzaufnahme in der Operationsplanung von Korrekturosteotomien der Beine. Z Orthop 112:344
4. Hilgenreiner H (1939) Zur angeborenen Dysplasie der Hüfte. Z Orthop 69:30
5. Lanz T von, Wachsmuth W (1972) Praktische Anatomie, Bd I/4. Bein und Statik, 2. Aufl. Springer, Berlin Heidelberg New York
6. Mikulicz J (1879) Die seitlichen Verkrümmungen am Knie und deren Heilmethoden. Arch Klin Chir 23:561
7. Müller ME, Ledermann KL (1962) Die Epiphysenlösung am Schenkelkopf. Ther Umsch 19/10:441–448
8. Müller ME (1971) Die hüftnahen Femurosteotomien, 2. Aufl. Thieme, Stuttgart
9. Müller ME, Allgöwer M, Schneider R, Willenegger H (1977) Manual der Osteosynthese. Springer, Berlin Heidelberg New York
10. Oest O (1970) Die kniegelenksnahe Korrekturosteotomie. Orthop Prax 4:102
11. Oest O (1973) Röntgenologische Beinachsenbestimmung. Z Orthop 111:497
12. Oest O (1978) Die Achsenfehlstellung als präarthrotische Deformität für das Kniegelenk und die röntgenologische Beinachsenbeurteilung. Unfallheilkunde 81:629–633
13. Oest O (1981) Radiodiagnostique dans l'évaluation de la déviation de l'axe de la jambe et son importance pour la préarthrose géniculaire. Rev Rhum Mal Osteoartic 752:
14. Oest O (1981) Spezielle Röntgentechniken in der Kniegelenksdiagnostik. In: Hohmann D (Hrsg) Praktische Orthopädie. Das Knie. Stork, Bruchsal

15. Oest O, Frank W (1974) Die Achsenfehlstellung als präarthrotische Deformität für das Kniegelenk. Z Orthop 112:632
16. Oest O, Sieberg HJ (1971) Die Röntgenganzaufnahme der unteren Extremitäten. Z Orthop 109:54
17. Oest O, Süssenbach F (1982) Achsenfehler der unteren Extremitäten nach Wachstumsfugenverletzung. In: Eichler J, Weber U (Hrsg) Frakturen im Kindesalter. Thieme, Stuttgart New York
18. Pauwels F (1935) Der Schenkelhalsbruch, ein mechanisches Problem. Enke, Stuttgart
19. Pauwels F (1965) Gesammelte Abhandlungen zur funktionellen Anatomie des Bewegungsapparates. Springer, Berlin Heidelberg New York
20. Spirig G (1967) Die Diagnose der Achsenfehler der unteren Extremität. In: Müller ME (Hrsg) Posttraumatische Achsenfehlstellungen an den unteren Extremitäten. Huber, Bern, S 17

Mechanical and Technical Principles of the Internal Fixation of Corrective Osteotomies

S. M. Perren

Proximal femoral osteotomies and their stabilization with an angled blade plate are common procedures. It is worthwhile to examine the mechanical and technical principles of the internal fixation of corrective osteotomies, using this operation as an example.

The specific problem of the fixation of osteotomies near epiphyses is that one of the two fragments created by the osteotomy consists largely of cancellous bone and thus provides a poor anchorage for plate-fixing screws. The holding strength of 6.5-mm screws in cancellous bone is only 1 – 2 kp/mm, as opposed to the 40 kp/mm provided by 4.5-mm screws in cortical bone (maximum holding strength is referred to 1 mm of screw length). Given the low specific load-bearing capacity of cancellous bone (less than 0.5 kp/mm^2 under fatigue conditions in vivo), it is necessary to use an implant that has a large area of contact with the bone. The angled blade plate satisfies this requirement owing to the large surface area of the blade. The present article deals with the principles of the use of the angled blade plate.

Use of the Angled Blade Plate as a Tension Band

For simplicity we shall assume that a varus bending load is acting on the proximal end of the femur in the frontal plane. This causes tension to be exerted on the lateral cortex and compression on the medial cortex. The internal fixation technique for a subtrochanteric osteotomy must transmit tension through the implant on the lateral side, while allowing the medial bone to absorb compression. Practically any implant from a wire to a screw to a plate is capable of absorbing tensile forces. The bending strength of the implant is immaterial. Thus, Pauwels was able to achieve satisfactory fixation of the proximal femur using a simple wire loop. However, this arrangement lacks significant strength reserves and may lead to problems during general use. Weak points are the anchorage of the wire in the bone and the fatigue strength of the wire, especially at sites where it is bent. The angled blade plate produces a tension band effect in which the part of the blade near the bend of the plate exerts pressure on the lateral cortex (Fig. 1). The length of the blade is unimportant in this type of fixation. The pressure-transmitting contact area between the plate and bone is oriented ideally at right angles to the direction of the compressive force.

During function, cyclic loads are exerted on the osteotomy site. By prestressing the plate longitudinally, it is possible to create a sustained

Corrective Osteotomies of the Lower Extremity
Edited by G. Hierholzer, K. H. Müller

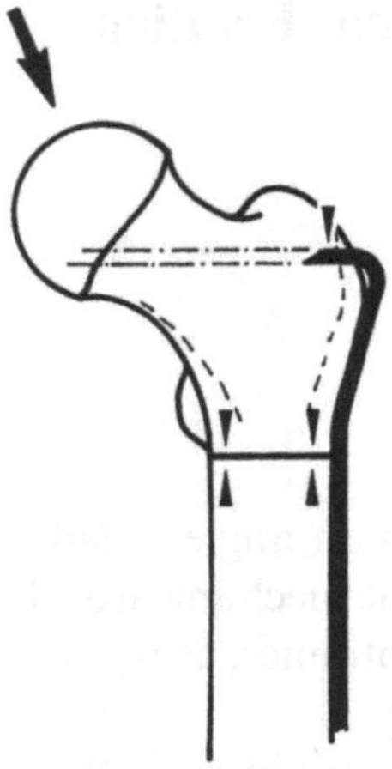

Fig. 1. Use of the angled blade plate as a tension band

compression that holds the plate against the bone and maintains rigid lateral apposition of the bone ends. This is made necessary by the tendency of the applied bending moment to open the osteotomy on the lateral side. In the absence of a countermoment, cyclic functional loads would cause a periodic gaping of the lateral osteotomy line. Static compression is virtually the only means the surgeon has for creating an effective countermoment. While this requires that an unnecessarily high compression be applied across the osteotomy primarily, this is not harmful owing to the biological pressure tolerance of the bone.

If the countermoment is temporarily too small relative to the applied bending load, the osteotomy will gape intermittently on the lateral side. The resulting motion induces a superficial resorption of bone, which aggravates the instability. This vicious cycle of motion, bone resoprtion, and aggravated motion is countered to some degree by motion-induced callus formation, which is effective in the metaphysis owing to the large interior bone surface (cancellous bone) and long lever arms.

We have spoken of the bending moment in connection with fixation mechanisms. Because the bending moment equals force times effective lever arm, the projected distance between the pressure-exerting part of the implant and the bony buttress is of major importance. The greater this distance, the less force has to be applied to the implant and bone buttress in order to "neuralize" a given bending load on the femoral head. We consider this when evaluating the moment-force relationships in a shaft osteotomy as opposed to a metaphyseal osteotomy. The smaller force needed to maintain stability makes it possible to transmit the force to the cancellous bone or a relatively small area of plate contact on the cortex.

Splinting an Osteotomy with the Angled Blade Plate

If the fragments of a transverse osteotomy of the femoral neck are connected using the blade of a 130° plate, the plate is functioning basically as a simple

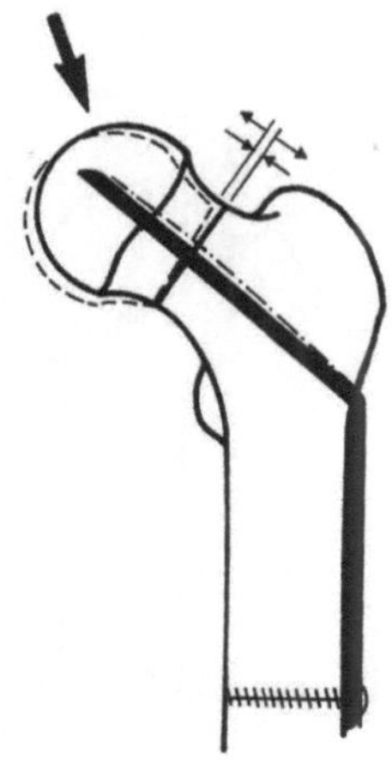

Fig. 2. Use of the angled blade plate as a simple splint

splint (Fig. 2). Like a wooden splint strapped to the outside of a limb for the temporary immobilization of a fracture, the plate lessens the mobility of the bone fragments. It is important to understand that a splint inhibits motion but does not eliminate it entirely. The reduction of motion is proportional to the stiffness of the splint, which in turn depends on the material (E modulus) of the splint and especially on the cross-sectional area of the splint (inertial moment). The magnitude of these last two factors is limited, however, and so, therefore, is the action of the splint. Any residual motion will inevitably stimulate bone resorption at the ends of the fragments, which is of less consequence in cancellous bone than in the cortical bone of the diaphysis. This is why an implant is able to splint a metaphyseal osteotomy more effectively than an osteotomy of the shaft.

Use of the Angled Blade Plate as a Gliding Splint

This function of the angled blade plate is similar to that of the intramedullary nail, a slotted, tubular implant introduced into the bone in such a way that motion and/or resorption of the bone ends allows appositional movement of the fragments.

A splint which bridges the bone fragments but does not entirely prevent interfragmental motion and resorption is useful only if adjunctive measures are taken to immobilize the fragments, or if the splint allows the fragments to come into contact. In the diaphyseal area, the lag screw is a common adjunctive measure to prevent interfragmental motion. In the area of the femoral neck, we prefer to utilize the second mechanism, i.e., an implant that permits appositional movement of the fragments in response to "inevitable" motion and resorption. This is made possible either by the proximal migration of the plate blade within the femoral neck (Fig. 3) or by the telescoping action of a specially designed implant (e.g., the dynamic hip screw of DHS, Fig. 4).

Shearing of the fragments at right angles to the blade axis is largely *prevented* by the blade if it has a good transverse seating in the bone. Of course, this may be difficult in loose cancellous bone even if the area of bone-blade

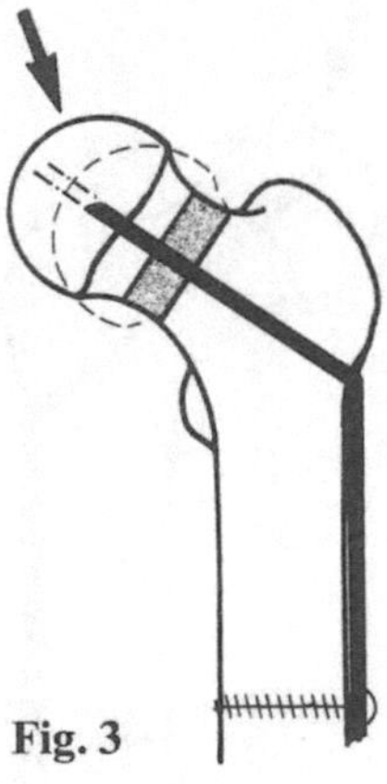

Fig. 3

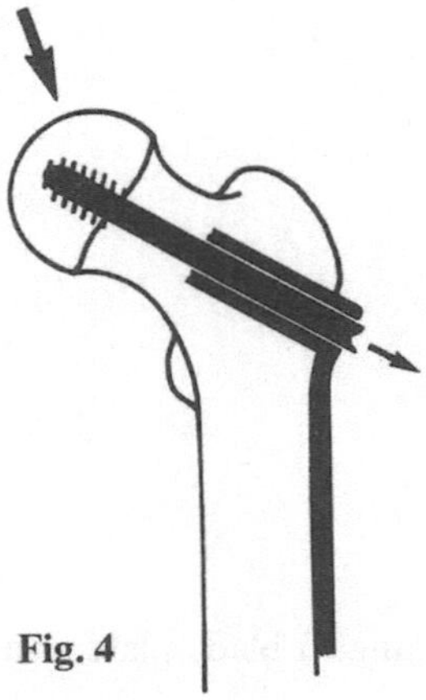

Fig. 4

Fig. 3. Approximation of the fragments through anterior migration of the plate blade in the femoral neck (gliding splint)

Fig. 4. Approximation of the fragments by a telescoping implant (dynamic hip screw)

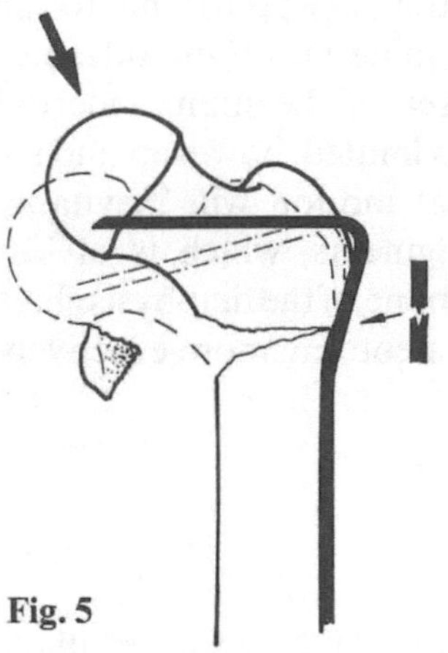

Fig. 5

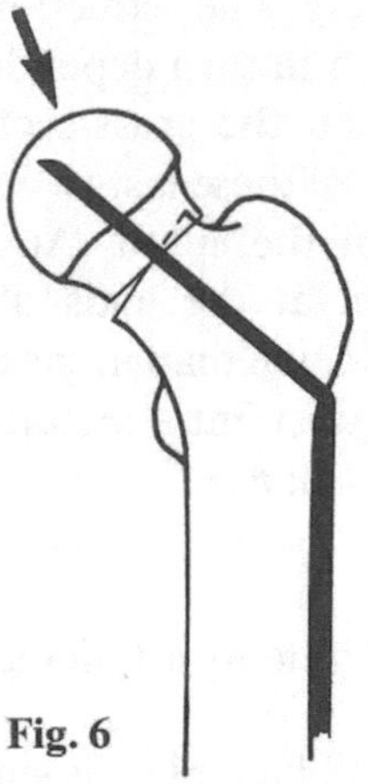

Fig. 6

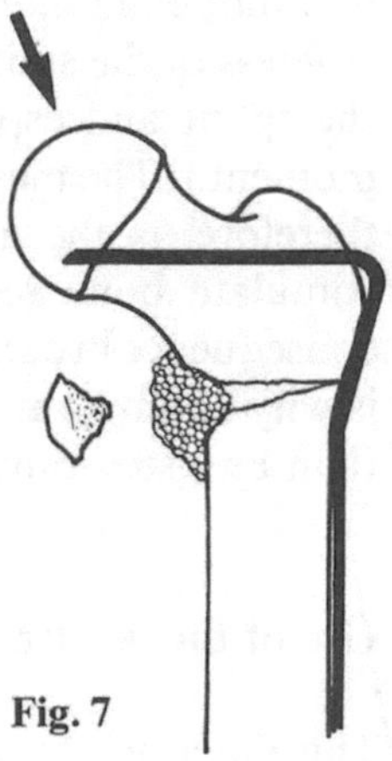

Fig. 7

Fig. 5. Buttressing with the angled blade plate alone: Without support on the compression side, varus displacement of the fixation is inevitable and may cause plate breakage (cf. Fig. 7)

Fig. 6. Impaction of the proximal fragment onto the distal fragment ("hat on hook" principle)

Fig. 7. Use of a cancellous bone graft to construct a medial buttress

contact is large. The splint can only *reduce* anterior and posterior movements of the fragment about an axis perpendicular to the long axis of the blade. Besides the aforementioned plate factors of material stiffness and cross-sectional geometry, the mobility of the fragments also depends on the magnitude of the applied bending moment. The more the cross-sectional plane of the blade is oriented perpendicular to the direction of the applied force, the smaller the bending action on the blade, and the better the stability.

As mentioned above, splinting alone can prevent gross displacement of the fragments, but it cannot provide a long-term, rigid fixation. It allows residual motion, which stimulates resorption of the bone ends. If the load-bearing ability of the fragments is poor, the bone ends may become mechanically overloaded and collapse.

The angled blade plate solves this problem by allowing the head fragment to glide over the blade in response to interfacial motion and resorption. With the dynamic hip screw (DHS), the implant consists of two telescoping parts. The gliding part of the device is screwed securely into the head fragment.

Buttressing with the Angled Blade Plate

The angled blade plate is also suitable for buttressing (Fig. 5). However, given the magnitude of the loads about the hip, it is apparent that buttressing cannot be adequately achieved with the relatively narrow blade alone. One way to solve this problem is to appose the medial fragment to the cranial part of the distal fragment (Fig. 6), creating an "imperfect" apposition. This increases the load-bearing capacity of the fixation, especially if the fragments are impacted in that position. If a medial buttress is absent, one can be constructed with grafted cancellous bone (Fig. 7).

Summary

Taking the internal fixation of proximal femoral osteotomies as an example, it is shown how the angled blade plate can act as a tension band, a neutralizing device, a buttressing device, and a "gliding splint." Bone grafts are used to construct a satisfactory buttress in cases where the implant alone is too weak.

Special Techniques of Internal Fixation for Corrective Osteotomies

G. Zeiler and U. Pfeiffer

Introduction

Even special techniques of internal fixation must be able to stabilize a corrective osteotomy securely enough to permit early postoperative mobilization of the joints and ambulation with partial weight bearing [1].

As the results from a large patient series indicate (Tables 1 and 2), these special techniques of internal fixation do provide adequate stabilization of the lower extremity, even though the stabilizing ability of the implants may appear questionable to the casual observer. This is because the fixation material consists entirely of semitubular plates, usually modified to a "hook plate" configuration (Fig. 1), one-third tubular plates in children, as well as Kirschner wires and screws, i.e., implants that are thin, easily deformed, and elastic [3–6]. This apparent contradiction is explained by the fact that in the examples presented here, the task of stabilization rests not on the implant alone, but to a large degree on the form of the osteotomy or the relative position of the osteotomy fragments. In some cases even soft-tissue structures are enlisted to enhance the fixation. The key to obtaining a stable osteotomy with a minimum of fixation material lies either in leaving an intact bridge of cortex opposite the base of the wedge (the part continuous with the apex of the wedge), or in creating a bony buttress which stabilizes the osteotomy against displacement and rotation and transmits purely compressive loads. The

Table 1. Supracondylar, Infracondylar and Supramalleolar Osteotomies Stabilized with a Semitubular Hook Plate or One-Third Tubular Plate

Closed wedge osteotomies	266
Open wedge osteotomies	111
Displacement osteotomies	45
Total	422

Table 2. Sites of the Osteotomies

High tibial osteotomies	304
Supracondylar osteotomies	94
Supramalleolar osteotomies	24
Total	422

Corrective Osteotomies of the Lower Extremity
Edited by G. Hierholzer, K. H. Müller

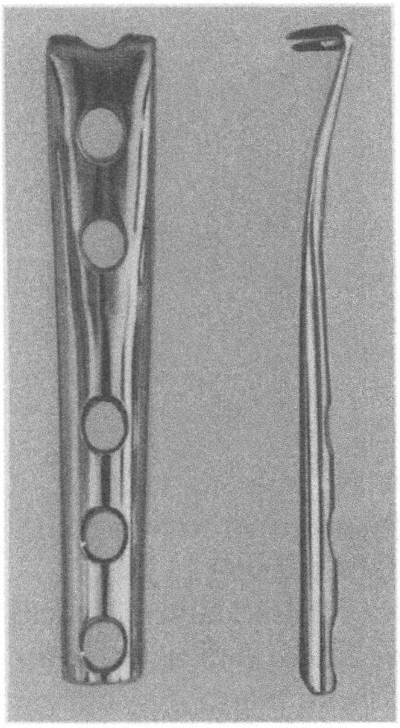

Fig. 1. The terminal screw hole in a semitubular plate is opened in V-shaped fashion with a side-cutting pliers. A flat-nosed pliers with smooth jaws is to adapt the plate to bony contours, and the two prongs are bent toward the concave side of the plate with round-nosed pliers

resulting decrease in the size and amount of internal fixation material has important advantages for the course of treatment and recovery.

Techniques of Osteotomy and Internal Fixation

Unilateral Closed Wedge Osteotomy and its Stabilization with the Semitubular Hook Plate

This type of osteotomy, which is particularly advantageous in the distal femoral metaphysis and the proximal and distal tibial metaphyses, requires that a wedge of bone be removed from the convex side of the axial deformity (Fig. 2). The wedge is cut close to but not through the opposite cortex, leaving it intact. The defect is bridged with a semitubular hook plate, which is attached to the juxta-articular fragment with one or two fully threaded cancellous bone screws and the terminal prongs of the plate. The wedge osteotomy is closed by

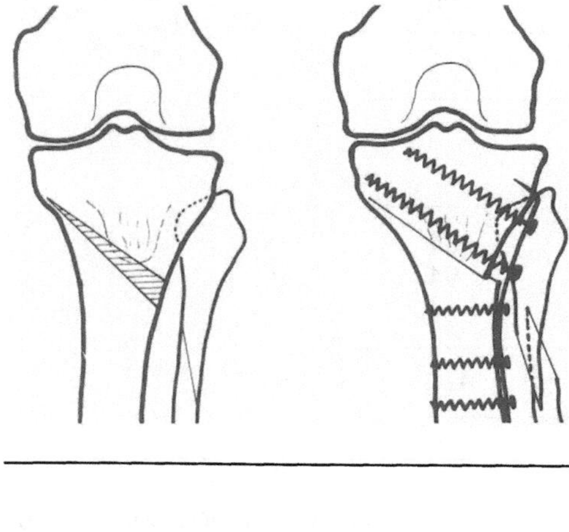

Fig. 2. Schematic drawing of an unilateral closed wedge osteotomy for varus deformity of the proximal tibia, stabilized with the semitubular hook plate. The resected wedge extends obliquely upward from below the tibial tuberosity to but not through the medial cortex, which is left intact

attaching a tension device to the main fragment and applying an incremental longitudinal tension to the plate. As the tension increases, the bone is slowly brought into the desired axial alignment. The apex of the removed bone wedge should closely approach the opposite cortex so that closure of the osteotomy will take place about an axis located within the cortex. If this axis were shifted toward the center of the bone, potentially damaging tensile forces would act on the surface of the intact cortex. We have obtained the best results by angling the osteotomy toward the epicondyle such that the apex of the wedge terminates in the thin, flexible cortex of the condyle. This bone yields elastically to the axial correction but has sufficient tensile strength to keep the osteotomy closed on the side opposite the plate. The tensile strength of the intact bone also ensures uniform compression of the large osteotomy surface by the thin, prestressed plate. If the residual bone is found to be excessively rigid when the correction is attempted, it can be perforated several times with a 2-mm drill bit to make it more pliable. Cracking of the cortex may occasionally occur toward the end of the correction, usually accompanied by an audible snap. With experience, the surgeon will be able to determine by clinical examination or image intensification whether the tensile strength of the affected structures is still intact. If gaping of the osteotomy is detected at that site, a cancellous bone screw generally can be inserted across the osteotomy line on the side away from the plate as a lag screw to restore apposition of the bone surfaces. After the correction is carried out, the plate is attached to the main fragment with two or three cortex screws, which are positioned eccentrically in the plate holes to maintain the longitudinal stress in the implant.

Open Wedge Osteotomy

The unilateral open wedge osteotomy is also stabilized with the semitubular hook plate. In this operation the bone is osteotomized obliquely from the concave side of the deformity to the juxta-articular part of the epicondyle on the opposite side. As in the closed wedge osteotomy, the cut closely approaches the opposite cortex without dividing it (Fig. 3). In the supracondylar and infracondylar areas, the osteotomy can in principle occupy any plane in space, and an intact cortical bridge can be left anywhere on the circumference of the bone. Hence, this osteotomy permits the correction of any deformity, though with varying degrees of difficulty. Even combined axial corrections, such as the simultaneous correction of a valgus and recurvatum deformity of the upper tibia, are possible. If desired, the osteotomy can be done from the postero-lateral aspect of the supracondylar area to correct a limitation of extension of the knee joint in the presence of a valgus deformity. The semitubular hook plate is contoured to the osteotomy side of the bone and is attached with a screw to the juxta-articular fragment. A Weller-type distraction device is attached to the diaphyseal end of the plate, and an incremental distractive stress is applied which gradually opens the osteotomy and realigns the limb. In some cases good results can be obtained with a bone spreader or direct manipulation by the surgeon.

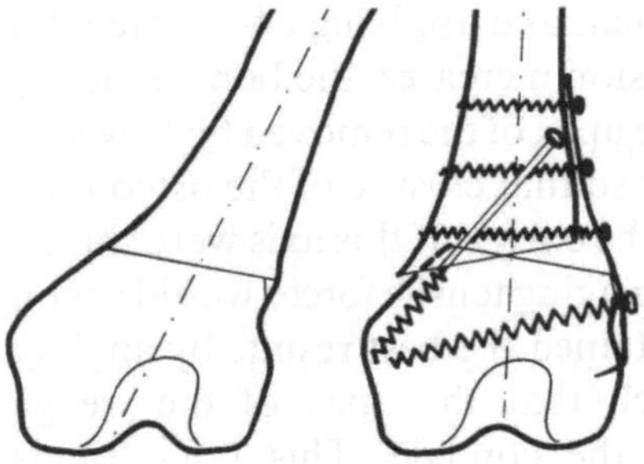

Fig. 3. Schematic drawing of a supracondylar lateral open wedge osteotomy. The osteotomy line extends obliquely downward to the elastic cortex of the medial epicondyle, leaving it intact. After alignment of the fragments and application of a semitubular hook plate to buttress the osteotomy, the lateral defect is packed with cancellous bone

The lengthening effect of this procedure, which is on the order of 1 to 2.5 cm, results from the length gained by straightening the limb axis and opening the osteotomy and therefore is dependent on the preexisting deformity and the possible extent of the correction. The resulting osseous defect should be packed with cancellous bone at sites crucial to union, i.e., sites where the cortical margins of the osteotomy surface gape the most widely. The necessary graft material is usually obtained from the osteotomy surface.

In this type of fixation, the semitubular plate is subjected to compressive loads and performs a buttressing function. The plate, when combined with an intact opposite cortex, can stabilize a 2- to 3-cm-wide osteotomy well enough to provide adequate exercise stability, maintain the new alignment, and promote rapid bone healing (Figs. 4 and 5). If cracking of the far cortex should occur following large axial corrections, an oblique lag screw will secure interfragmental contact (Figs. 6 and 7).

The open wedge osteotomy is excellently suited for multiple corrections necessitated by progressive axial deviations like those caused by unilateral epiphyseal plate injuries during growth. The timing of each operation depends on the current extent of the deformity, the possibility of secondary injuries, or the development of opposing deformities in neighboring epiphyses. With a careful evaluation of all relevant factors, one usually can greatly limit the number of operations and avoid the significant losses of limb length that may attend multiple corrective procedures. The selected technique of internal fixation has a very low association with significant structural changes and troublesome callus formation and thus permits several osteotomies to be performed at the same site without technical difficulty. Occasionally, bowing of the corrected bone segment may develop after multiple open wedge osteotomies. If this occurs, a final corrective osteotomy should be done after the epiphyseal plate has closed, at which time a normal shaft alignment is restored by appropriate displacement of the osteotomy surfaces.

Displacement Osteotomy

The two types of osteotomy discussed thus far are not indicated for the correction of rotational deformities or deformities that require a displacement of the fragments relative to each other. Many problems, such as the correction of femoral neck deformities, require varying degrees of relative displacement of the osteotomy fragments, possibly for the full width of the shaft, with or

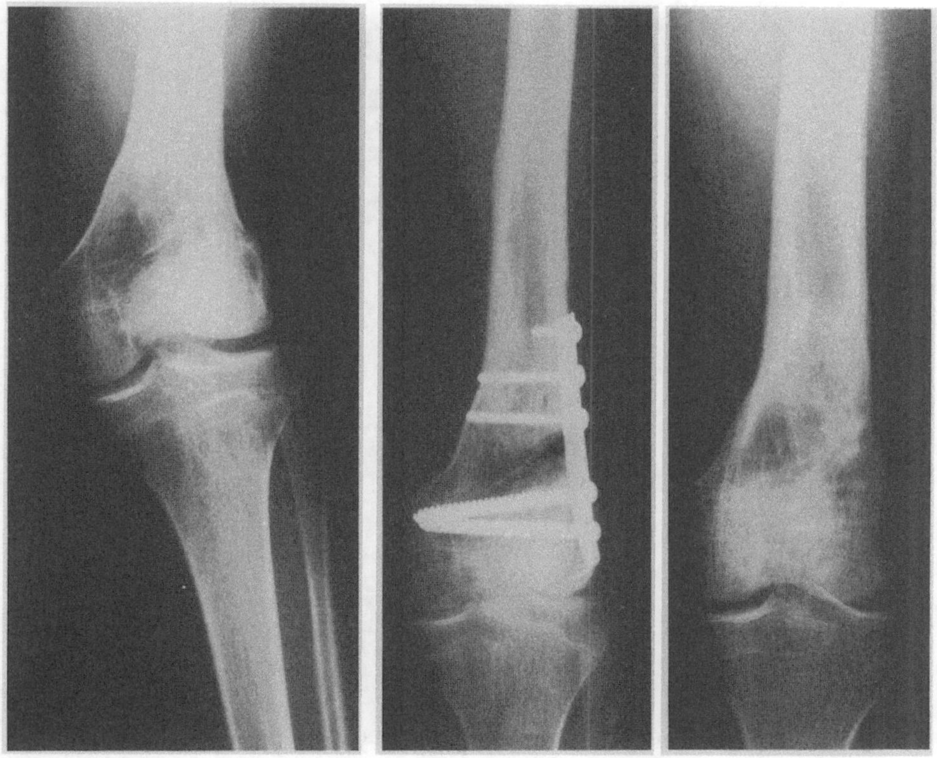

a b c

Fig. 4. a Supracondylar valgus deformity secondary to an epiphyseal plate fracture 3 years previously in a patient who is now 16 years old. **b** Supracondylar open wedge osteotomy with the semitubular hook plate. **c** Two years after the operation there is good axial alignment and normal osseous structure

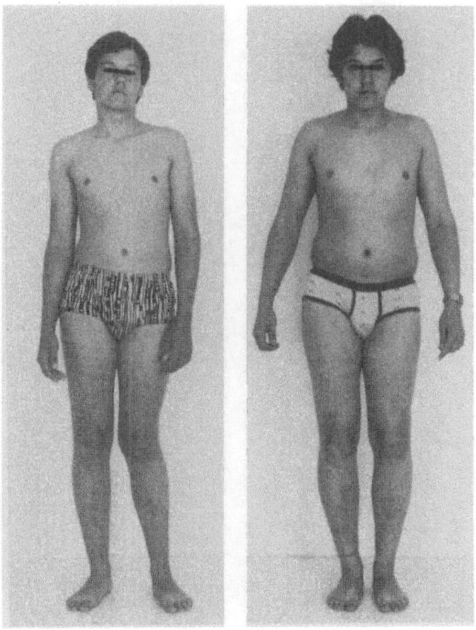

a b

Fig. 5 a,b. Same patient as in Fig. 4. **a** At 16 years of age, several days before corrective surgery: Supracondylar valgus deformity of the left femur with 4 cm of limb shortening. **b** Two years after surgery the leg axes are symmetrical, with a residual shortening of 2 cm

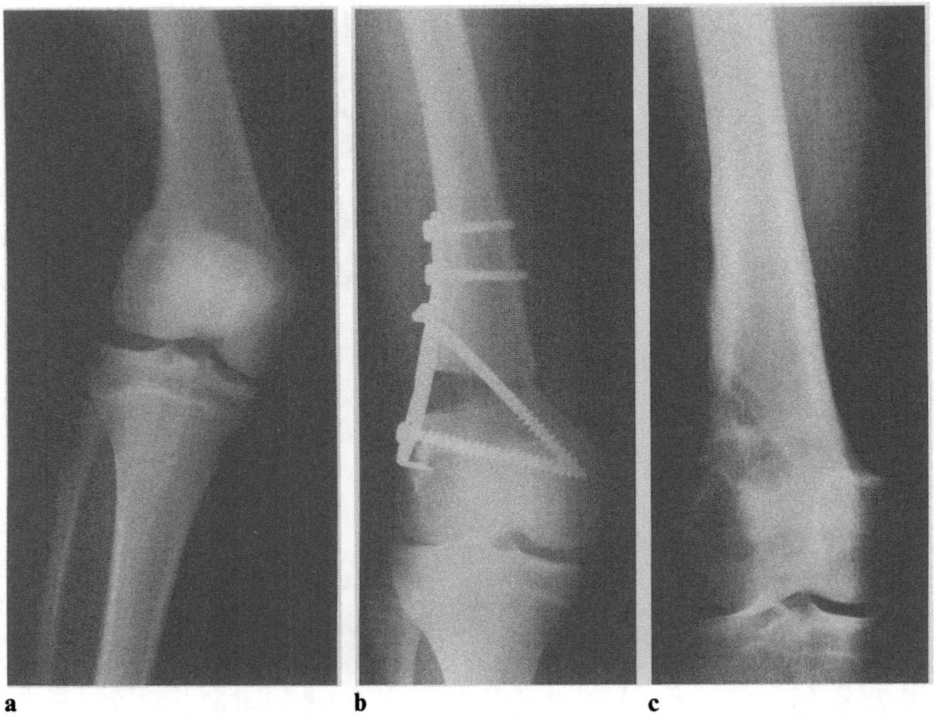

Fig. 6. a Roentgenogram of the knee joint of a 15-year-old patient 4 years after an epiphyseal plate injury of the distal femur. **b** The oblique osteotomy is made through the lateral cortex of the proximal part of the metaphysis. Cracking of the brittle medial cortex occurred when the bone was realigned, and so a compression lag screw was inserted obliquely to secure medial apposition. **c** Four years after operation

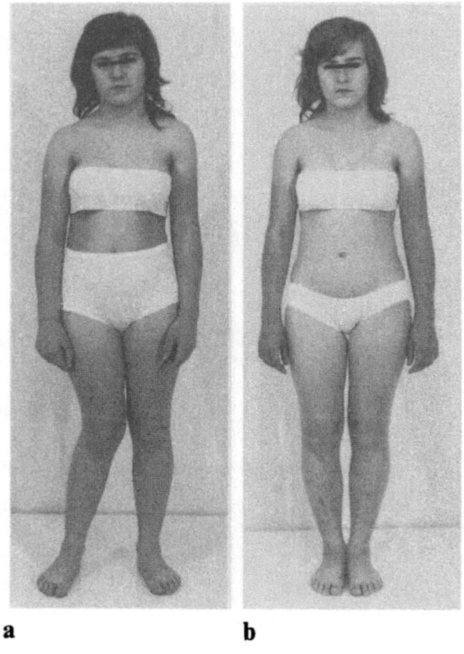

Fig. 7 a,b. Same patient as in Fig. 6. **a** At 15 years of age prior to surgery: 3 cm of limb shortening with a valgus angulation of 30°. **b** One year after surgery the leg axes are symmetrical, and the length discrepancy is corrected

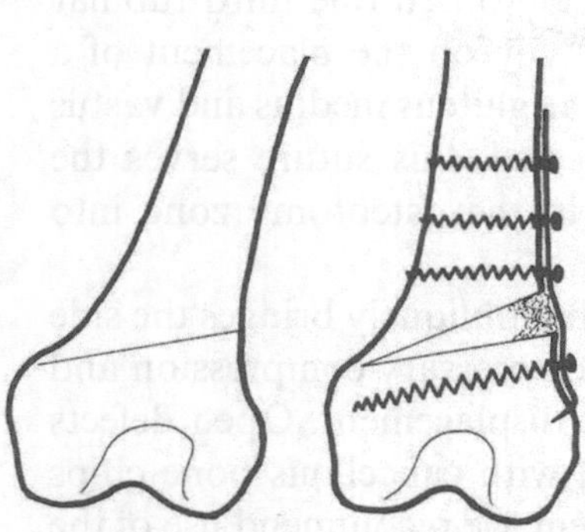

Fig. 8

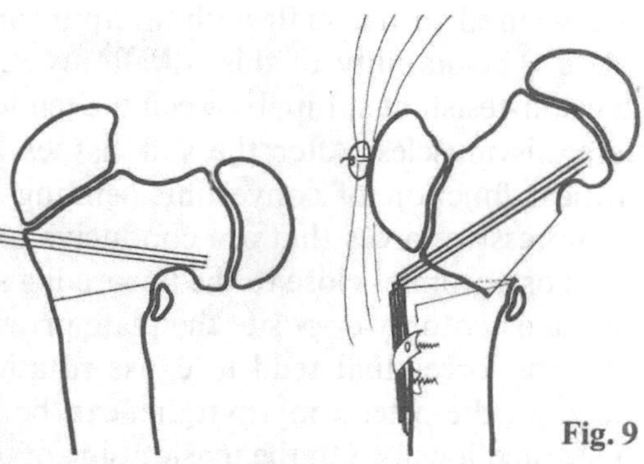

Fig. 9

Fig. 8. Schematic drawing of a supracondylar displacement osteotomy stabilized with the semitubular hook plate. The necessary amount of displacement is determined by the goal of aligning the femoral shaft axis over the center of the knee joint. An oblique lag screw stabilizes the medial buttress

Fig. 9. Diagram showing how Kirschner wires may be used to fix an intertrochanteric valgus osteotomy in a child. The medial bony buttress, which is spontaneously loaded in compression, is stabilized with a Kirschner wire against displacement and rotation. A contoured one-third tubular plate attached to the shaft with two small-fragment screws acts as a clamp to hold the angled Kirschner wires in place. A tension-band suture between the gluteus medius and vastus lateralis muscles contributes greatly to overall stability

without the resection of a bone wedge. This type of osteotomy is necessary in the supra- and infracondylar regions of the knee when there is bowing of the diaphysis or marked angulation in excess of 20°. Hinging the osteotomy on an intact bridge of medial or lateral cortex in such cases may move the tibial or femoral shaft away from the midline of the knee, causing stresses to become concentrated on one side of the joint (Fig. 8).

To maximize the stability of a displacement osteotomy, the bony buttress between the fragments should be as far from the fixation plate as possible. This buttress, which generally is on the medial side, should derive stability from the configuration of the fragments and the quality of the apposed bone surfaces. It should be placed on the compression side of the fixation whenever possible, as this will allow spontaneous compression. Ideally, a simple Kirschner wire joining the edges of the fragments stabilizes the buttress against displacement and rotation, as in an intertrochanteric osteotomy (Fig. 9).

If a valgus osteotomy must be performed on the pediatric femoral neck because of a malunited or nonunited fracture, the simple Kirschner wire fixation described by Wagner [7] gives adequate stability (Fig. 9). With great care taken to spare the growth plates, three 2- or 3-mm Kirschner wires are twisted into the femoral neck distal to the epiphyseal line of the greater trochanter. The bone is osteotomized above the lesser trochanter, and soft-tissue connections are freed between the medial edges of the fragments. Then the valgus correction is carried out on the proximal fragment, and the femoral shaft is displaced laterally as required. A medial bony buttress is produced and secured with a thin Kirschner wire that were previously inserted into the femoral neck are bent downward at the lateral margin of the osteotomy and are secured to the shaft with an appropriately contoured one-third tubular plate. The stability of this osteotomy relies heavily on the placement of a tension-resistant suture between the tendons of the gluteus medius and vastus lateralis muscles. After the soft tissues have healed, this suture serves the critical function of converting bending forces in the osteotomy zone into compressive forces that are conducive to union.

In osteotomies close to the knee, a lag screw that obliquely bridges the side of the osteotomy opposite the plate provides the necessary compression and absorbs forces that tend to cause rotation and displacement. Open defects between the osteotomy margins can be packed with cancellous bone chips harvested locally. On the tension side of the system, we recommend use of the semitubular hook plate described previously. This device makes an excellent tension band, and it can be easily molded to fit the strongly contoured bone surfaces in this type of osteotomy.

Advantages of the Methods Described

Bone Healing

The very site of the correction – the cancellous metaphyses of the femur and tibia – is promising in terms of rapid consolidation. Moreover, the oblique direction of the osteotomy creates relatively large osteotomy surfaces, which contribute to rapid union. A further advantage of the oblique osteotomy is that it places the level of correction very close to the joint, yet the margin of the juxta-articular fragment on the plated side of the bone is considerably longer than in a high transverse osteotomy. This makes it much easier to anchor the internal fixation material securely in the "short fragment." Even atrophic bone will provide sufficient anchorage for two fully threaded cancellous bone screws and the terminal hooks of the semitubular hook plate.

Open wedge osteotomies are performed most frequently in adolescents and young adults. With the selective use of cancellous bone, it should be possible to achieve rapid osseous bridging of defects in this population. Generally the cancellous bone is taken from the osteotomy surface with a gouge or sharp spoon. The amount required can be significantly reduced by filling central defects with a substitute material and using cancellous bone only in continuity with the cortex on the gaping osteotomy surface. However, the course and outcome of bone healing are influenced most decisively by the proper use of the nonrigid implant.

In the closed wedge osteotomy, where there is broad apposition of the bone ends, union is very rapid because the fixation technique ensures an even distribution of compression across the osteotomy line. The advantages of this technique are obvious in the open wedge and displacement osteotomies, which show initial signs of restored bony continuity only eight weeks after surgery. A particular advantage is the relatively short time required for the filling of osseous defects in the osteotomy zone. With rigid implants like the 130° plate, condylar plate, and broad plate of the ASIF, defects may persist for years, especially in proximity to the plate, and may necessitate secondary bone grafting or even replacement of the implants. This contrasts with the semitubular hook plate, which promotes the rapid obliteration of defects. Normalization of the newly formed bone with the development of a cortical structure and central cancellous tissue is generally complete within a few months. The nonrigid implant transmits only a small fraction of the stresses that traverse the osteotomy region. Even prolonged application of the plate causes few visible changes in the underlying cortical bone. Frequently the cortex grows up around the edges of the plate to form a peripheral ridge that enhances stability after implant removal and eliminates the danger of fatigue fracture (Table 3).

Table 3. Advantages of the Method in Terms of Bone Healing

Oblique and therefore large osteotomy surface in cancellous tissue
Rapid consolidation owing to broad interfragmentary contact
Rapid obliteration of osseous defects
Prompt normalization of osseous structure
Avoidance of fatigue fracture

Internal Fixation Technique

The semitubular plate offers a number of advantages in terms of the practical conduct of the internal fixation. First, its small volume occupies a minimum of space. This helps to reduce tension during closure of the soft tissues, even in a problem areas like the upper tibia. Second, the thin implant can be shaped intraoperatively to fit any surface using little force and relatively simple tools. This avoids unnecessary irritation of the soft tissues by projecting fixation material and facilitates postoperative mobilization. Third, the large screw holes in the semitubular plate give the surgeon great freedom in the use of different types of screws and in selecting the direction of screw insertion. In the upper tibia, this option can be of great value when it is necessary to insert fully threaded cancellous screws into structurally deficient bone. Even with severe bone atrophy, these screws will always hold securely in the dense subchondral bone just below the articular surface. Fourth, the excellent malleability of the semitubular plate makes it possible to avoid contact with epiphyseal plates in the growing skeleton and thus avoid potential damage to these critical areas. The plate hooks and a fully threaded cancellous bone screw provide very good anchorage of the implant in the hard metaphyseal cancellous bone of young patients. At the same time, the part of the fixation near the joint involves only a narrow segment of the metaphysis adjacent to the growth cartilage, enabling the bone to be corrected in close proximity to the joint. The danger of dislodgment of the cancellous bone screw, even when the osteotomy surface is very close to the implant, is far less than with an angled blade plate, for example, which requires that the osteotomy be at least 2.5 cm from the seating of the blade (Table 4, Fig. 10).

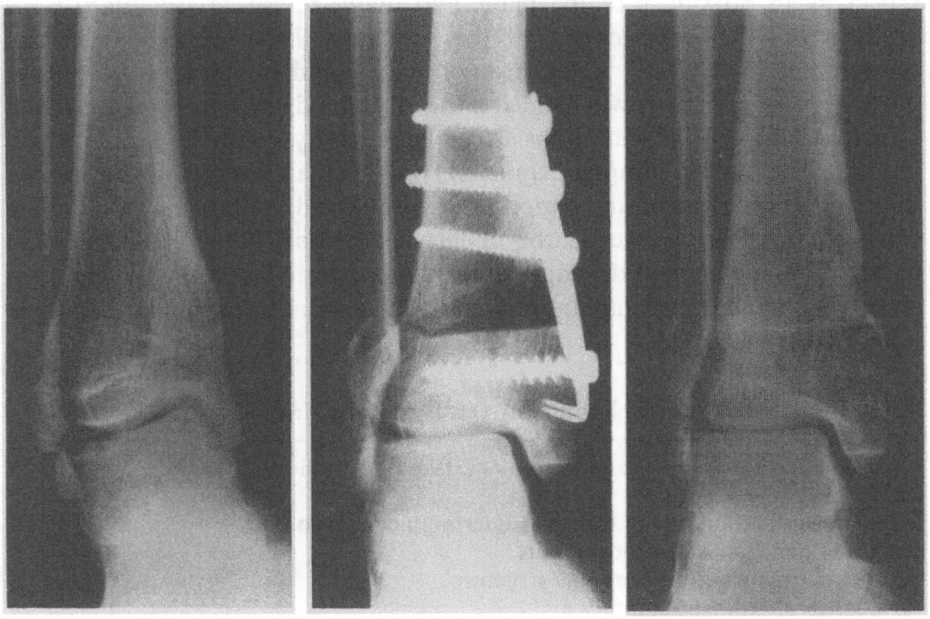

a b c

Fig. 10. a Ankle joint of a 20-year-old man who fell from a 3rd floor balcony, sustaining a comminuted fracture of the femur and an epiphyseal plate injury of the distal tibia. **b** Periarticular open wedge osteotomy with correction of the lateral malleolus. Narrow distal fragment stabilized with a cancellous bone screw and the semitubular hook plate. **c** Two years after surgery the osteotomy is consolidated, and there is good joint congruity with no limitation of motion

Table 4. Advantages of the Semitubular Hook Plate

Small volume
Causes minimal soft-tissue irritation
Is adaptable to any situation
Permits variable directions of screw insertion
Facilitates osteotomies near joints
Is resistant to dislodgment

Avoidance of Over- or Undercorrection

A major problem in the surgical correction of angular limb deformities is the difficulty of determining the optimum amount of correction preoperatively. The evaluation of roentgenograms carries significant potential for error. An accurate determination becomes even more difficult if corrections in multiple planes are desired, especially since the correction of a deformity in one plane can affect alignment in another. A further difficulty is that the correction is performed in the recumbent patient, but the corrected limb will have to function in the upright, weight-bearing position. What is more, the amount of correction is not just a skeletal problem, and so it cannot simply be measured on radiographic tracings with a protractor. Besides osseous factors, the functional result depends on the congruity of the joint surfaces and the stability of the ligaments.

With the semitubular plate, the surgeon is able simply to estimate the necessary extent of the correction beforehand and shape the implant accordingly. The plate is first secured to the short, juxta-articular fragment, which is the more difficult in terms of anchorage. Once this is done, there will be no need to modify the anchorage afterward, because the elastic implant will spontaneously alter its shape as needed as the limb is brought into alignment. When the tension or distraction device is used, the surgeon can test the alignment of the limb in the unloaded state and under axial loading using a Verbrugge forceps under the protection of the free end of the plate, adjusting the correction as needed until the result is optimal (Figs. 11 and 12).

Another feature of the techniques described is that both the amount and the dimensions of the internal fixation material are in the "borderline" area of what is necessary for adequate stability. The challenge is to design the fixation so as to achieve a rapid, problem-free consolidation for a given type and location of osteotomy, bone quality, and patient age [8]. If there is doubt as to the ability of the patient to restrict weight bearing voluntarily, as is often the case in the elderly, a plaster splint can be strapped to the posterior aspect of the limb to assist ambulation.

The described techniques of osteotomy and internal fixation place high demands on the experience and manual skills of the operator. But with a meticulous execution, the risks are very small.

Among the 304 upper tibial osteotomies that we have performed to date, there have been only 4 cases of delayed consolidation – 3 in closed wedge osteotomies and 1 in a displacement osteotomy. In one case the technique of the internal fixation had been faulty. Three patients bore full weight on the limb a short time after surgery, causing a depression of the osteotomy surface

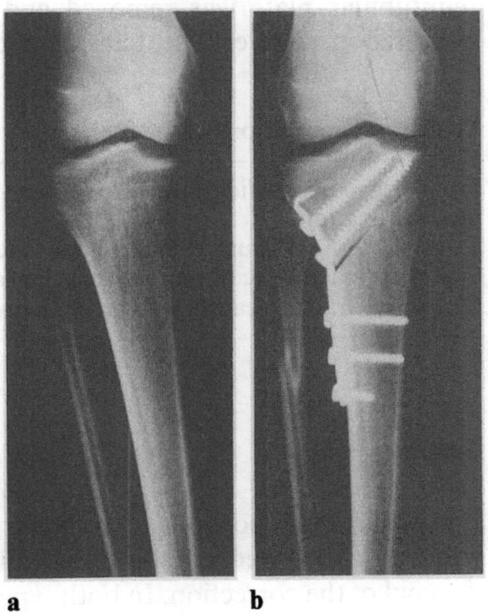

Fig. 11 a,b. Unilateral closed wedge osteotomy of the tibia with an intact opposite cortex. Roentgenograms of the patient in Fig. 12 **a** before and **b** after corrective osteotomy

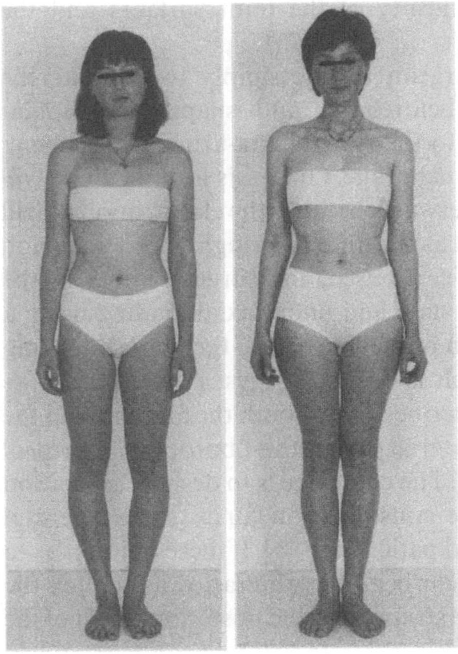

a b

Fig. 12 a,b. Applying the appropriate degree of correction is especially important in patients with bilateral angular deformity. This is readily achieved with the semitubular hook plate. **a** The 17-year-old patient before and **b** after the operation D

which compromised the stability of the osteotomy/internal fixation system. In two of the four cases the internal fixation had to be repeated. In the remaining two, delayed union ensued after a plaster splint was strapped to the limb. A total of two infections were recorded. In one case with a supramalleolar osteotomy, the infection led to a delay of consolidation. In the second case, a fistula formed after the osteotomy had united. Among the 422 cases in which a semitubular or one-third tubular plate was used to stabilize an osteotomy, there was only 1 instance of a plate fracture. In this case the fractured semitubular plate was removed and a new one applied. A cortex screw fractured in another case, but this had no adverse consequences (Table 5).

Table 5. Complications and Problems Encountered in Our Series

Four delayed consolidations, two requiring revision of the internal fixation
Two infections, 1 causing delayed consolidation
One plate fracture requiring replacement of implant
One screw fracture causing no adverse consequences

Summary

The periarticular portions of the femur and tibia can be osteotomized in open wedge or closed wedge fashion, depending on the nature of the deformity and the goal of the correction. In both types of osteotomy an area of cortex is left intact near the apex of the osteotomy wedge. In the closed wedge operation, this continuity of bone ensures an even pressure distribution across the osteotomy site; in the open wedge operation, it provides a stabilizing bone bridge on the side opposite the plate.

In a displacement osteotomy, the surgeon must create an area of secure interfragmental contact, which should be located as far from the plate as possibel ("medial buttress") on the compression side of the bone. A single implant is used to stabilize the area of contact.

Interfragmental contact opposite the implant moderates the demands placed on the stabilizing ability of the implant. This enables the semitubular plate or even the one-third tubular plate (in children) to withstand the tensile stresses of a closed wedge or displacement osteotomy and to bridge up to 3 cm of an open wedge osteotomy without difficulty.

In addition, use of the semitubular hook plate offers significant advantages over other devices in terms of fixation technique, precision of correction, and progress of bone healing.

References

1. Müller ME, Allgöwer M, Willenegger A (1969) Manual der Osteosynthese. Springer, Berlin Heidelberg New York
2. Wagner H (1976) Indikation und Technik der Korrekturosteotomie bei der traumatischen Arthrose des Kniegelenkes. Hefte Unfallheilkd 128:155–174 (1976)
3. Wagner H (1977) Prinzipien der Korrekturosteotomien am Bein. Orthopäde 6:145
4. Wagner H (1978) Femoral osteotomies for congenital hip dislocation. Orthop Surg 2:85–105
5. Wagner H (1978) Die operative Behandlung beim Altersknie. Prakt Orthop 8:247
6. Wagner H (1982) Orthopädische Probleme nach Schenkelhalsfrakturen im Kindesalter. Hefte Unfallheilkd 158:241–247
7. Zeiler G (1977) Korrekturosteotomien am Arm. Orthopäde 6:121–144

Summary: Principles of the Surgical Correction of Posttraumatic Deformities of the Lower Extremities

G. Hörster

Normal function of the extremities depends as much on proper joint anatomy as on the presence of normal functional loads. Every surgical correction of posttraumatic deformities must be aimed at normalizing both of these factors in order to avoid local cartilage damage leading to painful restriction of motion. The lower extremity is unique in that its major points are positioned eccentrically with respect to the axis of weight bearing (in the stance phase of gait, this axis extends downward and outward at an angle of about 3° from the partial center of gravity S5). As a result, the level of the joint load depends basically on the body weight and the distance of the joint center from the weight-bearing axis. Because the distance of the weight-bearing axis from the joint center decreases from the hip to the ankle, the body must generate different intrinsic countermoments in the various joints in order to distribute the pressure loads more evenly. The "mechanical axis" of the lower extremity should not be confused with the weight-bearing axis. The mechanical axis is a straight line connecting the centers of the hip and ankle joints and is simply a graphic means of representing the loads on the knee. Deviation of the mechanical axis from the center of the knee can indicate no more than a qualitative alteration of loading; it cannot be used as a quantitative measure of joint loads.

Pathophysiology

Any alteration of joint anatomy or functional loading causes excessive, unphysiologic loads to be placed on parts of the joint, leading to cartilage damage and local joint destruction. This process may result from changes in the margins of the articular surfaces or from deformities that are more distant from the joint. Because we are not yet able to analyze unphysiologic joint loads associated with limb deformities in quantiative terms, the magnitude of an abnormal load must be assessed indirectly based on the distance between the center of the joint and the weight-bearing axis. Changes in this distance have no pathologic significance *per se*, because initially they can be neutralized through increased activity of compensatory structures. This results in a general increase of pressure in the affected joint. A local overload does not occur until compensatory mechanisms fail (decompensation). Age, body weight, the condition of the cartilage and ligaments, and the position of the joint during function all play a role in this process.

Corrective Osteotomies of the Lower Extremity
Edited by G. Hierholzer, K. H. Müller

In the *hip joint*, a varus deformity tends to relieve pressure on the joint, while a valgus deformity increases joint pressure by lengthening the lever arm of the attached muscles, creating the danger of a local overload. The medial compartment of the *knee joint* is at particular risk for excessive loads associated with posttraumatic deformity. While a valgus deformity will cause the mechanical axis to deviate the same distance from the joint center as an equivalent varus deformity, the initial result is a reduction of the bending moment imposed on the joint. Decompensation will occur in valgus only if the weight-bearing axis actually crosses the center of the knee joint, because the medial side of the joint lacks the effective compensatory structures found on the lateral side. In the *ankle joint*, the relative proximity of the weight-bearing axis and joint center removes the danger of significant local overloading of the medial or lateral joint space. The principal effect of a tibial deformity is to cause obliquity of the talar baseline. If the deformity is near the ankle joint, corrective surgery is necessary to permit a flat landing of the foot. Given the functional anatomy of the subtalar joint and its limited range of pronation, decompensation is a danger when varus deviation of the talar baseline reaches approximately 5°.

Indication

The indication for corrective surgery is based largely on pathophysiologic considerations. Surgery on purely cosmetic or functional grounds is conceivable, but the great majority of these cases will also have a pathophysiologic rationale.

Surgery for an unphysiologic joint load secondary to deformity may be prophylactic or therapeutic. Prophylactic surgery is done with the intent of preventing degenerative joint changes secondary to pathologic loads. It follows empirically established values due to a lack of measurable data on joint loads. Therapeutic surgery attempts to relieve functionally disabling complaints, which in the early stage are caused by overloading of the muscles and in later stages by local cartilage degeneration. Age, body weight, and the level of functional demands placed on the joint play an important role in the selection of patients for surgery.

In this section we shall present average values for the principal angular deviations of the lower extremity that are considered to represent an indication for corrective surgery. In the *hip joint*, the projection of the femoral neck axis in the frontal and lateral planes is used to measure the degree of angular deformity. Rotational alignment is evaluated in anteversion films. An isolated varus deformity *per se* does not warrant surgical correction, because in this situation pressure on the joint is reduced and there is not exorbitant risk of degenerative change. Functional aspects such as limitation of abduction and disturbance of gait are the primary concern. An isolated valgus deformity of more than about 20° should be corrected, because the altered lever arms significantly increase compressive forces in the joint. Varus repositioning following a prior valgus operation (e.g., for the internal fixation of a nonunited femoral neck fracture) should be considered. In posttraumatic osteoarthritis of the hip without significant angular deformity, the osteotomy is planned on the basis of function studies to achieve the best possible seating of the femoral head in the acetabulum. Isolated rotational deformities of more than about 20° should be corrected on functional grounds. This particularly applies to external rotation deformities, which often cause painful contractures of the internal rotators.

In the *knee joint*, the indication for corrective surgery is based on the distance between the mechanical axis and joint center and on the degree of inclination of the joint surface in the frontal plane. For a given degree of deformity, the danger to the knee increases with the proximity of the deformity to the joint, because this greatly influences the amount by which the mechanical axis is shifted from the center of the knee. A varus deformity of more than 5–10° and a valgus deformiy of more than about 10–15° should be corrected when located close to the knee. Inclination of the knee baseline of more than 10° should be avoided, as this subjects the cartilage to unphysiologic shear stresses. The close interrelationship between instability and degenerative change should always be kept in mind in the region of the knee. In the sagittal plane, corrective surgery is indicated for periarticular deformities of 15–20° or more to improve ambulatory ability and remove excessive loads from the femoropatellar joint.

In the *ankle joint*, a deformity-related inclination of the joint axis is the most important factor in the development of osteoarthrities. Given the limited range of pronation, surgical correction is indicated for distal varus deformities of 5° or more, and for distal valgus deformities of about 10° or more. In the sagittal plane, deformities of more than 15° require correction because of impaired ankle joint mobility and unphysiologic loads on the anterior or posterior part of the joint. Internal or external rotation deformities of the tibia require intervention when the deformity reaches or exceeds 15–20°.

Preoperative Planning

In preparing the operation, it is necessary to obtain long roentgenograms of the injured and uninjured legs. It is best to do this with the patient standing, as this posture can affect the apparent degree of diaphyseal deformities, including those near joints. The roentgenographic images are then transferred to tracing paper, on which the longitudinal axes, axial intersections, mechanical axis and articular baselines are drawn. The principles were described by Oest in detail. With knowledge of local clinical findings, it is possible to prepare and evaluate the various alternatives with regard to the location, form and stabilization of the osteotomy. Ideally, a simple diaphyseal deformity is corrected by osteotomizing the bone at the level of intersection of the partial axes (the longitudinal axes of the bone segments adjacent to the deformity). In combined deformities, the axial intersection does not coincide with the level of bone injury. The advantage of this is that the osteotomy can be performed at a site with better osseous and soft-tissue conditions. If local conditions make it necessary to osteotomize the metaphysis for the correction of a shaft deformity, the angle of correction should be such that the mechanical axis is centered in the knee joint, and the knee baseline and talar baseline are made horizontal. Even for osteotomies of the proximal femur, it is recommended that the entire limb axis be considered, because varus or valgus operations about the hip secondarily alter the loads on the knee.

Operative Technique

Diaphyseal deformities are generally managed with a wedge resection osteotomy. The danger of delayed union can be reduced by making an oblique osteotomy to enlarge interfragmental contact. A stepped osteotomy may also be considered. With regard to outcome, both the amount of the correction and the level of the center of rotation of the osteotomy have a critical bearing on the final position of the mechanical axis. This center of rotation should be as close as possible to the point of axial intersection. In addition, the osteotomy should be designed in such a way that it corrects or improves leg length discrepancy while normalizing the mechanical axis.

In principle, a corrective osteotomy can be stabilized with the same implants used for fractures in the same location. With proper technique and a strong bony buttress, most corrective osteotomies can be fixed securely enough to allow postoperative exercise. Supplementary fixation with one or more lag screws enhances stability and should be used whenever possible. If osseous and soft-tissue conditions are poor, external fixation devices offer a low-risk method of stabilizing tibial osteotomies.

II. The Proximal Femur

Indications, Localization and Preoperative Planning of Proximal Femoral Osteotomies in Posttraumatic States

M. E. Müller

Indications

Nonunions of the femoral neck with a viable head and deformities secondary to fractures are the most frequent indications for posttraumatic osteotomies of the proximal femur. Corrective osteotomy may also be indicated for partial avascular necrosis of the femoral neck, for contractures secondary to pelvic fractures, and after the healing of an avascular femoral head necrosis in which the articular cartilage is reasonably well preserved. Traumatic separation of the epiphysis in young patients may also be mentioned in this context.

Localization

The proximal femur may be osteotomized in the subtrochanteric region, intertrochanteric region, or through the femoral neck. *Subtrochanteric osteotomies* have been largely abandoned, because the abduction produces a medialization of the shaft which decreases the angle between the mechanical axis and anatomic axis to zero, producing a marked genu valgum, and also because a corrective osteotomy will be necessary prior to a proposed total hip replacement. Another factor to be considered is the relatively long healing time of diaphyseal osteotomies compared with osteotomies performed through the cancellous bone of the intertrochanteric region. *Femoral neck osteotomies* are reserved for epiphyseal plate separations with more than 50° posterior slip of the femoral head.

In the *intertrochanteric region*, which is the site of choice, it is easy to perform any desired angular correction in the frontal, sagittal and horizontal plane and to displace the distal fragment laterally, medially, anteriorly or posteriorly as needed. In this type of osteotomy the length of the femur and the position of the greater trochanter and weight-bearing part of the head should always be evaluated before and after the procedure.

Preoperative Planning

Pre-requisites

An accurate diagnosis based on clinical and roentgenographic findings, a clear understanding of the goal of the chosen procedure, and the selection of a

Corrective Osteotomies of the Lower Extremity
Edited by G. Hierholzer, K. H. Müller

satisfactory operating technique and reliable implant are necessary preliminaries to the preoperative planning of the end result and the tactical steps necessary to achieve it.

These points will be illustrated in the planning of an intertrochanteric osteotomy for treatment of a nonunion of the femoral neck.

Nonunion of the Femoral Neck

It is known that every reactive "elephant-foot" type of nonunion will unite after relative micromotion between the fragments has been eliminated, allowing mineralization of the interposed fibrocartilage and its invasion by bone-forming vascular tissue [7].

In 1927 Pauwels [6] recognized that a nonunion of the femoral neck would consolidate within a few months if shear stresses acting on the nonunion were transformed into compression. Even today, Pauwels' principle of reorienting the nonunion at right angles to the resultant force R by resecting a laterally based wedge of bone retains its validity.

Pauwels used an abduction cast to stabilize his osteotomies. Since 1959 we have used a 120° double-angled blade plate to fix the osteotomy internally, and we do not apply plaster after surgery. In a nonunion, appositional movement

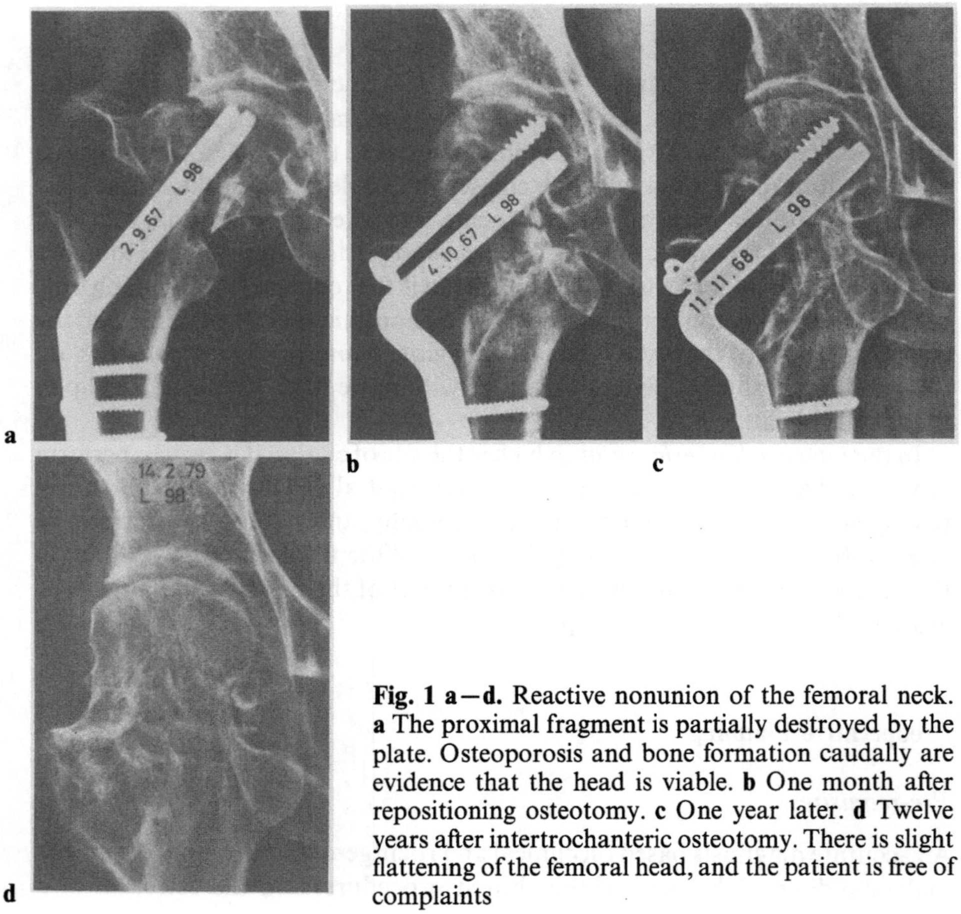

Fig. 1 a–d. Reactive nonunion of the femoral neck. **a** The proximal fragment is partially destroyed by the plate. Osteoporosis and bone formation caudally are evidence that the head is viable. **b** One month after repositioning osteotomy. **c** One year later. **d** Twelve years after intertrochanteric osteotomy. There is slight flattening of the femoral head, and the patient is free of complaints

of the fragments is not desired, and mineralization of the fibrocartilage depends on absolute immobilization under axial compression.

To preserve the blood supply and structure of the femoral head in the area of greatest axial loading, it is necessary for the end of the blade to engage the caudal half of the head. This is not possible if the blade is oriented at right angles to the plane of the nonunion!

A viable femoral head is essential to a good long-term result. General sclerosis and a loss of head roundness are indicative of necrosis, while a uniform density of the femoral head and trochanter and reactive sclerosis at the bone ends similar to that in an elephant-foot nonunion are evidence of viability. With extensive avascular necrosis in adults, the repositioning osteotomy may well promote ossification of the nonunion, but collapse of the femoral head shortly thereafter will spoil the result. If the patient is relatively young and the necrosis involves only the weight-bearing part of the head, repositioning osteotomy is the procedure of choice. Some compaction of the head may occur, but the situation will usually stabilize thereafter (Fig. 1).

The plane of the nonunion relative to a line perpendicular to the femoral axis is determined on x-rays. Sometimes abduction and adduction films or even tomograms will be required. Pauwels calculated that the resultant force R acting across the hip forms an angle of 16° with the vertical body axis. The angle between the body axis and the anatomic axis of the femur is 8 – 10° (Fig. 2). Therefore, a plane of nonunion that forms an angle of 25° with the femoral shaft perpendicular will come under pure axial compression. The difference between the plane of nonunion and this 25° angle equals the desired angle of correction in the frontal plane. External rotation deformities measured in the prone position determine the correction in the horizontal plane, and the extension deficit measured in lateral decubitus determines the correction in the sagittal plane.

Pauwels performed a simple closed wedge osteotomy in ordinary cases and used a Y-shaped osteotomy when there was caudal displacement of the

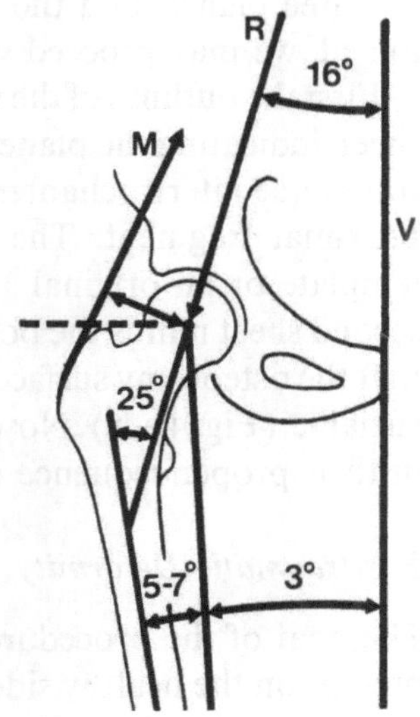

Fig. 2. The resultant force **R** of Pauwels: The R line extends from the intersection of the muscular force **M** and vertical gravitational force to the center of the femoral head. It forms a 16° angle with the vertical **V**. The anatomic axis of the femur forms an angle of 8° with the vertical in men and an angle of 10° in women. Thus, the angle between the extended R line and shaft axis is 25°

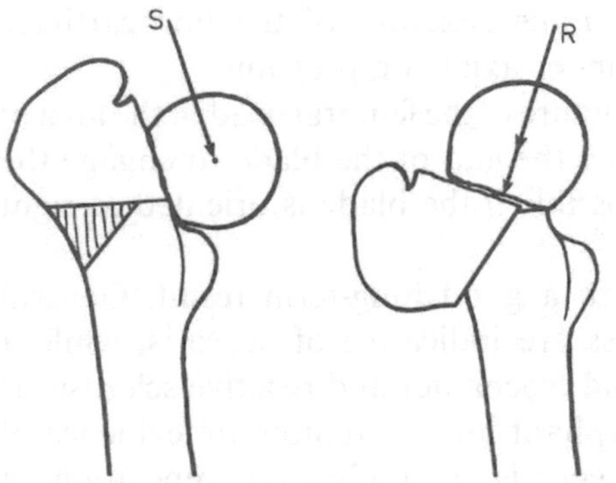

Fig. 3. The Y-shaped osteotomy of Pauwels. The purpose of this operation is to transform the shear stress **S** into pure axial compression **R**. The repositioned proximal fragment is supported by the horizontal plane of the Y-shaped osteotomy

femoral head. In the latter case he placed the medial femoral cortex under the projecting part of the head as a means of buttressing it (Fig. 3). His osteotomies were unable to correct limb shortening and produced a marked medial displacement of the femoral axis, resulting in significant genu valgum. By using the 120° angled blade plate, it is possible not only to lateralize the axis of the femur but also to correct or improve leg length discrepancy and allow early postoperative mobilization.

We always begin our periarticular corrective osteotomies with a cut at right angles to the shaft. Of course, the first step following transverse osteotomy of the femur is to correct rotational alignment. If a 120° plate is to be used, a 30° wedge of bone is resected from the distal fragment (90° + 30° = 120°). Additional abduction, if needed, is accomplished by the resection of a proximal wedge. Later the blade of the plate will be inserted parallel to the cranial osteotomy surface.

The plane of the osteotomy is stabilized under compression as described in the ASIF Manual, i.e., the plate is attached distally to the femoral shaft with screws, and the upper end of the shaft is approximated to the plate with a long screw (see ASIF Manual [5]).

After the diagnosis is made, goals defined, the angle of correction defined in all three planes, and the operative procedure and fixation technique determined, we may proceed with the preoperative drawings.

First the outlines of the proximal femur are traced onto a transparent plastic sheet, indicating the plane of the nonunion, the femur axis, and the lines of the transverse intertrochanteric osteotomy and wedge resection in the shaft and proximal fragment. The selected implant is also drawn using the ASIF template or an original 120° plate. Next the femoral shaft is traced onto a second sheet minus the bony wedge, and the proximal fragment is traced such that the osteotomy surfaces are in apposition. The size of the resected wedge is variable (Fig. 4 a,b). Now the various steps of the procedure can be indicated in their proper sequence on the first drawing (Fig. 4 c) [3].

Posttraumatic Deformity

The goal of the procedure is to restore the same anatomic relations as are present on the healthy side. The outlines of the healthy and affected proximal

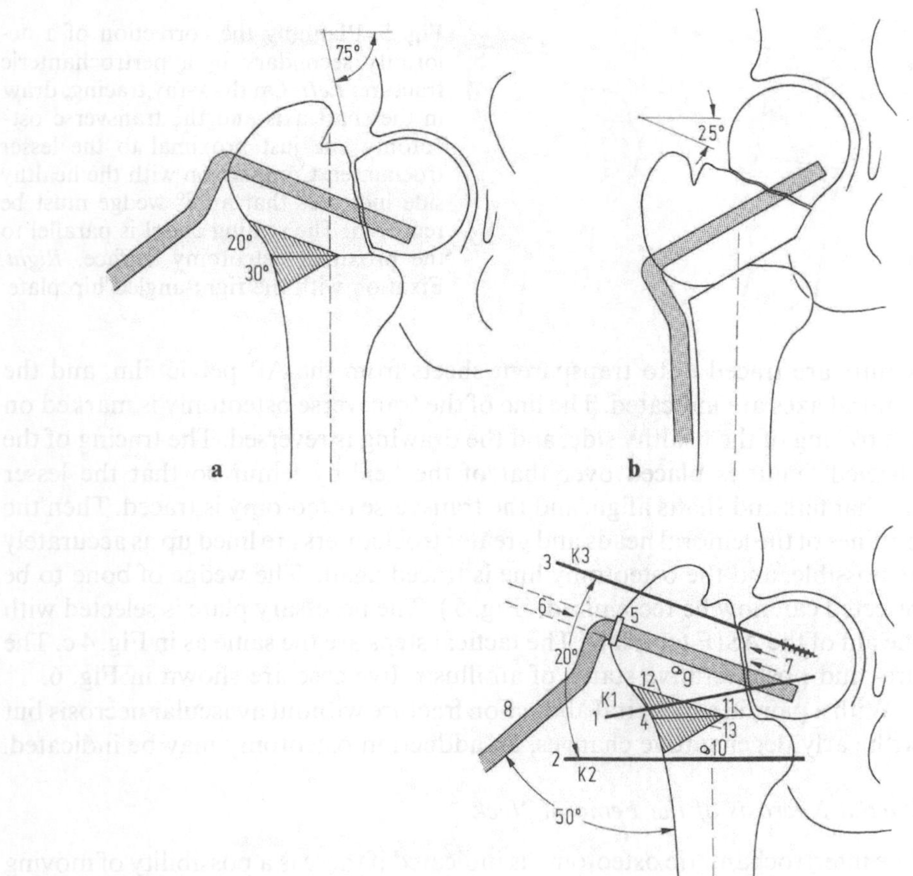

Fig. 4 a – c. Repositioning osteotomy for nonunion of the femoral neck with a viable head: planning the end result. **a** Tracing prepared from the roentgenogram of the nonunion, showing the femoral axis, the transverse osteotomy, the calculated angle between a perpendicular to the shaft and the line of nonunion (here 20° and 30°), and the implant in position. **b** After excision of the wedge, the osteotomy lines are apposed and the plate is attached to the femoral shaft. **c** Tactical steps of the operation: **1** Insert K1 (2mm diam.) through the femoral neck. **2** Insert K2 (2 mm diam.) perpendicular to the shaft axis at the level of the lesser trochanter. **3** Insert K3 (2.5 mm diam., threaded) through the apex of the greater trochanter at a 20° angle to K2 and parallel to K1 in the sagittal plane; remove K1. **4** Mark the level of the osteotomy with a saw. **5** Make an opening for insertion of the seating chisel. **6** Drive in the seating chisel parallel to K3 and angled 10° posteriorly to allow for subsequent extension; its tip should enter the caudal half of the femoral head. **7** Withdraw the seating chisel. **8** Insert the selected angled blade plate. **9, 10** Insert 2 Kirschner wires at right angles to the shaft to define rotational correction. **11** Make the transverse intertrochanteric osteotomy and rotational correction (horizontal plane). **12** Make the cranial osteotomy parallel to the seating chisel in the frontal and sagittal planes. **13** Make the distal osteotomy at an angle of 30°. Abduct the limb, insert the short distal screw, compress the osteotomy, and insert the remaining plate screws

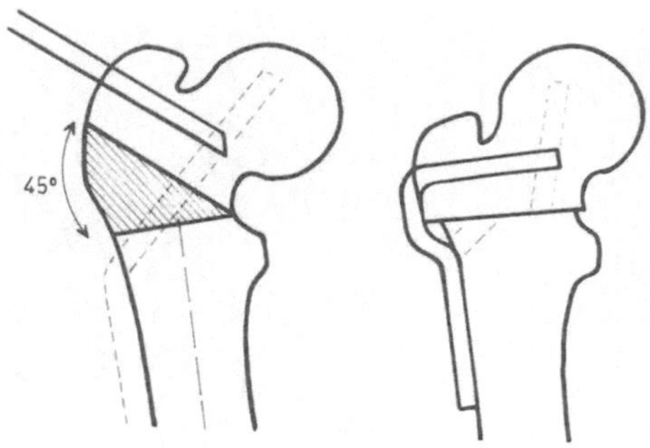

Fig. 5. Planning the correction of a deformity secondary to a pertrochanteric fracture. *Left:* On the x-ray tracing, draw in the shaft axis and the transverse osteotomy line just proximal to the lesser trochanter. Comparison with the healthy side indicates that a 45° wedge must be removed. The seating chisel is parallel to the proximal osteotomy surface. *Right:* Fixation with the right-angled hip plate

femurs are traced onto transparent sheets from the AP pelvic film, and the femoral axes are indicated. The line of the transverse osteotomy is marked on the tracing of the healthy side, and the drawing is reversed. The tracing of the affected femur is placed over that of the healthy femur so that the lesser trochanters and shafts align, and the transverse osteotomy is traced. Then the outlines of the femoral heads and greater trochanters are lined up as accurately as possible, and the osteotomy line is traced again. The wedge of bone to be resected can now be recognized (Fig. 5). The necessary plate is selected with the aid of the ASIF template. The tactical steps are the same as in Fig. 4 c. The pre- and postoperative status of an illustrative case are shown in Fig. 6.

With a painful subcapital abduction fracture without avascular necrosis but with early degenerative changes, an adduction osteotomy may be indicated.

Partial Necrosis of the Femoral Neck

The intertrochanteric osteotomy is indicated if there is a possibility of moving the necrotic part of the femoral head out of the weight-bearing zone. Planning

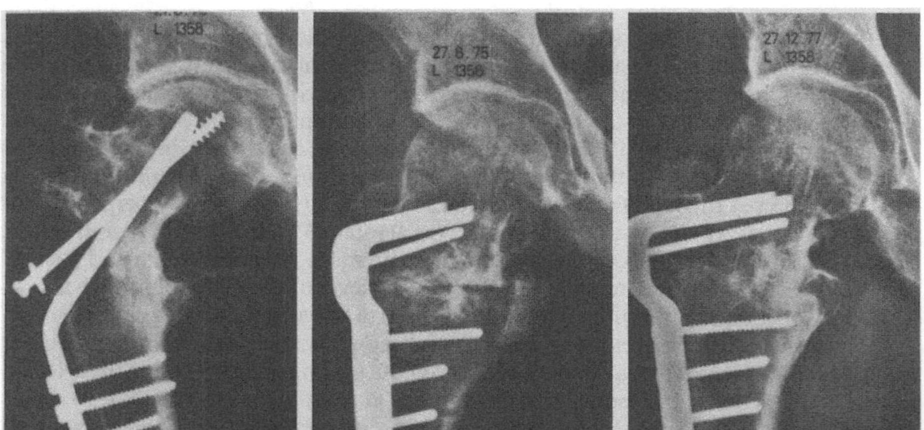

a **b** **c**

Fig. 6. a 47-Year-old patient, 1 year after his pertrochanteric fracture was treated with a 130° blade plate, which has penetrated the posterior surface of the femoral neck. **b** Status immediately after corrective osteotomy. The limb is rotated externally. **c** Two years later the hip shows nearly physiologic relations, as calculated preoperatively

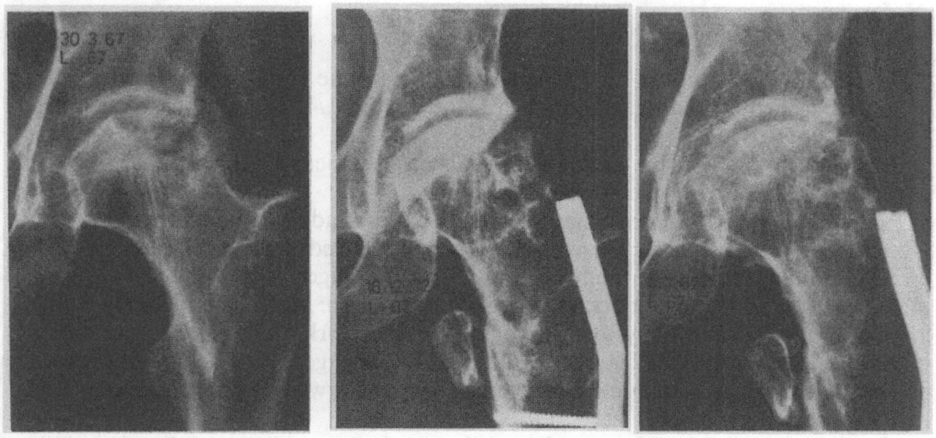

a b

Fig. 7. a Partial avascular necrosis of the femoral head two years after a subcapital abduction fracture. **b** Status after intertrochanteric osteotomy with 20° of abduction, 30° of extension, detachment of the lesser trochanter, fenestration of the femoral neck, cancellous bone grafting of the necrotic area, and fixation with a 160° plate. Eleven years later there is evidence of early posttraumatic osteoarthritis. The patient is free of complaints but tires easily

is based on roentgenograms in flexion and in te oblique projection [8]. Usually the proximal fragment has to be rotated 20–60° about its axis (Fig. 7).

Adduction Osteotomy for an Abduction Contracture after a Pelvic Fracture

The planning is the same as that for any varus osteotomy [4].

Slipped Capital Femoral Epiphysis

With an acute, "traumatic" slipped capital femoral epiphysis that shows more than a 50° slip of the femoral head, a simple reduction and fixation is almost invariably followed by avascular necrosis. A subcapital resection osteotomy is indicated, therefore [2]. First the caudal osteophyte is excised to restore the original neck angle. Care is taken to spare the blood supply to the femoral head during resection of the subcapital wedge. The size of the wedge is calculated on AP and axial orthograde filme [2]. This procedure is very demanding technically and should be performed by an orthopedic surgeon who specializes in hip surgery.

Conclusions

Preoperative drawings are a necessary preliminary to corrective procedures on the proximal femur [3–5]. Often the planning phase is much more time-consuming that the operation itself, but it forces the surgeon to give careful attention to clinical and radiologic diagnosis, goals, angular corrections and axial displacements, and it enables him to develop a clear concept of operative tactics and technique.

References

1. Lanz T v, Wachsmuth W (1938) Praktische Anatomie. Ein Lehr- und Hilfsbuch der anatomischen Grundlagen ärztlichen Handelns Bd 1/4. Bein und Statik. Springer, Berlin
2. Müller ME (1971) Die hüftnahen Femurosteotomien, 1. Aufl. 1957. 2. Aufl. mit Anhang: 12 Hüfteingriffe. Thieme, Stuttgart
3. Müller ME (1975) Intertrochanteric osteotomies in adults: Planning and operating technique, chapter 6. In: Cruess RL, Mitchell NS (eds) Surgical management of degenerative arthritis of the lower limb. Lea & Febiger, Philadelphia.
4. Müller ME (1983) Intertrochanteric osteotomies. In: McCollister C (ed) Surgery of the musculoskeletal system. Livingstone, New York
5. Müller ME, Allgöwer M, Schneider R, Willenegger H (1977) Manual der Osteosynthese. AO-Technik. 2. neubearbeitete und erweiterte Aufl. Springer, Berlin Heidelberg New York
6. Pauwels F (1973) Atlas zur Biomechanik der gesunden und kranken Hüfte. Prinzipien, Technik und Resultate einer kausalen Therapie. Springer, Berlin Heidelberg New York
7. Schenk RK, Müller J, Willenegger H (1968) Experimentell-histologischer Beitrag zur Entstehung und Behandlung von Pseudarthrosen. Hefte Unfallheilkd 94:15–24
8. Schneider R (1979) Die intertrochantere Osteotomie bei Coxarthrose. Springer, Berlin Heidelberg New York

Osteotomies of the Proximal Femur: Forms and Techniques

G. Muhr

Osteotomies of the proximal femur are relatively simple procedures when they are predicated on accurate, thoughtful planning. Modifying the neck-shaft angle, improving the seating of the femoral head in the acetabulum, altering the tension on the pelvitrochanteric muscles, improving blood flow (e.g., by reducing venous pressure), and the stable fixation of osteotomies have become integral parts of reconstructive surgery of the hip.

A number of measures must be implemented in order to achieve the desired effect.

Preparation

A careful clinical and radiologic examination is an essential part of preparation. The radiologic examination may include special roentgenograms (rotation films, contour films, tomograms), isotope scans, or even a CT scan. When muscle contractures are present, intensive preoperative physical therapy is strongly recommended, as it facilitates postoperative mobilization and fosters patient cooperation in rehabilitation.

It is also important that the nature and objective of the procedure be fully explained to the patient so that his expectations will be in line with the prospective result. Despite the favorable long-term prognosis, the early result will probably be inferior to that of a total hip replacement in cases where disease of the hip joint is advanced.

Operative Techniques

Except in special techniques, the hip joint is approached through a lateral incision with the patient supine. A flat cushion under the buttocks hyperextends the hip joint slightly and facilitates intraoperative manipulations. The leg should be draped so that it is free to move, and facilities should be available for intraoperative roentgenograms or fluoroscopy. After the fascia is divided, it is generally necessary to cut around the vastus lateralis muscle in L-shaped fashion and reflect it off the proximal femur. In the cranial part of the field, above the innominate tubercle, the tendinous insertions of the gluteal muscles are notched or retracted together with a small piece of periosteum.

The femoral neck axis is marked with a Kirschner wire laid alongside the neck and anchored in the hip capsule. The level of the lesser trochanter is

Corrective Osteotomies of the Lower Extremity
Edited by G. Hierholzer, K. H. Müller

determined by digital palpation. Together with the innominate tubercle, these sites represent the three major landmarks used for preoperative planning.

Twelve types of correction are possible in the intertrochanteric region of the femur: valgus or varus, internal or external rotation, flexion or extension (i.e., anterior or posterior angulation), lengthening or shortening, medial or lateral displacement of the shaft, and anterior or posterior displacement of the shaft. Rotation of the femoral neck is also possible. Recently, there has been increasing interest in revascularizing procedures using free or pedicle bone grafts (Table 1).

Table 1. Types of Proximal Femoral Osteotomy

Valgus	Displacement
Varus	Shortening
Extension	Lengthening
Flexion	Neck rotation
Rotation	Revascularizing

Fixation of the osteotomies is accomplished with angled blade plates that have a preset blade angle.

As a rule, four screws are sufficient to attach the plate to the shaft. A range of blade lengths are available. The rightangled hip plates offer the additional option of controlling medial displacement of the femoral shaft.

Types of Osteotomy

The *valgus osteotomy* is important in the management of posttraumatic as well as degenerative hip changes. Besides reorienting the plane of a subcapital fracture or nonunion with respect to the line of compression across the hip, the procedure is of value in osteoarthritis with a large medial or caudal osteophyte that can be used to increase the weight-bearing area of the femoral head. This removes excessive loads from the lateral part of the acetabulum and improves the distribution of joint pressure. Valgus osteotomy is also useful for correcting adduction deformity of the hip. During planning, it is important to consider that the valgus osteotomy lengthens the extremity, and that a planned resection may be necessary to counter this effect. The operation also produces lateral displacement of the mechanical axis of the limb, which can cause valgus overloading of the knee joint if the correction is excessive. This is why lateralization of the femoral shaft is desired. As a rule, varus osteotomies are stabilized with a double-angled 120° plate, especially in cases of posttraumatic deformity (Fig. 1). Given the fixed angle of the plate, the osteotomy is always performed in the intertrochanteric region. If the blade of the 120° plate is driven into the femoral neck at right angles to the shaft, a 30° wedge of bone must be removed. Other angles of insertion may be used depending on the amount of valgus correction desired. Even the 90° hip plate is suitable for a valgus osteotomy, especially if there is preexisting limb

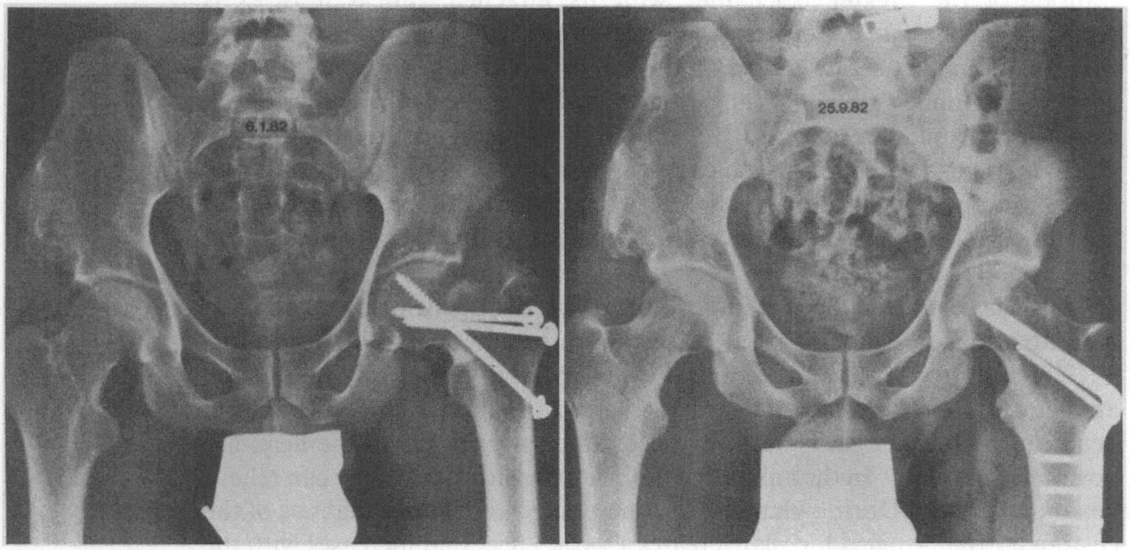

Fig. 1. Posttraumatic coxa vara following the fixation of a subcapital fracture with screws. Axial deformity and length discrepancy corrected by intertrochanteric valgus osteotomy (with 120° plate)

shortening and the blade does not have to engage the head fragment as securely as in a subcapital nonunion. The classic valgus osteotomy in trauma surgery is the correction of a nonunion of the femoral neck with a steep plane of nonunion (Fig. 2).

The *varus osteotomy* is rarely indicated after trauma. It, too, is a classic type of osteotomy, but it was developed less for posttraumatic deformity than for degenerative joint disease. The purpose is to center the femoral head within the acetabulum. Varus osteotomy shortens the extremity and relaxes the pelvitrochanteric muscles, providing an immediate reduction of joint pressure. Because gluteal insufficiency results in a pronounced and refractory limp, a

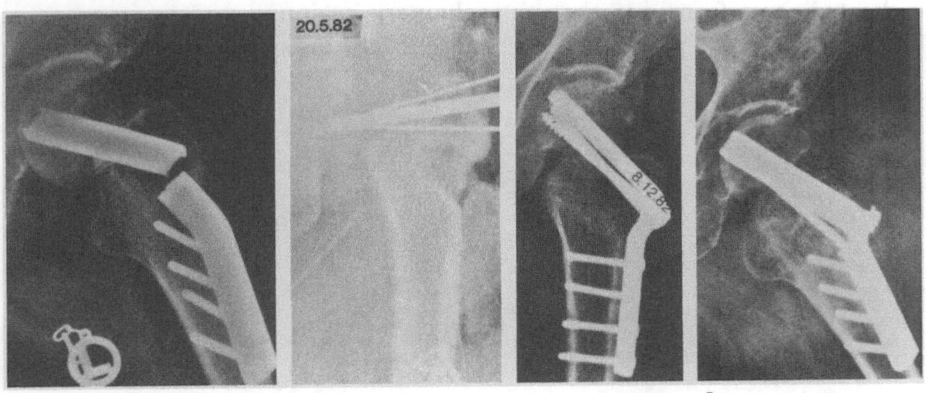

a b c d

Fig. 2 a–d. a Nonunion of the femoral neck with breakage of the implant. **b–d** After 50° introchanteric valgus osteotomy, the nonunion consolidated without difficulty (130° plate)

transfer of the greater trochanter with its attached gluteal muscles is recommended in cases where the varus correction is 20° or more. Also, because the osteotomy can cause a prominence of bony hip contours that is cosmetically undesirable in young women, a shortening of the femoral neck should be included in preoperative plans. This is readily combined with the trochanteric osteotomy, in which case a 15-mm disc of bone is removed from the femoral neck before the trochanter is reattached. All varus osteotomies lead to varus overloads on the knee, and so medial displacement of the femoral shaft is necessary.

The *extension osteotomy* is important in the treatment of posttraumatic osteoarthritis of the hip or partial avascular necrosis of the femoral head (Fig. 3). The intertrochanteric resection of a wedge based posteriorly relaxes the abductor muscles and reduces joint pressure. At the same time, the femoral head can be rotated such that previously anterior portions of the head are positioned cranially. In the ankylosed hip, the extension osteotomy can relieve flexion deformity. During planning, it is necessary to consider that use of the customary right-angled hip plate creates a varus effect that increases with the proposed degree of posterior angulation. Also, because the blade must be inserted somewhat anteriorly in order to appose the plate to the shaft, penetration of the greater trochanter by the blade is a danger.

In the *flexion osteotomy* the resected wedge has an anterior base, causing posterior portions of the femoral head to face cranially. Because flexion contractures are relatively common following trauma, extension of the hip joint may be lost. In this case a psoas tenotomy and anterior capsulotomy are indicated (Fig. 3)

Displacement osteotomies in posttraumatic hip surgery are usually a side-effect of varus or valgus operations done to correct the mechanical limb axis. Only a medial displacement osteotomy of the femoral shaft should be considered as an isolated procedure, with the object of relaxing the ilipsoas and other muscles.

Rotational osteotomies are of practically no importance in posttraumatic hip surgery. With rotational deformity of the femoral shaft, the operation, if indicated, is performed in the subtrochanteric region.

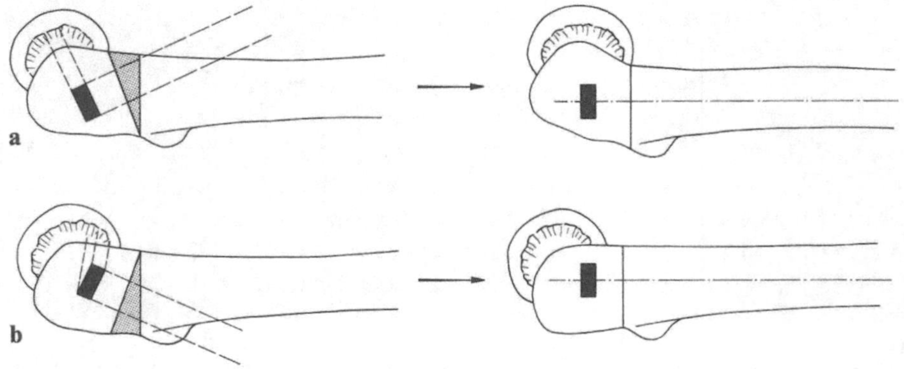

Fig. 3. a Flexion osteotomy with intertrochanteric wedge based anteriorly. **b** Extension osteotomy with wedge based posteriorly

In the *correction of leg length discrepancies*, intertrochanteric osteotomies are mainly used for limb shortening. The intertrochanteric region is osteotomized such that the attachment of the lesser trochanter to the proximal fragment is preserved. After this cut is made, up to 4 cm of shaft may be resected distally. The upper end of the distal fragment is then tapered slightly and pressed into the proximal fragment. Allowance for impaction of the fragments should be made during planning.

Limb lengthening generally can be achieved in valgus osteotomies for nonunions of the femoral neck when there is marked concurrent lateralization of the shaft. The lengthening in this case is relative and results from apposition of the oblique osteotomy surfaces.

The technique for all intertrochanteric osteotomies is similar: After surgical landmarks are defined, the seating chisel for the blade plate is driven into the femoral neck at the planned site. At this time we generally make a transverse intertrochanteric osteotomy at a level just cranial to the lesser trochanter. This creates a proximal and distal fragment from which individual bone wedges may be resected as needed. If rotational correction is desired, it is carried out before the distal wedge is removed. If a proximal wedge is to be resected, this may be done before rotating the distal fragment. The apex of the wedges should not extend past the center of the shaft to avoid excessive shortening. After corrections have been carried out, the seating chisel is removed and the selected blade plate is inserted. The plate is held against the shaft with a self-retaining bone clamp. At this time the blade is driven the last 5 mm into the trochanteric region. Before the plate is definitively attached to the shaft, the function of the hip joint is carefully tested, and the position of the limb is checked. In horizontal osteotomies and when the right-angled plate is used, the tension device of the ASIF is essential. This device may also be used with 120° and 130° blade plates if the proximal fragment is secured with an additional screw. In oblique osteotomies, the screws are inserted and tightened in a distal to proximal sequence to effect compression of the oblique osteotomy surfaces.

Hematomas are flushed from the wound, suction drains are placed, and the vastus lateralis muscle is reattached. The fascia is closed, a subcutaneous Redon drain is inserted, and the skin is sutured.

Further details on individual operating techniques may be found in the ASIF Manual.

With posttraumatic avascular necrosis involving no more than one-third of the cranial part of the head, the *transtrochanteric rotation osteotomy* of Sugioka may be performed. The procedure requires careful planning and is done with the patient in the lateral position. After division of the fascia, the joint capsule is approached anteriorly between the vastus lateralis and gluteal muscles. The greater trochanter is osteotomized parallel to the superior margin of the femoral neck, taking care not to injure the vessels supplying the femoral head.

The gluteals are reflected to expose the joint capsule, which is incised circumferentially at its attachment to the acetabular labrum. A transtrochanteric osteotomy is made at a right angle to the femoral neck axis, angling the

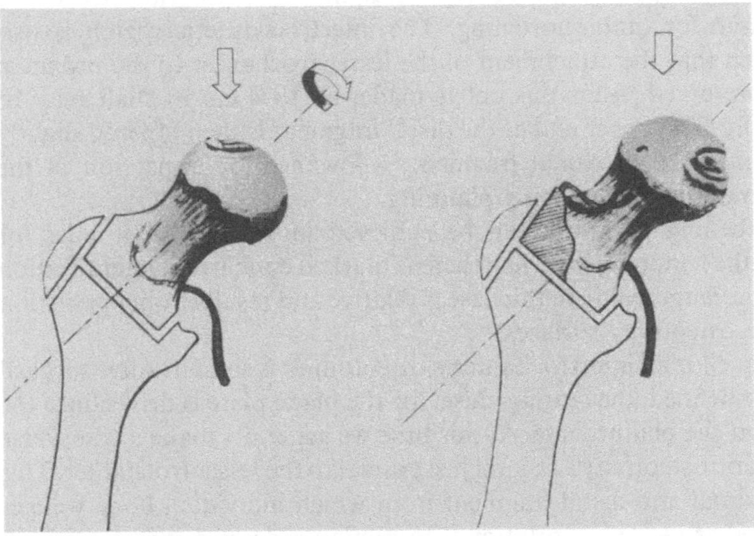

Fig. 4. Schematic drawing of the transtrochanteric rotational osteotomy of Sugioka

osteotomy line 90° medially just above the lesser trochanter. Two Steinmann pins are inserted into the femoral neck and trochanter at right angles to the neck axis, and the proximal pin is rotated anteriorly to the desired angle of correction. The osteotomy is then fixed in position with three or four cancellous bone screws inserted through the lateral femoral cortex, and the greater trochanter is reattached with lag screws (Figs. 4 and 5). Usually the osteotomy surface above the lesser trochanter forms an additional support for the proximal fragment. Postoperatively, skin traction is applied for two weeks, followed by six weeks in a plaster splint. With meticulous technique and preservation of blood supply, the results are generally good.

Another localized procedure for the treatment of avascular necrosis involves the transplantation of a *muscle pedicle corticocancellous bone graft* from the intertrochanteric crest. With the patient prone, the proximal end of the femur is exposed through a posterior approach. The quadratus femoris muscle is isolated and snared, and the bony attachment of this muscle is chiseled from the intertrochanteric crest to form a rectangular graft measuring $3 \times 1.8 \times 5$ cm. The posterior part of the joint capsule is incised, necrotic tissue is scraped out, and the muscle pedicle graft is impacted into a prepared slot with chips of cancellous bone. A nonunion, if present, is fixed with a screw. The joint capsule is sutured, the wound is closed, and the joint is immobilized for six weeks in a plastic or plaster splint with no weight bearing.

Recently there have been reports of several cases treated by the *microvascular transplantation of autogenous bone grafts* to revascularize necrotic portions of the femoral head. So far there has been relatively little experience with this obviously very difficult procedure.

a b c d

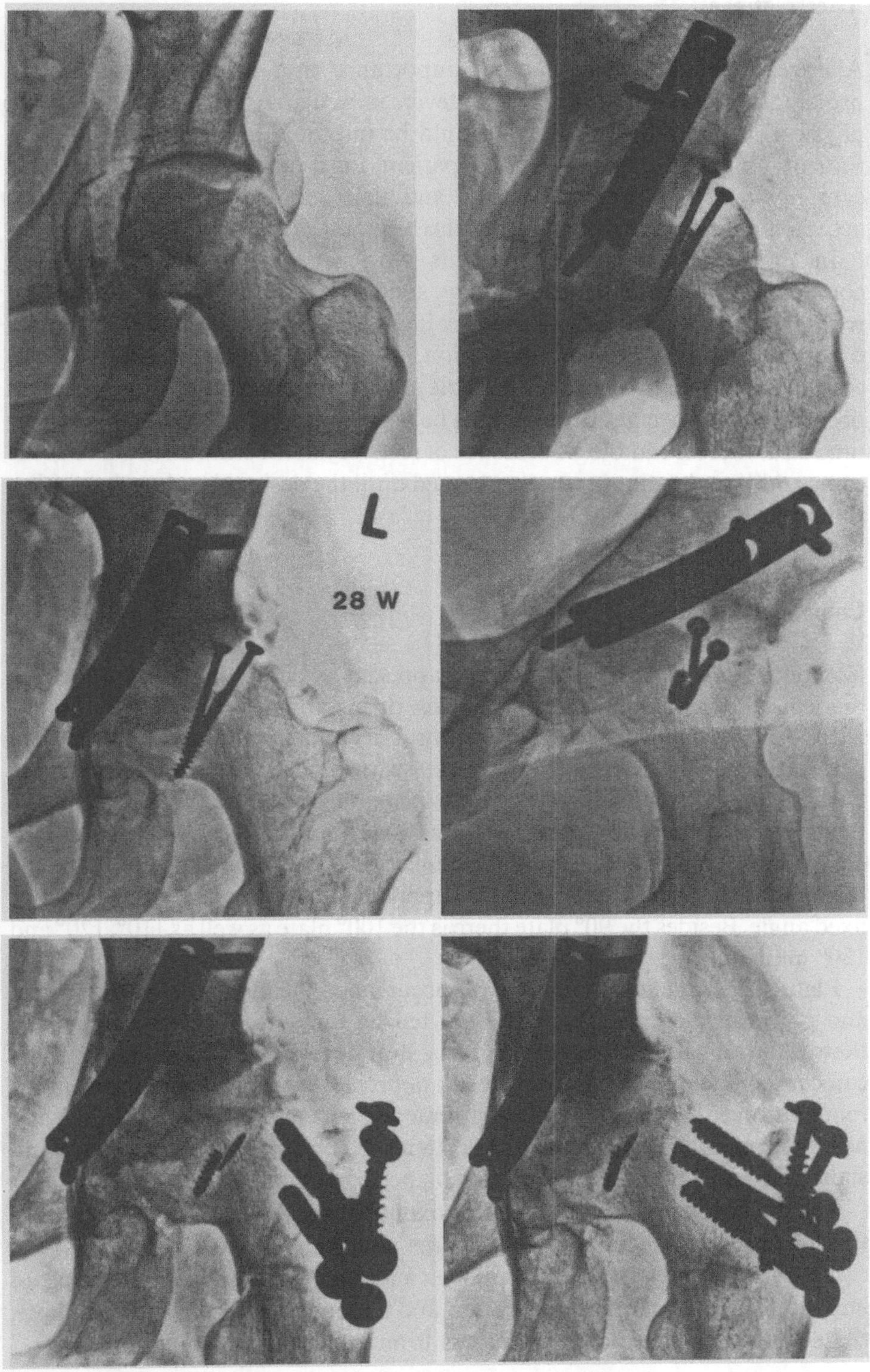

Fig. 5 a – d. a Acetabular fracture with an associated shear fracture of the cranial part of the femoral head. **b** Original postoperative roentgenogram at two weeks postinjury. **c** Seven months later there was marked necrosis of the head fragment. **d** Eight weeks after 70° transtrochanteric rotational osteotomy, the position of the femoral head is good

Aftertreatment

Aftertreatment is of fundamental importance in patients who have had proximal femoral osteotomies. With severe muscular atrophy or contractures, physical rehabilitative measures should be initiated prior to the operation. Patient cooperation is vital. The patient must understand the need for carefully restricted weight bearing, and that certain complaints must be accepted as the price of preserving the hip joint.

In unreliable patients or patients with severe osteoporosis, a spica composed of plastic bandages may sometimes be necessary. Follow-up roentgenograms at three- to four-week intervals will demonstrate the progress of bone healing or revascularization. With most intertrochanteric osteotomies, full weight bearing is possible after three months. In revascularizing procedures, non-weight bearing must be maintained for a considerably longer time until there is radiologic evidence of recovery of the femoral head. In some cases additional sittings must be planned until the desired head-neck position is achieved and the head is viable.

Complications

Complications of the aseptic type may present as blood flow disturbances of the femoral neck, angular discrepancies, or instabilities.

Blood flow disturbances of the femoral neck most commonly result from perforation of the cortex by the plate seating chisel, destroying the main nutrient vessel, and from incisions of the joint capsule. It is also conceivable that overcorrection with torsion of the capsule might cause a venous statis that compromises blood flow. Discrepancies between the planned position and the postoperative status are remedied by applying a new implant with a different fixed angle. Besides the 90° plate there is the 100° plate as well as 110°, 120° and 130° implants.

Plate dislodgment is most likely to occur when the blade is near the cortex, and powerful muscular forces are exerted on the area of the fixation. Then there is the long lever of the leg versus the short lever of the femoral neck, which can cause plate dislodgment as a result of premature passive mobilization. At reoperation either the old implant is removed and a new implant inserted at a new site, or, preferably, a refixation is attempted by applying a second implant, such as a hook plate, at an anterior or posterior site.

The foundation of any successful proximal femoral osteotomy is preoperative planning which takes into account anatomic surgical landmarks, the corrective options that are available, and the most appropriate type of implant. Through careful preparation and a meticulous operating technique, there should be little danger of errors from a mechanical standpoint.

References

1. Baksi DP (1983) Treatment of posttraumatic avascular necrosis of the femoral head by multiple drilling and muscle-pedicle bone graft. J Bone Joint Surg [Br] 65:268
2. Ganz R, Jakob RP (1980) Partielle avaskuläre Hüftkopfnekrose: Flexionsosteotomie und Spongiosaplastik. Orthopädie 9:265
3. Meyers MH, Harvey JP, Moore TM (1973) Treatment of displaced subcapital and transcervical fractures of the femoral neck by muscle-pedicle-bone graft and internal fixation: a preliminary report of one hundred and fifty cases. J Bone Joint Surg [Am] 55:257
4. Müller ME, Allgöwer M, Schneider R, Willenegger H (1977) Manual der Osteosynthese. Springer, Berlin Heidelberg New York
5. Schneider R (1979) Die intertrochantäre Osteotomie bei Coxarthrose. Springer, Berlin Heidelberg New York
6. Sugioka Y (1978) Transtrochanteric anterior rotational osteotomy of the femoral head in the treatment of osteonecrosis affecting the hip. Clin Orthop 130:191

The Intertrochanteric Osteotomy for Posttraumatic States: Reports of Selected Cases

R. Schneider

The indications for corrective osteotomies of the proximal femur after trauma can be discussed only in general terms. Preoperative constraints, the technically and biomechanically correct conduct of the operation, and the morphologic and clinical course form a unique pattern that is unlikely to be repeated from one case to the next. Thus, the presentation of individual case histories is as important in a didactic sense as is the knowledge of general rules.

The situation is simple with isolated, posttraumatic lesions of the femoral head. Contour films are obtained to localize the damaged head area, and an extension or flexion osteotomy is performed to rotate this area out of the zone of greatest pressure. The benefit of this procedure is illustrated by three examples:

- A 19-year old man sustained a fracture-dislocation of the left hip with shearing of a cranionaterior fragment. A 30° flexion osteotomy was performed; 7 1/2 years later the patient was free of complaints and active athletically.
- A 19-year-old man sustained multiple injuries that included fractures of the pelvic ring and femoral shaft. After union of the fractures, he was left with a painful right hip. Contour films demonstrated a compression fracture of the cranioposterior part of the femoral head. Symptoms regressed following a 40° extension osteotomy.
- A 9-year–old girl suffered a severe contusion of the left groin with subsequent septic thrombosis of the femoral vein. Thrombectomy was followed by avascular necrosis of the femoral head. A varus osteotomy at 14 months postinjury was unsuccessful due to a cranioposterior osteophyte that caused a painful snapping in the hip. A 30° extension, 25° valgus and 15° external rotation osteotomy was performed, and 5 1/2 years later the girl was free of complaints.

The situation is more complex in acetabular fractures with associated bony and cartilaginous lesions of the femoral head, which often go unrecognized. Fig. 1 shows an example: In 1961 I performed an intertrochanteric osteotomy in a 45-year-old woman with severe osteoarthritis of the left hip secondary to a compression fracture. The correction involved 40° of extension and 15° of valgus. Twenty-two years later the woman is still free of complaints and enjoys unrestricted ambulation. Her range of flexion was increased from 50° to 80°, she has full extension compared with a 10° limitation preoperatively, and she has a 30° range of rotation compared with a complete blockage of rotation before surgery. She can tie her shoes and climb stairs normally. The operated limb is stable, and the gait is free of limp despite 1.0 cm of shortening. While

Corrective Osteotomies of the Lower Extremity
Edited by G. Hierholzer, K. H. Müller

this case is unusual, it nonetheless demonstrates the capabilities of corrective osteotomies in the sagittal plane.

The situation becomes extremely difficult in young patients with extensive avascular necrosis of the femoral head, especially if the height of the patient contraindicates an arthrodesis.

The case presented in Figs. 2–6 clearly demonstrates how individual case histories and selective surgical measures cannot be fitted into statistical classifications or into a scheme of generally valid principles:

– A 20-year-old man and 182 cm tall underwent a valgus-extension osteotomy of the proximal femur. At 17 months there was adduction deformity with 5.5 cm of shortening, 90° of flexion, and a 10° loss of extension (Fig. 2). Arthrotomy and joint debridement were performed with extirpation of a large medial head sequestrum (Fig. 3). Three weeks in an abduction cast relieved the adduction contracture. This was followed by intensive physical therapy to mobilize the hip, which had only 10° of motion, and the allowance of sufficient time for the medial part of the femoral head to regenerate. Sixteen months after arthrotomy, regeneration of the head was

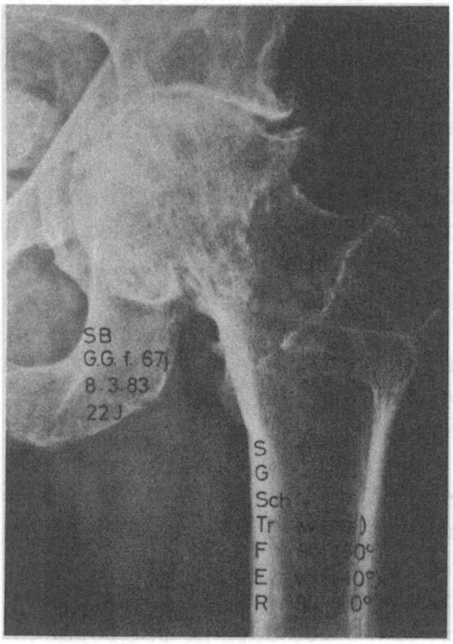

Fig. 1

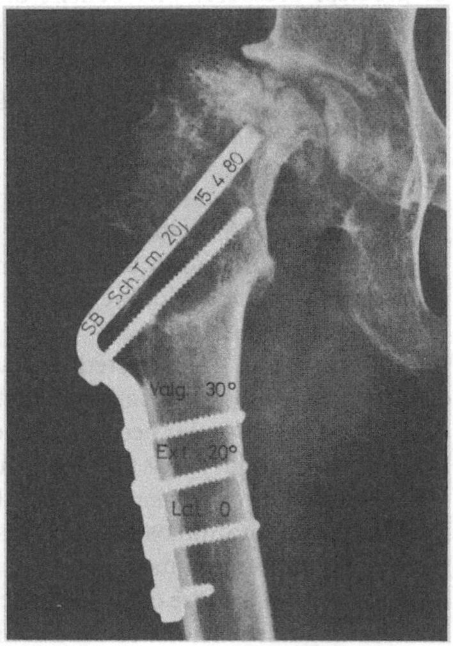

Fig. 2

Fig. 1. 67-year-old woman 22 years after 40° extension and 15° valgus osteotomy for osteoarthritis of the hip secondary to a compression fracture of the acetabulum and probable femoral head lesion with asymmetric narrowing of the joint space by 0–3 mm Today the hip is painless, and walking distance is unlimited. The patient has 80° of flexion (vs. 50° preoperatively), full extension, and 30° of rotation (vs. 0° preoperatively)

Fig. 2. Avascular necrosis of the femoral head after screw fixation of a femoral neck fracture in a man 20 years of age. Poor result 17 months after 30° valgus and 20° extension osteotomy with large medial sequestrum; 5.5 cm of limb shortening

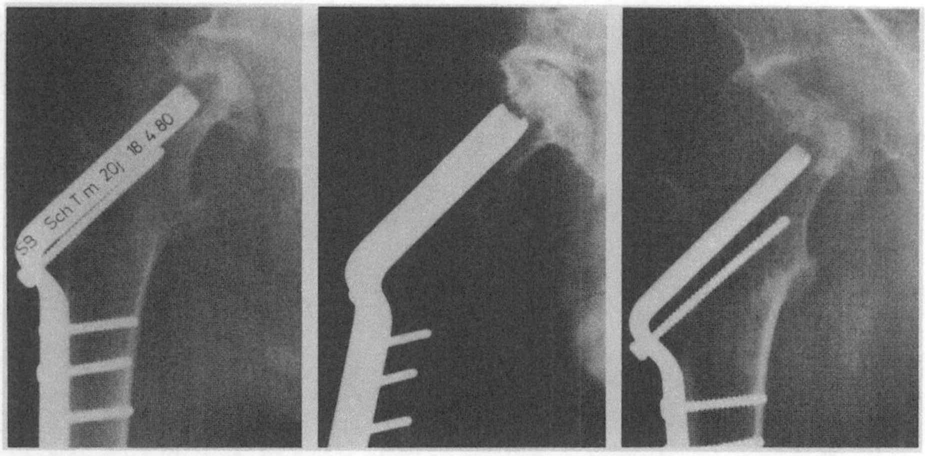

Fig. 3. Very severe incongruity following arthrotomy with sequestrectomy, "head debridement" and relief of abduction contracture

in progress (Fig. 4), and 2 years later joint congruity was improved by a second, 30° valgus osteotomy with 2.3 cm of lateralization (Fig. 5). Eight months later the hip is painless, and the limb is stable with 0.5 cm of shortening. The legs can by symmetrically abducted to a malleolar distance of 135 cm and crossed to a malleolar distance of 20 cm. The patient has 60° of flexion, full extension, and 30° of rotation (Fig. 6).

When faced with avascular necrosis of the femoral head in the young patient, we try to rotate a viable part of the head into the weight-bearing zone.

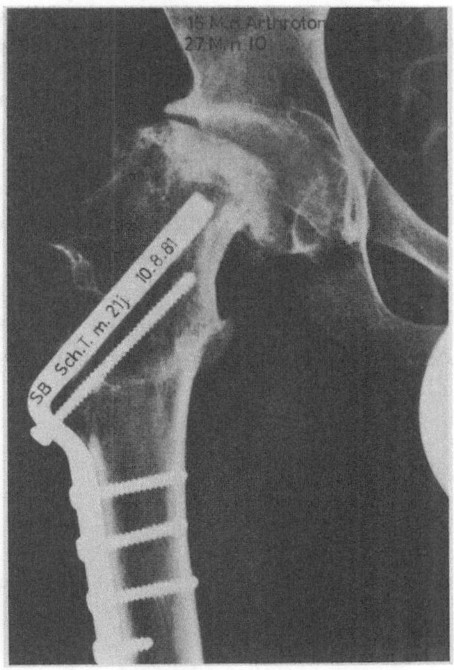

Fig. 4. Regeneration of the femoral head is evident 16 months after arthrotomy and 27 months after intertrochanteric osteotomy

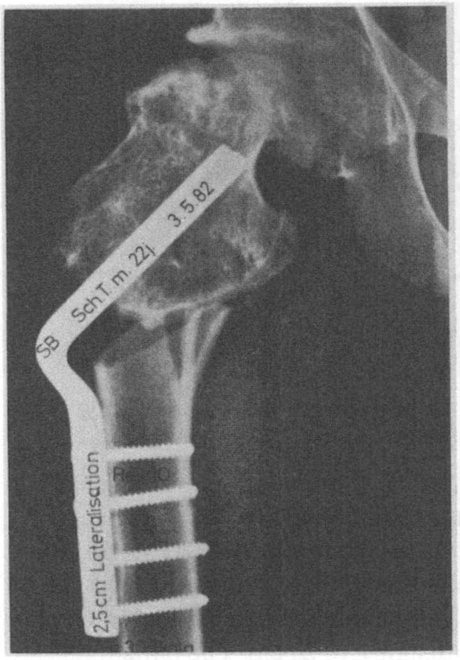

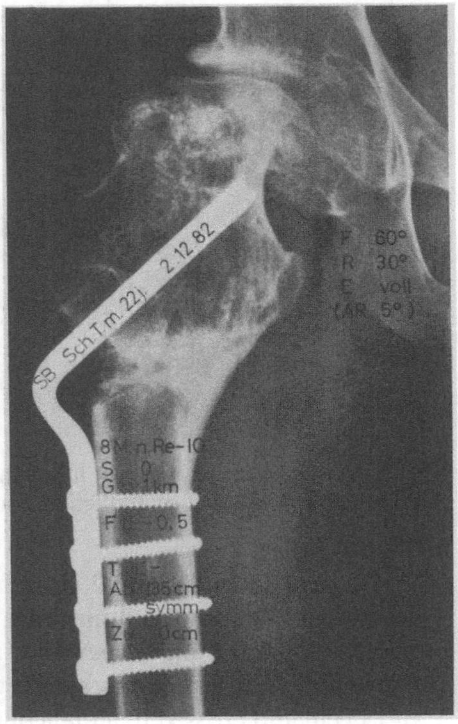

Fig. 5 **Fig. 6**

Fig. 5. Second valgus correction of 30° with lateralization of the shaft 2 years after arthrotomy

Fig. 6. Status 8 months after the 2nd osteotomy. Congruity is improved, and new cartilage is forming in the joint space. The patient is free of pain, has a negative Trendelenburg sign, has 0.5 cm of limb shortening, 60° of flexion (10° after plaster fixation to relieve adduction contracture), full extension, 30° of rotation, full abduction, and 1/2 the adduction of the left side. Acetabuloplasty is indicated unless there is spontaneous improvement of head coverage

If this fails, we carry out joint debridement and relieve deformity through physical therapy, using anesthesia and casting as required. We then wait for the head to regenerate and perform a secondary osteotomy to improve joint congruity.

My intention has been to illustrate the value of the intertrochanteric osteotomy in the management of posttraumatic hip disease.

Results of Proximal Femoral Osteotomies Following Trauma

A. Lies and I. Scheuer

Corrective osteotomies offer an effective means of managing problem cases following the operative and conservative treatment of femoral neck fractures, including nonunions and malunions [4–7]. While the frontal-plane valgus osteotomy, used by Pauwels to change shear forces into compressive forces, will promote the healing of virtually any nonunion [4], other options are available for the treatment of posttraumatic osteoarthritis of the hip and malunited fractures [1,7] (Fig. 1). In such cases it is usually necessary to combine the valgus correction with a flexion, extension or rotation osteotomy. Accurate preoperative planning is the key to a successful outcome [1,3,7].

In reviewing our patients, we found 67 who had undergone proximal femoral osteotomies following trauma. Fifty-eight of these patients were available for follow-up – 16 females and 42 males. The average age of the patients at the time of corrective osteotomy was 37.3 years, with a range from 13 to 69 years.

The osteotomies were performed to correct fractures about the hip that had united in a faulty position or had progressed to nonunion. Most of these fractures were caused by accidents at work, in motor vehicles or at home; few were the result of athletic or war injuries. Fifty of the fractures were closed and 8 were open; 34 involved the left hip and 24 the right hip. Primary treatment had been operative in 39 patients and nonoperative in the remaining 19. The injuries consisted mostly of femoral neck fractures. Lateral and pertrochanteric fractures were less common in this series.

The indications for corrective osteotomy were deformity in 22 cases, deformity with nonunion in 28 cases, the course of the fracture line in 4 patients, and osteoarthritis or partial avascular necrosis in the remaining 4.

The decision to undertake corrective osteotomy was based chiefly on subjective complaints, clinical findings, and roentgenologic findings, in that order.

Only 8.6% of the patients rated the result of their primary treatment as good, 60.3% rated it as fair, and 31.1% rated it as poor (cf. Fig. 2). We evaluated hip function according to our modification of the scheme of Merle d'Aubigné [2] (Table 1).

With regard to function, hip mobility was good in 16 patients, fair in 25, and poor in 17.

Walking distance was only 100 m in 27 patients, 1000 m in 21 patients, and more than 1000 m in only 10 patients.

Eighteen patients walked with a normal gait or had a slight limp. Fourteen patients required one or two crutches (Table 2). Eight patients had additional

Corrective Osteotomies of the Lower Extremity
Edited by G. Hierholzer, K. H. Müller

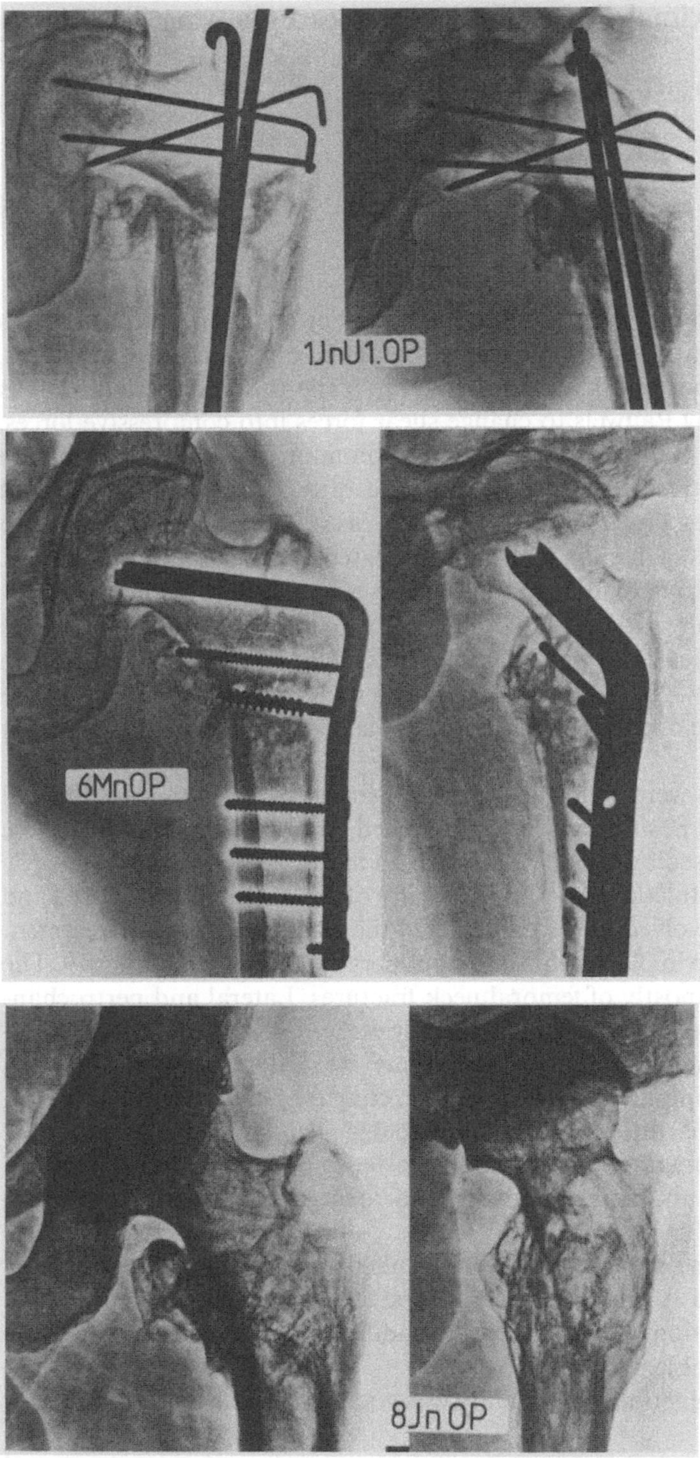

Fig. 1. Malunited sub- and pertrochanteric fracture in a 20-year-old man that healed in excellent position following corrective osteotomy. *Top*: 1 year after injury, 1st operation; *middle*: 6 months after corrective osteotomy; *bottom*: 8 years after corrective osteotomy

complaints referrable to back pain, coexisting fractures, or traumatic nerve lesions.

Limb shortening in excess of 1 cm was present in 63.8% of the trauma patients; 37.9% had an external rotation deformity of 10° or more.

Roentgenograms demonstrated the presence of a nonunion in 28 cases (48.2%). Six patients exhibited partial avascular necrosis of the femoral head. Mild osteoarthritis of the hip was evident in 27 patients (46.5%), moderate osteoarthritis was present in 20.7%, and severe osteoarthritis was present in

Table 1. Modified Merle d'Aubigné Scheme for Evaluation of Hip Function

	Pain	Active mobility		Gait
Good	Little or no pain and no functional disability	Flexion Abduction Contracture Internal and external rotation	>90° >25° <10° 20°	Normal or slight limp, crutch not required
Fair	Mild to severe pain during walking, none at rest, moderate functional disability	Flexion Abduction Contracture Internal and external rotation	>40° >10° <20° 10°	Limp, one crutch required
Poor	Severe pain that interferes with sleep, severe functional disability	Flexion Abduction Contracture Ankylosis	<40° 0° >20°	Patient is unable to walk or requires two crutches

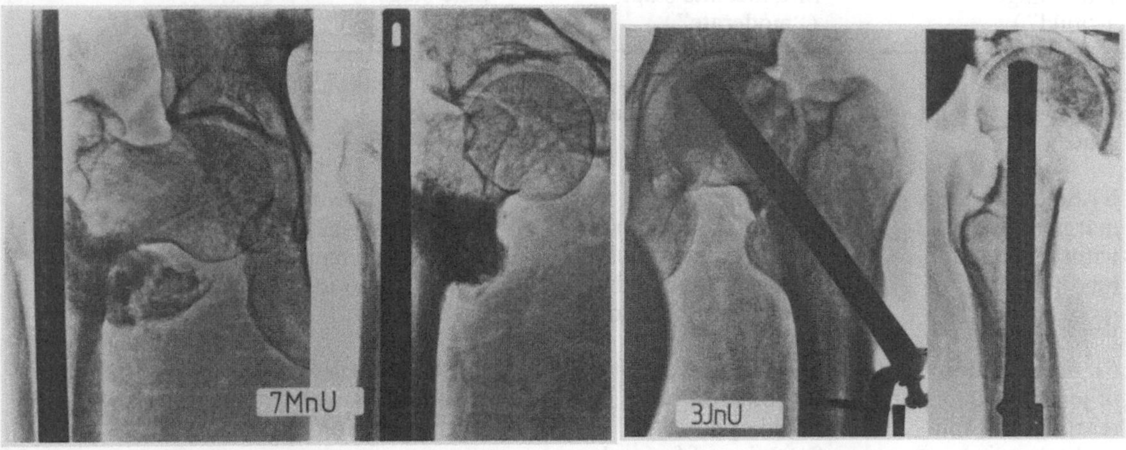

Fig. 2. Examples of poor result following inadequate primary treatment: *Top*: 44-year-old man with deformity 7 months after injury; *bottom*: 40-year-old man with nonunion 3 years after injury

Table 2. Clinical Evaluation before Corrective Osteotomy (n=58, Bergmannsheil Bochum)

Mobility of the affected hip	n
Good	16
Fair	25
Poor	17
Quality of gait	**n**
Good	18
Fair	16
Poor	24
Walking distance	**n**
100 m	27
1000 m	21
2000 m	7
5000 m	3

3.4% (Fig. 3). In all patients the severity of osteoarthritis was assessed on the basis of a specially developed evaluation scheme (Table 3).

A varus deformity was diagnosed in 60.3% of all cases, and a valgus deformity in 8.6% (Table 4).

We conducted follow-up examinations in 58 patients who had undergone corrective osteotomies on the proximal femur (Table 5). The osteotomies were of the varus, valgus, extension, and flexion types (Fig. 4). The rate of postoperative complications was low (Table 6).

Table 3. Stages of Osteoarthritis of the Hip

Early stage ("mild")	Intermediate stage ("moderate")	Late stage ("severe")
a) Little or no narrowing of joint space	a) Narrowing of joint space in weight-bearing zone	a) Obliteration of joint space
b) Slight marginal exostosis without extension, mild porosis	b) Osteophytes in marginal areas, on femoral head, at junction of head and neck and at fovea, "double fond"	b) Heavy lipping of joint margins, possible anomalies of joint position
c) Accentuation of joint lines, reactive subchondral sclerosis	c) Increased density of subchondral bone, occasional cysts, slight flattening of femoral head	c) Marked sclerosis of subarticular bone, formation of cysts or necrotic areas, head deformity

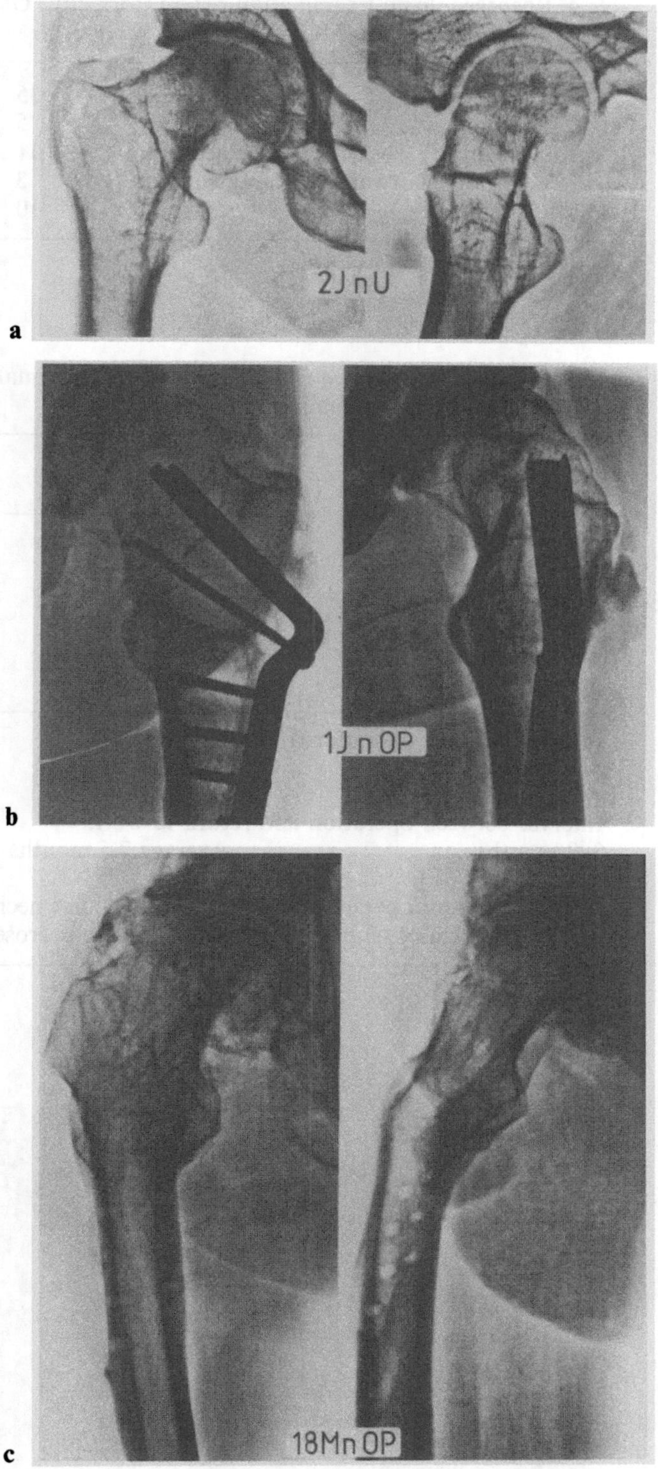

Fig. 3 a–c. Examples of the stages of osteoarthritis described in Table 3. **a** 50-year-old man 3 years after injury; **b** 56-year-old man 1 year after surgery; **c** 48-year-old man 18 months after surgery

Table 4. Roentgenologic Examination *before* Corrective Osteotomy (n = 58, Bergmannsheil Bochum)

Varus deformity	35
Valgus deformity	5
Extension deformity (backward displacement)	11
Flexion deformity (forward displacement)	3
Rotational deformity	10

Table 5. Results of Corrective Osteotomies of the Proximal Femur after Trauma (n = 58, Bergmannsheil Bochum)

Sex			
Male: 42		Female: 16	
Age: 13–69		Average: 37.3 years	
Right hip	24	Left hip	34
Closed fracture	50	Open fracture	8
Primary treatment			
Operative:	39	Nonoperative:	19

1. Interval between operation and follow-up
   5–8 years Average 3.6 years
2. Interval between operation and return to work
   3–8 months Average 7.5 months
3. Interval between operation and onset of avascular necrosis
   1–3 years: 10 cases (3 partial necroses, 7 severe necroses)

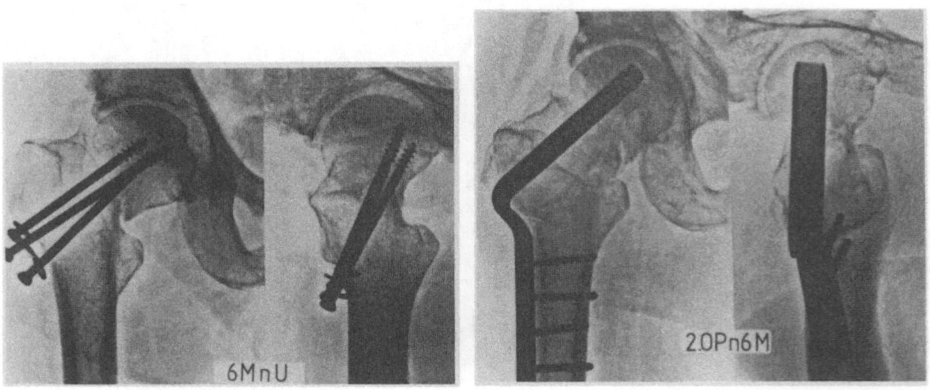

Fig. 4. Screw fixation of a Pauwels type III fracture in this 53-year-old man resulted in nonunion with deformity (*top*, 6 months postinjury). Six months after repositioning osteotomy (*bottom*) bony consolidation is progressing well

Table 6. Complications
(n = 58, Bergmannsheil Bochum)

1. Hematoma	3
2. Soft-tissue infection	2
3. Infection	0
4. Thrombosis	2
5. Pulmonary embolism	1
6. Cardiovascular disorders	3

While our follow-up examinations confirm the efficacy of modern internal fixation methods in the treatment of nonunions, avascular necrosis of the femoral head continues to be a significant problem [1]. Of the 58 patients who were reviewed, 7 (12.1%) developed avascular necrosis within 1 to 3 years after surgery and required a total hip arthroplasty (Fig. 5). Three patients developed partial necrosis; one case improved slightly, and findings remained stationary in the other two.

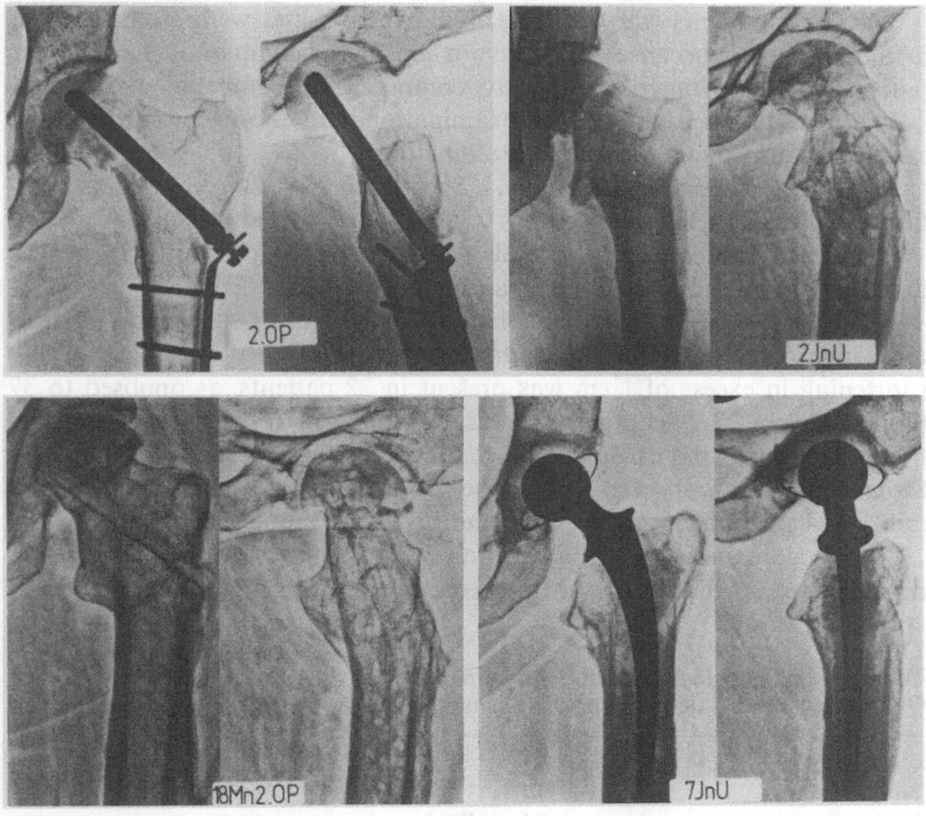

Fig. 5. Repositioning Osteotomy was performed in this 51-year-old-man following inadequate primary fixation. Avascular necrosis of the femoral head ensued, and total hip arthroplasty was necessary

Table 7. Clinical Evaluation *After* Corrective Osteotomy (n = 58, Bergmannsheil Bochum)

Mobility of the affected hip		
Good	35	68.7%
Fair	14	27.4%
Poor	2	3.9%
Quality of gait		
Good	39	76.5%
Fair	11	21.6%
Poor	1	1.9%
Walking distance		
100 m	0	
1000 m	23	45.1%
2000 m	8	15.7%
5000 m	20	39.2%

The seven patients who had total hip arthroplasties were excluded from further follow-up, because they were not considered comparable to the other patients in terms of function, subjective complaints or roentgenologic findings.

The procedure for our follow-up examinations after the osteotomies was the same as that in the preoperative examinations.

Following corrective osteotomy, 35 patients (68.7%) showed a good functional result, as compared with 27.6% before corrective surgery.

Significant improvements were also noted in walking distance, leg length discrepancy, rotational deformity, and quality of gait (Table 7).

While only 31% of the patients had a normal gait or slight limp prior to corrective osteotomy, this percentage rose to 76.5% after surgery. Limb shortening in exeess of 1 cm was present in 22 patients, as opposed to 37 preoperatively. On roentgenographic examination it was found that all nonunions were solid except for those that culminated in avascular necrosis. Seventeen patients showed no evidence of osteoarthritis. Osteoarthritis was mild in 24 patients, moderate in 8, and severe in only 2 (Table 8).

As the data indicate, the operation was able to slow the rate of the degenerative process, and even to effect improvement in some cases.

Table 8. Roentgenologic Examination *After* Corrective Osteotomy (n = 51, Bergmannsheil Bochum)

Osteoarthritis	
None	17 = 33.3%
Early-stage	24 = 47.1%
Intermediate-stage	8 = 15.7%
Late-stage	2 = 3.9%

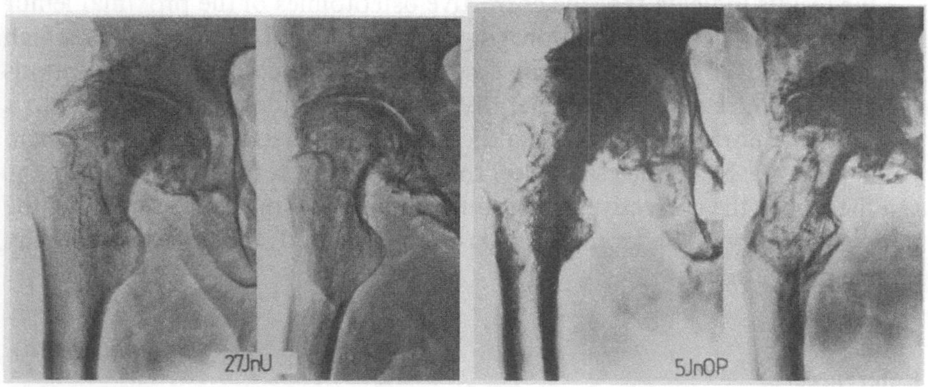

Fig. 6. 48-Year-old man 5 years after a repositioning osteotomy of the right hip: The joint space is widened, and there is a marked slowing of the osteoarthritic process

The most decisive factor, however, is the subjective evaluation of the result by the patients themselves: 38 (74.5%) rated the result of the corrective osteotomy as good, 12 (23.6%) rated it as fair, and only 1 (1.9%) rated it as poor. Thirty-four patients (58.6%) were able to return to their jobs without restriction, 11 (18.9%) returned to work with lighter duties, and 13 (22.5%) had to change their occupation.

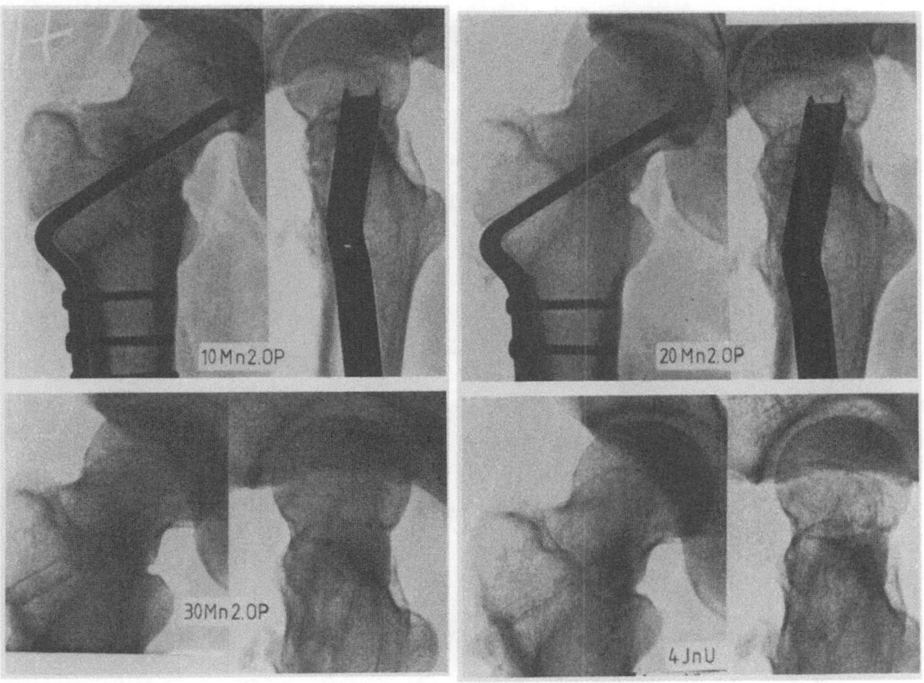

Fig. 7. 30-Year-old man who underwent a repositioning osteotomy for a nonunited fracture. At 4 years after surgery (bottom right) the nonunion is consolidated, and there is no evidence of osteoarthritis

Our results indicate that the corrective osteotomies of the proximal femur were remarkably effective in improving the prognosis of these fractures, which are notorious for their unfavorable courses and outcomes. The operations usually cannot reverse the degenerative changes that develop secondary to a malunited femoral neck fracture, although they often are able to arrest them [1,7] (Fig. 6). Nevertheless, we feel that the present results are encouraging. On the whole, the corrective osteotomies in this series markedly improved the patients' quality of life, even at the cost of a long and sometimes demanding course of treatment.

References

1. Ganz R, Noesberger B (1978) Die posttraumatische Koxarthrose und ihre Behandlungsmöglichkeiten. Unfallheilkunde 81:238–247
2. Merle d'Aubigné R (1949) Bewertung der Hüftgelenkfrakturen. Rev Orthop 35:541
3. Müller ME (1971) Die hüftnahen Femurosteotomien. Thieme, Stuttgart
4. Müller ME, Allgöwer M, Schneider R, Willenegger H (1977) Manual der Osteosynthese, 2. Aufl. Springer, Berlin Heidelberg New York
5. Pförringer W, Rosemeyer B (1977) Schenkelhalsfrakturen bei Jugendlichen. Arch Orthop Unfallchir 90:169–185
6. Raaymakers E (1981) Schenkelhalsfraktur und Pseudarthrose, Pauwels-Osteotomie oder Alloarthroplastik? Hefte Unfallheilk 153:173–178
7. Schneider R (1977) Die intertrochantäre Extensions- und Flexionsosteotomie bei traumatischen Hüftkopfdefekten. Unfallheilkunde 80:177–181

Repositioning Osteotomies for Malunited Fractures Near the Hip

E. Ludolph, G. Hierholzer and M. Strigl

During the period from 1977 to 1981 a total of 69 posttraumatic repositioning osteotomies of the proximal femur were performed in 65 patients at the Duisburg-Buchholz Trauma Clinic. In 33 of these patients, surgery was done for the correction of malunited fractures about the hip. Thirty of these patients were male and 13 were female, with average ages of 41 and 56 years, respectively.

All the osteotomies were performed in the intertrochanteric region of the femur, and all were stabilized according to ASIF principles. In all cases stability was adequate to permit postoperative exercise.

Twelve of the osteotomies were of the valgus type, 4 were varus, 6 were rotational, and 11 were combined types (Table 1).

With regard to the rotational osteotomies, it should be noted that these do not include osteotomies for femoral shaft fractures that united with rotational deformity.

The combined osteotomies almost always included a valgus correction.

Complications were as follows: one loose plate that necessitated revision of the fixation, one hematoma that required open evacuation, two instances of delayed union of the osteotomy site that necessitated cancellous bone grafting, and one deep infection that resolved after early operative revision (Table 2).

Table 1. Types of Repositioning Osteotomy Performed in the Present Series (n=33)

	n
Valgus osteotomy	12
Varus osteotomy	4
Rotational osteotomy	6
Combined osteotomy	11

Table 2. Complications after Repositioning Osteotomies (n=33)

	n
Plate loosening	1
Hematoma	1
Delayed union of osteotomy	2
Infection	1

Corrective Osteotomies of the Lower Extremity
Edited by G. Hierholzer, K. H. Müller

Twenty-five patients were available for follow-up – 16 men and 9 women. The average age of the men at follow-up was 39 years, and the average age of the woman was 54 years.

The average interval between corrective osteotomy and follow-up was 40 months.

The follow-up examination was both clinical and roentgenologic. The latter included one standard projection of the pelvis and axial projections of both hips.

The patients presenting for follow-up had undergone a total of 10 valgus osteotomies, 2 varus osteotomies, 4 rotational osteotomies, and 9 combined osteotomies (Table 3).

The results of the follow-up examinations were evaluated according to the criteria in Table 4.

Measurements of the neck-shaft angle of the femur showed that of the 25 osteotomies performed, the planned angle of correction was achieved in 12 cases and was accurate to withing 5° in 10 cases.

Table 3. Osteotomies Performed in the Patients Who Were Followed after Surgery (n=25)

	n
Valgus osteotomies	10
Varus osteotomies	2
Rotational osteotomies	4
Combined osteotomies	9

Table 4. Criteria Used to Evaluate the Results

Good or excellent	Essentially unrestricted hip motion, no subjective complaints
Fair	Up to 1/3 limitation of the hip motion, occasional subjective complaints; sensitivity to weather changes and pain on prolonged exertion
Poor	Severe limitation of motion, severe subjective complaints

Table 5. Results of Follow-up Examination (n=25)

	n
Good or excellent	16
Fair	7
Poor	2

Summary

This article reports the results of 25 follow-up examinations in patients who underwent proximal femoral osteotomies for the correction of posttraumatic deformities.

The examinations were both clinical and roentgenologic. The result was excellent or good in 16 cases, fair in 7 cases, and poor in 2 cases.

References

1. Gierse H, Schramm W (1981) Spätergebnisse nach Umstellungsosteotomien des Hüftgelenkes. Orthop Prax 17:656
2. Müller ME (1971) Die hüftnahen Femurosteotomien, 2. Aufl. Thieme, Stuttgart
3. Müller ME, Allgöwer M, Schneider R, Willenegger H (1977) Manual der Osteosynthese-AO-Technik. Springer, Berlin Heidelberg New York
4. Schmied H, Kaufmann L (1971) Indikation und Kontraindikation zur intertrochanteren Osteotomie. In: Morscher E (Hrsg) Die intertrochantere Osteotomie bei Coxarthrose. Huber, Bern

Results of Corrective Osteotomies after Trauma about the Hip. Causes and Treatment of Posttraumatic Deformities

G. Ritter, H. Weigand and J. Ahlers

Despite modern techniques of internal fixation, posttraumatic deformities about the hip are still not uncommon. They confirm the clinical observation that more than a few fractures of the proximal femur are difficult to manage and require special surgical experience and expertise, and that defects which seem trivial initially often progress to serious complications due to the peculiar stresses that act on the skeletal system in the region of the hip.

We have reviewed cases from the past five years in an effort to evaluate the outcomes of internal fixations of fractures about the hip, and especially to analyze the causes of posttraumatic deformities that required corrective surgery.

As Table 1 indicates, pertrochanteric fractures of the femur were by far the most common precursors of deformity. Taken together, the pertrochanteric and subtrochanteric fractures and their combinations account for a much greater proportion of posttraumatic and postoperative deformities than do medial femoral neck fractures.

We were also interested in identifying the technical deficiencies of the primary internal fixations that were responsible for the poor results. The internal fixation devices that were used in the primary operations are listed in Table 2. In almost all cases, roentgenograms disclosed the presence of at least one and usually several errors or deficiencies that had contributed to the poor result. It should be added, of course, that fractures about the hip can be

Table 1. Analysis of 31 Posttraumatic Deformities of the proximal Femur by Fracture Type and Fracture Healing (Mainz Trauma Surgery Department, 1978–1982)

	n	Deformity with fracture union	Deformity with nonunion
Medial femoral neck fractures	6	1	5
Pertrochanteric femoral fractures	16	6	10
Subtrochanteric femoral fractures	3	2	1
Per-and subtrochanteric femoral fractures	6	3	3
Total	31	12	19

Corrective Osteotomies of the Lower Extremity
Edited by G. Hierholzer, K. H. Müller

Table 2. Types of Primary Internal Fixation Performed for 31 Posttraumatic Deformities of the Proximal Femur (Mainz Trauma Surgery Department, 1978–1982)

Internal fixation device	n
130° Blade plate	16
Condylar plate	6
Nail and plate	6
Straight plate	1
Medullary nail	2
Total	31

Table 3. Most common Technical Deficiencies of Primary Internal Fixation in 31 Proximal Femoral Deformities (Mainz Trauma Surgery Department, 1978–1982)

	n
I. Improper selection of implant	8
II. Faulty placement of the implant	22
III. Poor reduction with fixation in faulty position	35
Total	65

Table 4. Improper Selection of Implant for Primary Internal Fixation (Mainz Trauma Surgery Department, 1978–1982)

		n
Condylar plate	instead of 130° blade plate	3
130° Blade plate	instead of condylar plate	3
Straight plate	instead of angled blade plate	1
Medullary nail	instead of angled blade plate	2
Total		9

extremely challenging therapeutically, and that an increased rate of complications often can be expected on the basis of the fracture configuration alone.

Analysis of our cases indicates that three deficiencies of operating technique were chiefly responsible for the unfavorable outcomes: improper selection of the implant, faulty placement of the implant, and poor reduction with fixation of the fragments in a faulty position (Table 3).

In most of the 31 cases reviewed, we were able to identify the presence of more than one technical deficiency. Improper selection of the implant, as shown in Table 4, was mainly based on inadequate preoperative planning from a biomechanical standpoint, such as the decision whether to use a condylar plate or 130° angled blade plate.

Table 5. Faulty Placement of the Implant during Primary Internal Fixation (Mainz Trauma Surgery Department, 1978–1982)

	n
Blade seated too far proximally in the femoral neck	13
Perforation of the femoral neck or head	5
Exclusion of biomechanically important fragments	4
Total	22

Table 6. Poor Reduction with Fixation in a Faulty Position during Primary Internal Fixation (Mainz Trauma Surgery Department, 1978–1982)

	n
Improper varus angulation of the femoral head	24
Anteversion of the femoral head	3
Rotational malalignment of the femoral shaft	5
Lateralization of the femoral shaft	3
Total	35

In 22 of the 31 cases, moreover, we found that the implant had been improperly placed during the primary fixation. The most common error was placing the blade of the angled blade plate too high in the femoral neck so that it failed to engage the central, most stable part of the femoral head. This caused the blade to penetrate the head and neck when weight was borne. Other serious placement errors included anterior or posterior perforation of the femoral neck by the blade, and failure to stabilize biomechanically important fragments, especially on the medial, compression side of the bone (Table 5).

The third main cause of posttraumatic deformity was malreduction of the fracture with fixation of the fragments in a faulty position. Our analysis showed that improper varus angulation of the femoral head was by far the most common error. Other less common errors were anteversion of the femoral head and rotational malalignment or lateralization of the femoral shaft (Table 6).

Below are several case reports which illustrate the technical deficiencies in Table 3, their role in the pathogenesis of serious posttraumatic deformities and complications, and the correction of these problems by osteotomy.

Case 1 (Fig. 1):
A 77-year-old woman sustained a segmental pertrochanteric and subtrochanteric fracture of the proximal femur that was treated primarily with a long, straight plate. The long distal length of the plate did not enhance the proximal stability of the fixation, which was unable even to with stand muscle-strengthening exercises in bed. The inevitable result was extreme varus deformity and nonunion in the region of the femoral neck. Four months after surgery the patient was referred to our care. We performed a valgus repositioning osteotomy using the 120° osteotomy plate of the

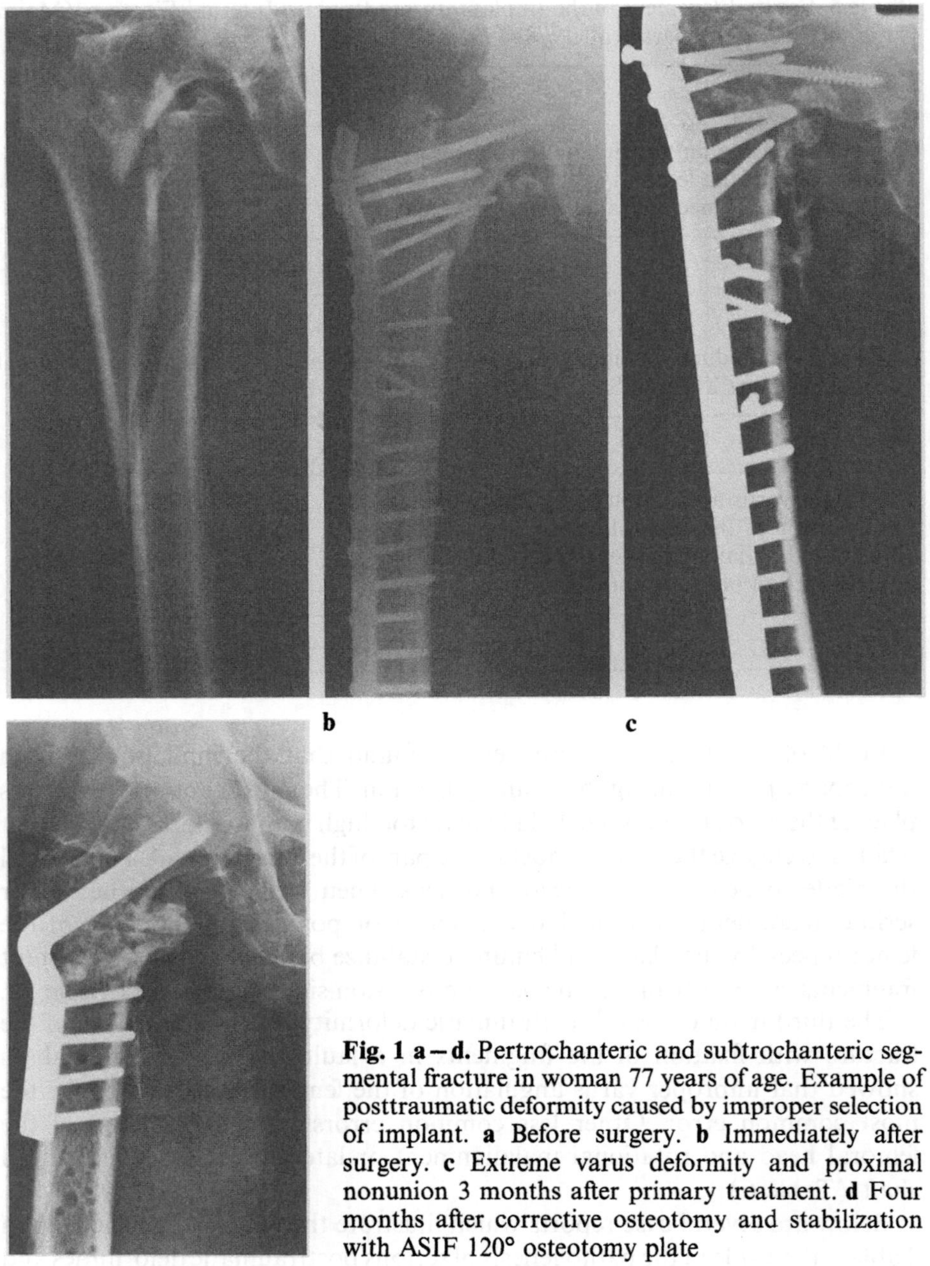

a b c d

Fig. 1 a – d. Pertrochanteric and subtrochanteric segmental fracture in woman 77 years of age. Example of posttraumatic deformity caused by improper selection of implant. **a** Before surgery. **b** Immediately after surgery. **c** Extreme varus deformity and proximal nonunion 3 months after primary treatment. **d** Four months after corrective osteotomy and stabilization with ASIF 120° osteotomy plate

ASIF. The patient's progress illustrated the rapidity with which a nonunion can be made to consolidate when normal biomechanics are restored. By six months the fracture had united in an ideal position. A long, 130° angled plate should have been used for the primary internal fixation of this fracture (Fig. 1a – d).

Case 2 (Fig. 2):
A 64-year-old man with a segmental pertrochanteric fracture was treated primarily with a 130° angled blade plate and cancellous lag screw. The main deficiency of the procedure was that the fracture was fixed in a faulty position that left a large defect on

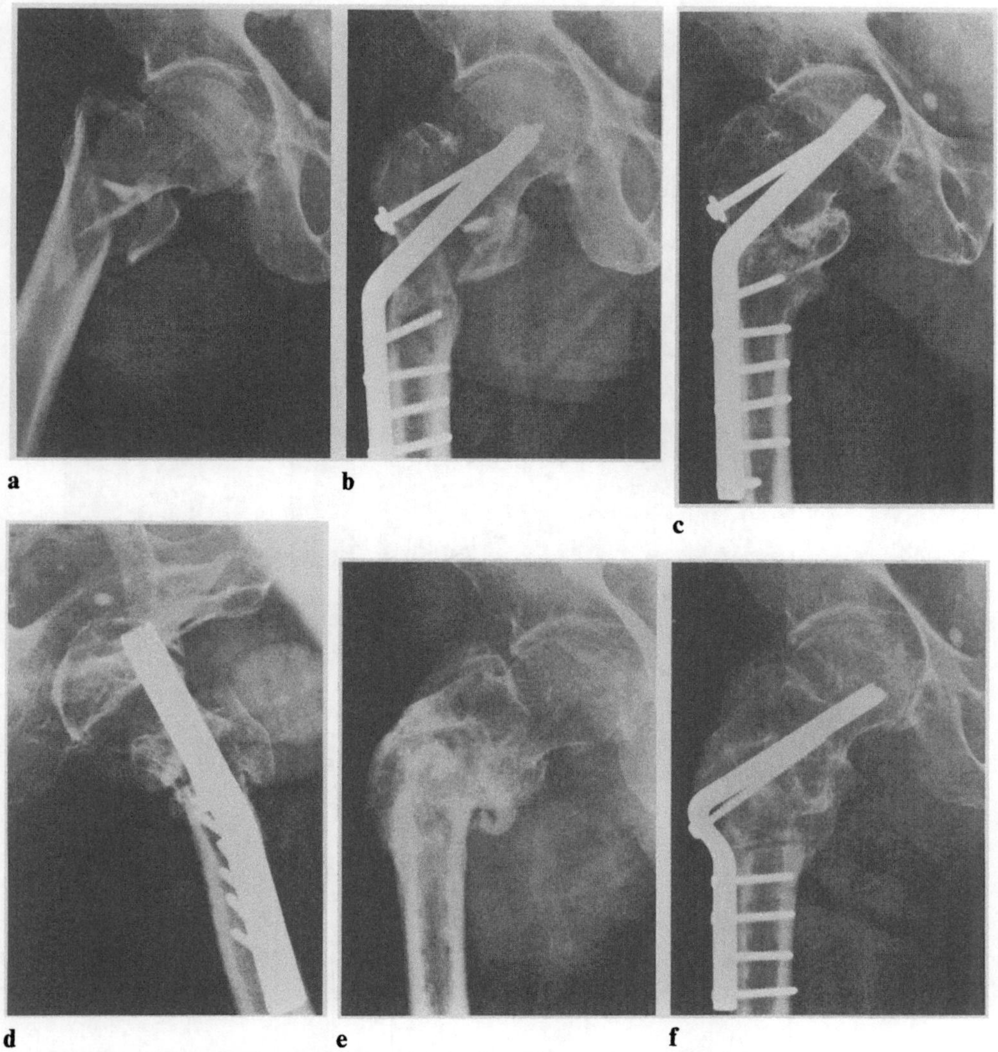

Fig. 2 a–f. Pertrochanteric segmental fracture in man 64 years of age. This case demonstrates the causal role of malreduction in deformity. **a** Before surgery. **b** After treatment with 130° blade plate and long cancellous bone screw: fixation in faulty position with large medial bone defect. **c,d** The fracture has collapsed, the head is tipped anteriorly, and the blade has perforated through the femoral head into the acetabulum. **e** Removal of the implant was followed by the development of a persistent subtrochanteric nonunion with marked varus angulation. **f** Repositioning osteotomy 3 years later led to rapid consolidation with good joint function

the medial side. At six months the fracture was not yet solid and showed evidence of collapse. Perforation of the displaced head fragment by the plate blade is clearly seen in the axial view. This necessitated removal of the implant, whereupon a nonunion developed in association with extreme varus deformity. Because of this bad experience, three years passed before the patient consented to corrective surgery. At that time we performed a subtrochanteric valgus osteotomy stabilized with an ASIF 120° blade plate. A few months later the nonunion was solid, and joint function was very good (Fig. 2 a–f).

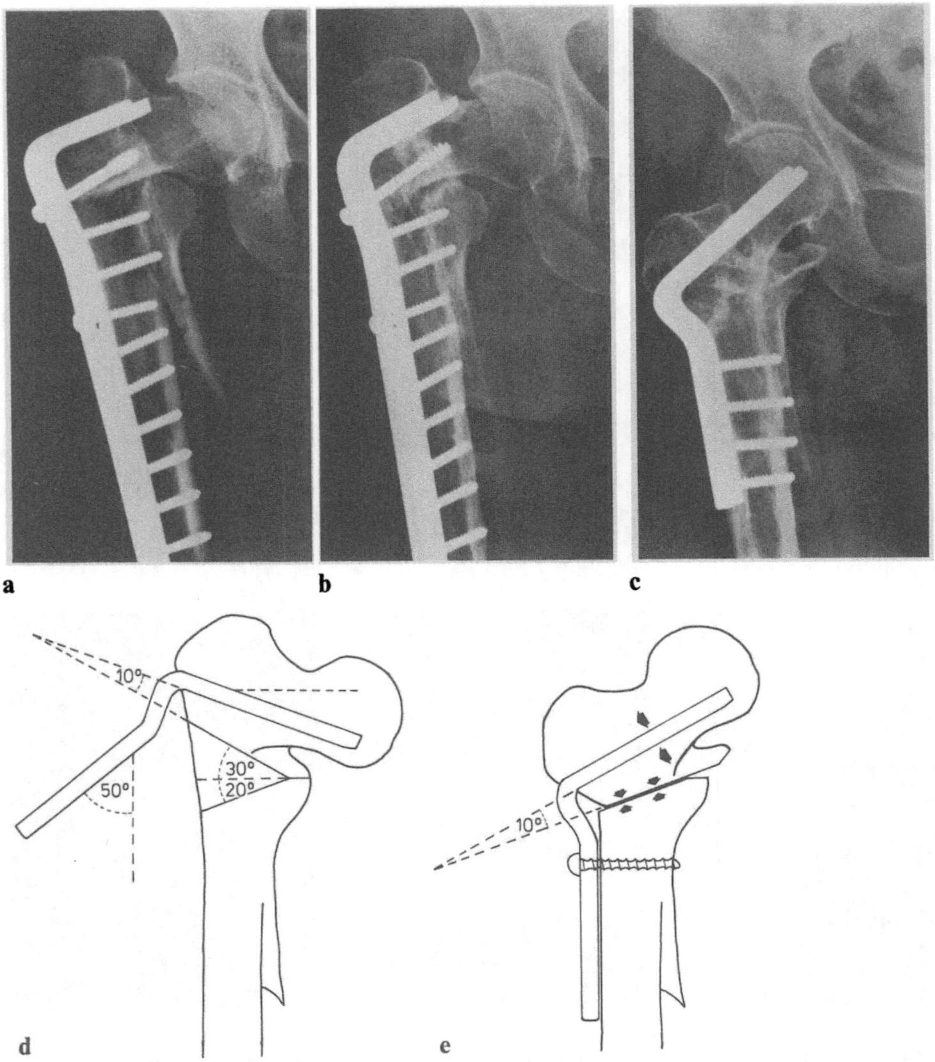

Fig. 3 a – e. Subtrochanteric femoral neck fracture with large medial fragment in woman 62 years of age. Example of faulty reduction and failure to include biomechanically important fragments in the fixation. **a** Primary surgery produced an extreme varus deformity with an unstabilized medial fragment. **b** After 17 months the medial fragment has united, but there is a nonunion of the femoral neck. **c** Six months after corrective valgus osteotomy the nonunion is solid and joint function is excellent. **d** Preoperative planning of the osteotomy: First the shaft is transversely osteotomized, rotational deformity is corrected, and then wedges are resected proximally and distally. **e** The angle between the osteotomy line and plate blade creates interfragmentary compression when the proximal fragment glides laterally on the blade

Case 3 (Fig. 3):
A 62-year-old woman sustained a segmental subtrochanteric fracture of the femur. In this case the fracture was improperly reduced and was fixed in extreme varus. This prevented the large, biomechanically important medial fragment from being incorporated into the fixation (Fig. 3 a). The patient was referred to us 17 months later. At operation we confirmed the roentgenologic suspicion of a proximal nonunion (Fig.

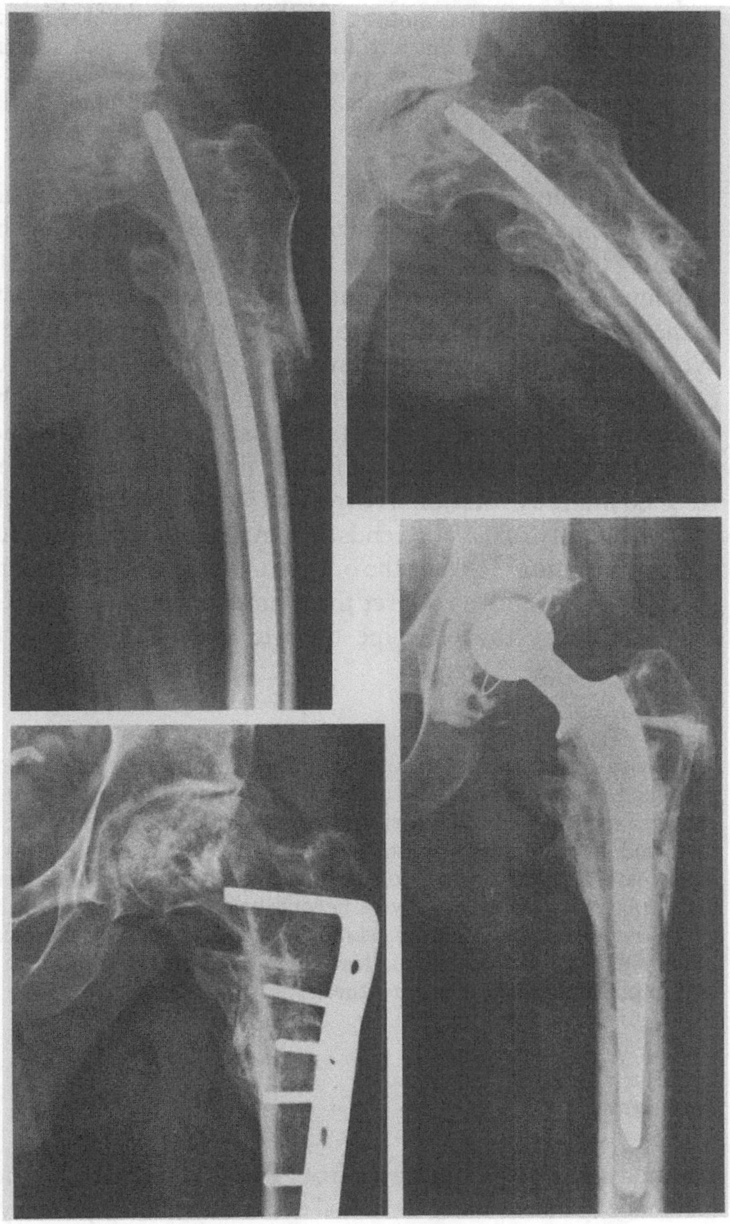

Fig. 4 a–d. An external rotation deformity developed in this 49-year-old man whose subtrochanteric fracture was fixed with an Ender nail in the presence of preexisting avascular necrosis. This case demonstrates the causal relationship between faulty implant selection and deformity. This type of fracture should have been treated primarily with a condylar plate. **a,b** One year after the injury and before corrective osteotomy. **c** Subtrochanteric rotational osteotomy stabilized with a prestressed ASIF condylar plate bent to approx. 87°. The osteotomy is firm 6 months after surgery. **d** After consolidation of the osteotomy and correction of posttraumatic deformities, a total hip had to be implanted because of severe avascular necrosis

3 b). The preoperative drawings of the repositioning osteotomy are shown in Fig. 3d. A final roentgenogram six months after surgery shows good consolidation of the nonunion (Fig. 3c). Clinically the joint shows excellent function. This example demonstrates that even with extreme deformity and a poor initial status, the restoration of normal biomechanics can ensure rapid union and a good long-term result.

In performing the osteotomy, we employ a slight modification of the usual technique: instead of osteotomizing the bone parallel to the blade of the plate, we make the cut at a slight angle to the blade, creating a slightly wedge-shaped proximal fragment. This will automatically compress the osteotomy surfaces in the event that the proximal fragment glides laterally on the blade (Fig. 3 e). We have used this technique for years and have found it very effective. The osteotomy should always begin with a transverse cut through the center of the wedge to be removed; then rotation can be corrected as needed before the oblique proximal and distal cuts are made. If the entire bone wedge were resected first, any rotational correction would create an angular deformity due to the obliquity of the bone ends. When planning the procedure, it is helpful in difficult situations to trace the outline of the healthy femur onto a clear plastic sheet, invert it, and lay it over the roentgenogram of the affected side. This is the easiest way to determine the site and configuration of the necessary osteotomy (Fig. 3 d,e).

Case 4 (Fig. 4):
A 49-year-old man with preexisting idiopathic avascular necrosis of the femoral head sustained a subtrochanteric fracture which was "stabilized" with an Ender nail. An extreme external rotation deformity of 80° ensued. This case should have been managed with a condylar plate, which would have prevented this complication. The extensive avascular necrosis of the femoral head made it apparent that a total hip arthroplasty would eventually be needed, and in anticipation of this we performed a corrective rotational osteotomy stabilized with a prestressed condylar plate bent to just under 90°. Nine months later, following union of the osteotomy, we removed the metal and implanted a long-stem prosthesis (Fig. 4 a–d).

Summary

On analyzing 31 of our cases from the past 5 years, we noted a very high incidence of one or more technical deficiencies in the primary internal fixation of fractures about the hip. The three principal errors were: improper selection of the implant, improper placement of the implant, and malreduction of the fragments.

It must be considered that fractures of the proximal femur and femoral neck can be extremely difficult to manage and require an experienced surgeon who is familiar with biomechanical principles and is able to visualize in three dimensions. The latter faculty is especially important in partially closed fixations performed with the aid of an image intensifier. Given the large loads on the hip, it is imperative that an internal fixation system in that region meets stringent biomechanical requirements; otherwise it is virtually certain that complications will arise. All the complications that occurred in the present series were predictable.

Our results also indicate that a corrective osteotomy, when carefully planned and executed, can still provide an excellent end result even in very difficult cases where deformity and nonunion are of long duration. In evaluating the results, one naturally must distinguish between the effects of the trauma and the actual result of the osteotomy, In the 31 cases reviewed here, we were able to achieve consolidation in an excellent position and obtain a result that was good to excellent compared with the preoperative status of the limb. These results clearly demonstrate the place of the planned corrective osteotomy in the management of posttraumatic deformities.

Posttraumatic Repositioning Osteotomies of the Proximal Femur

U. Pfister and A. Wentzensen

We performed a total of 314 proximal femoral osteotomies at the Tübingen Trauma Clinic from 1975 to 1982. Ninety-seven of these osteotomies were necessitated by posttraumatic changes. This series does not include primary repositioning osteotomies for vertical fractures of the femoral neck.

An analysis of the preoperative diagnoses indicates that nonunion of the femoral neck was by far the most common indication for repositioning osteotomy (29 cases). In nine cases the principal diagnosis was avascular necrosis of the femoral head, and in five cases, advanced osteoarthritis. The most frequent deformity was varus angulation, which occurred in 31 cases. External rotation deformity was presented in 11 cases and was usually severe. Excessive internal rotation was present in only two patients. A valgus deformity was corrected in only 7 cases, and in 2 cases it coexisted with excessive external rotation. There were 12 cases in which a flexion contracture of the hip was the principal indication for surgery. Twenty-two patients had a pure rotational deformity – 17 external and 5 internal. Four of these deformities developed after the conservative treatment of femoral shaft or pertrochanteric fractures, and 18 developed after the operative treatment of these fractures – 12 after medullary nailing.

Operative Technique

The operative technique was reasonably uniform. Ordinarily the osteotomies were performed in the intertrochanteric region; subtrochanteric osteotomies were done only for pure rotational deformities of the shaft exceeding 30°. In no case was the femoral neck shortened, and transfers of the greater trochanter were infrequent. The varus osteotomies were stabilized with an osteotomy plate in four cases and with a condylar plate in three. In valgus osteotomies the 120° or 130° plate was used in 45 cases and a modified condylar plate in 12. The degrees of correction are indicated in Tables 1 and 2.

When we consider that 68 of the cases had been operated upon previously, the number of complications following the osteotomies is relatively small. Hematomas had to be evacuated in two cases, and in one case the plate loosened following an abduction osteotomy of a stiff hip, and an infection developed after the fixation was revised. Of 29 nonunions, 2 failed to consolidate after valgus osteotomy. From 1975 to the present, 6 of the operated patients received total hip replacements – 2 only 3 months after the osteotomy, 1 after 7 months, 1 after 18 months, and 2 after 4 years. In each case

Corrective Osteotomies of the Lower Extremity
Edited by G. Hierholzer, K. H. Müller

Table 1. Valgus Osteotomy (n=57)

Wedge	20°	25°	30°	40°	>40°
No. of cases	12	7	26	11	1
+ Extension	1		2	4	
+ Flexion		2			
+ Derotation	3	1	4	1	
+ Rotation			2		

Table 2. Varus Osteotomy (n=7)

Wedge	10°	15°	20°	25°	30°
No. of cases	1	1	2	2	1
+ Extension			1		
+ Derotation	1				

the arthroplasty was necessitated by avascular necrosis secondary to a medial femoral neck fracture.

A roentgenologic evaluation of 24 repositioning osteotomies that were performed at least 3 years ago indicates complete healing with no significant osteoarthritis in 18 cases, partial and apparently progressive avascular necrosis of the femoral head in 2 cases, 3 cases of partial avascular necrosis that is beginning to consolidate, and 1 very severe case of osteoarthritis. All of the avascular necroses were secondary to medial femoral neck fractures. It is interesting to note that while the osteotomy does not always promote the consolidation of a necrotic femoral head, such consolidation is achieved in some instances.

In the most recent follow-up examinations performed an average of 39 months after the operation, hip mobility has improved relative to immediate postoperative mobility in 7 cases, it has become worse in 3 cases, and it remains unchanged in 14 cases.

Summary: Surgical Correction of Posttraumatic Deformities about the Hip

H. Zilch

Corrective osteotomies of the proximal femur require a highly accurate pathophysiologic analysis during the planning stage.

The following are considered potential indications for corrective osteotomy of the proximal femur after trauma: 1) nonunions of the femoral neck, 2) malunited fractures, 3) unstable pertrochanteric fractures (to obtain a flat weight-bearing surface), and 4) partial and resolved posttraumatic avascular necrosis of the femoral head (to alter the weight-bearing area of the femoral head).

At present, the site of choice for corrective osteotomies is the intertrochanteric region. Osteotomies in that region permit changes of axial alignment as well as displacements of the femoral shaft.

Corrective osteotomies for the treatment of *nonunions* utilize Pauwel's principle of converting shear forces into compressive forces. A repositioning osteotomy of this type should be regarded as the first-line treatment for nonunions and should be attempted before a total hip arthroplasty is considered, provided the femoral head is viable. Reactive osteophytes provide useful confirmation of head viability and often can be utilized surgically. In addition, the osteoporosis of the head should match that of the unaffected side.

When calculating the angle of correction, the direction of the resultant pressure force R and the anatomic axis of the femur must be known. Because the nonunion should come under pure compression after the repositioning osteotomy, the plane of the nonunion should form a 25 to 30° angle with a line perpendicular to the shaft axis after surgery. If the nonunion has a Pauwels angle of 75°, the angle of correction is 50°.

Internal fixation with the 120° angled blade plate of the ASIF had proved particularly effective in repositioning osteotomies.

The correction may be effected by means of a closed wedge osteotomy or Y osteotomy. In the closed wedge osteotomy, the two osteotomy surfaces should intersect at the level of the medial cortex. Due to the obliquity of the osteotomy line, the distal fragment should be displaced laterally to minimize shortening. The Y osteotomy allows for slipping of the femoral head and provides the head fragment with an area of support oriented at right angles to the resultant R. Otherwise the force would tip the head fragment caudally. The planning and steps of this osteotomy have been perfected by Müller (cf. p. 65).

In the *correction of deformities*, the object is to restore normal anatomic relations. Most deformities are the result of fractures that have united in a varus position. Theis may coexist with external rotation and flexion deformities. Correction in multiple planes can be difficult, for the plate blade often has

Corrective Osteotomies of the Lower Extremity
Edited by G. Hierholzer, K. H. Müller

an eccentric seating in such situations and can easily penetrate the bone. A varus osteotomy is rarely indicated after trauma. It may be used to revise a previous, excessive valgus osteotomy. Malunions of the proximal femur are most common after subtrochanteric and pertrochanteric fractures. They are caused by improper selection of the implant, faulty placement of the correct implant (e.g., blade seated too far cranially), and by faulty reduction (e.g., in varus) prior to internal fixation.

In *unstable pertrochanteric fractures*, an osteotomy may be used to create broad apposition of the fragments to permit early ambulation with weight bearing in older patients.

In *posttraumatic avascular necrosis of the femoral head*, a biologic problem, a varus or valgus osteotomy can be used to rotate a partially necrotic area out of the weight-bearing zone. In some cases extension or flexion osteotomies will also be necessary and must be based on accurate preoperative roentgenograms in various planes to obtain a satisfactory position of the femoral head. These osteotomies have been used for some time to treat idiopathic osteoarthritis of the hip. If degenerative changes are present, and especially if these changes involve the acetabular roof, the valgus extension osteotomy of Bombelli may be beneficial. However, this operation is based on other biomechanical considerations than the osteotomies mentioned above.

We do not feel that cancellous bone grafts have been particularly successful in the treatment of early avascular necrosis of the femoral head. It remains to be seen what value corticocancellous grafts or free microvascular pedicle grafts will have in the treatment of this condition.

Proximal femoral osteotomies can also be useful in the treatment of *posttraumatic leg length discrepancies*. The femur can be shortened by up to 3 cm in the intertrochanteric region and stably fixed with a condylar plate.

Reports from various clinics on the results of corrective osteotomies of the proximal femur after trauma are encouraging.

III. The Diaphyses

Corrective Osteotomies of the Femoral Shaft

L. Gotzen, H. Tscherne and A. Illgner

Introduction

Physiologic symmetry of the lower extremities is essential for normal leg function on a long-term basis [6]. Deformities secondary to shaft fractures frequently shorten the limb and thus interfere with the normal biomechanics of both the lower extremity and the spine.

Functional disturbances are primarily a result of abnormal forces, altered patterns of joint movement, and excessive muscular loads and are only secondarily a product of osteoarthritic disease [7].

The number of corrections available in the region of the shaft is smaller than the number of deformities that require correction. Not infrequently, the corrections are carried out in the metaphyseal bone adjacent to the deformity, or even in the contralateral leg if shortening has occurred. The overall prevalence of posttraumatic deformities of the femoral shaft has been decreased by operative fracture treatment [4].

Indications

A severe, complex deformity of the shaft is always corrected at the site of the deformity. Even with simple or fairly inconspicuous deformities, which are particularly common in the young, one will frequently elect to osteotomize at the site of th deformity in order to restore the shape of the femur.

With shaft deformities in the frontal plane, the main consideration is the effect on the knee joint, since the effect on the hip is very minor. The mechanical axis of the lower limb (line connecting the centers of the hip joint and ankle joint) provides a useful parameter for evaluating the loads on the knee. Even a small shift of this axis away from the center of the knee, especially toward the medial side, can produce a stress concentration that will cause degeneration in a portion of the knee [1–3].

Besides the magnitude of the angular deformity, the site of the deformity also influences the position of the mechanical axis, as Fig. 1 a demonstrates. Fig. 1 b shows that a 5° deformity of the distal shaft produces a great medial shift of the mechanical axis than does a proximal shaft deformity with 15° of varus.

Corrective Osteotomies of the Lower Extremity
Edited by G. Hierholzer, K. H. Müller

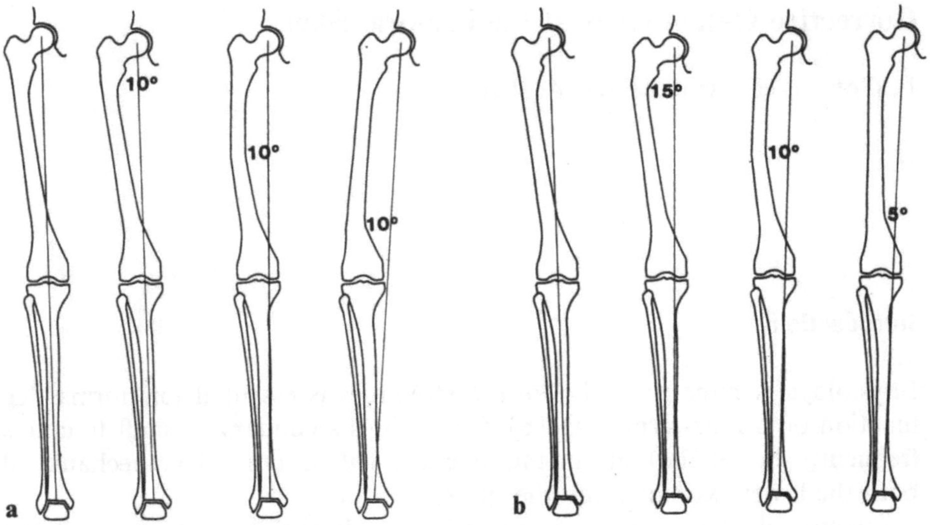

Fig. 1 a, b. Effect of the level of the deformity on the position of the mechanical axis. **a** Equal varus deformities; **b** different varus deformities

Clinical Material

Twenty-five corrective osteotomies of the femoral shaft were performed at our clinic from 1975 to 1981. Twenty-one patients had been previously treated elsewhere. Most of the patients were under 30 years of age (Table 1), and the average age was 25 years. The vast majority were male. The deformities involved the proximal third of the shaft in 6 patents, the middle third in 15, and the distal third in 4.

Most deformities developed after conservative therapy (11 cases) and after medullary nailing (10 cases). Only two were preceded by plate osteosynthesis. Two children developed a severe varus deformity following internal fixation with a Rush pin in one case and cerclage wiring in the other.

A breakdown of the 25 cases by type of deformity shows that only 8 patients had a single deformity, 11 had a double deformity, and 6 had a triple deformity. Five of the latter patients exhibited the typical triad of varus-shortening backward displacement (Table 2).

Table 1. Corrective Osteotomies of the Femoral Shaft for Posttraumatic Deformities (n=25, 1975–1981, Trauma Surgery Clinic, Medizinische Hochschule Hannover)

Age distribution		Other parameters	
<10 years	5	Age range	8–60
10–10 years	7	Males	23
10–30 years	7	Females	2
30–40 years	2	Proximal shaft	6
40–50 years	3	Midshaft	15
>50 years	1	Distal shaft	4

Table 2. Types of Deformity

	n
External rotation	3
Shortening	3
Varus	2
Varus and shortening	2
Varus and backward displacement	2
Varus and forward displacement	1
Shortening and external rotation	3
Shortening and backward displacement	1
Valgus and external rotation	2
Valgus –shortening –external rotation	1
Varus –shortening –backward displacement	5

Table 3. Number of Simple Deformities and their Average Values

Deformity	n	Average/cm
Shortening	15	3.5
Varus	12	22°
External rotation	9	25°
Backward displacement	8	18°
Valgus	3	12°
Forward displacement	1	10°

The most common deformity was limb shortening, with an average value of 3.5 cm. This was followed by varus (average 22°), external rotation (average 20°), and backward displacement (average 18°) (Table 3).

An average interval of 3 1/2 years elapsed between the injury and corrective surgery, with a range from 3 months to 30 years. Most deformities were corrected within two years after the fracture.

Preoperative Planning

Posttraumatic deformities of the femoral shaft present a highly variable picture and are often complicated by the displacement of fragments and callus formation. A mastery of all aspects of bone and reconstructive surgery is necessary to achieve an optimum result in a given case.

The indication for corrective surgery is based on a thorough clinical and roentgenologic evaluation. Prior to surgery, tracings should be made from the roentgenograms indicating the location and amount of the correction, the procedure for performing and stabilizing the osteotomy, and the end result of the correction.

In selecting the most appropriate techniques for the osteotomy and its stabilization, the surgeon must take into account the nature of the deformity, the configuration and quality of the bone at the site of the deformity, and the condition of the soft tissues. The techniques chosen will be those that are most likely to restore normal anatomic relations and secure consolidation.

The following osteotomy techniques are available:

- Transverse osteotomy
- Transverse or oblique closed wedge osteotomy
- Oblique displacement osteotomy
- Step-cut displacement osteotomy
- Lengthening osteotomy

Complex deformities will usually require a combination of osteotomy techniques to obtain satisfactory length, alignment and rotation.

A successful correction relies on the stable fixation of the osteotomy fragments. The fixation must secure the position of the osteotomy, provide the immobilization necessary for bone healing, and should be stable enough to permit active postoperative exercise. These requirements must be considered during the planning of surgery.

Almost all corrective osteotomies of the diaphyses are fixed by one of two methods: plate osteosynthesis or intramedullary nailing.

The major advantage of the plate is its universal range of application. Its main disadvantage is its relatively low bending strength, which is a problem in the bridging of large defects.

The intramedullary nail is limited in its applications. Its advantages are its high bending strength and its efficacy as an axial splint. In many cases intramedullary stabilization fails due to the absence or bony obstruction of portions of the medullary canal. Often the intramedullary nail must be supplemented with a plate to prevent undesired rotation.

Correction and Stabilization

The simple transverse osteotomy is used for derotation and for straightening. The advantage of the open wedge osteotomy is that it provides axial correction without sacrifice of length. The medullary fixation of this osteotomy usually must be supplemented with an antirotation plate (Fig. 2). Cancellous bone is packed into the osteotomy defect to assist consolidation. When plate fixation is used, it is recommended that a corticocancellous bone graft be interposed on the medial side as a buttress.

The closed wedge osteotomy is the technique most commonly used for axial corrections. If the osteotomy is plated, the plate must be adequately pre-bent to enhance stability and promote union [5]. If intramedullary fixation is used, a small plate should be added to prevent rotation (Fig. 3).

The oblique closed wedge osteotomy is more favorable biomechanically. With plate fixation, stability is effectively enhanced by inserting a lag screw either separately or through the plate, depending on the position of the osteotomy plane. With intramedullary fixation, the oblique osteotomy surface obviate the need for an antirotation plate (Fig. 4).

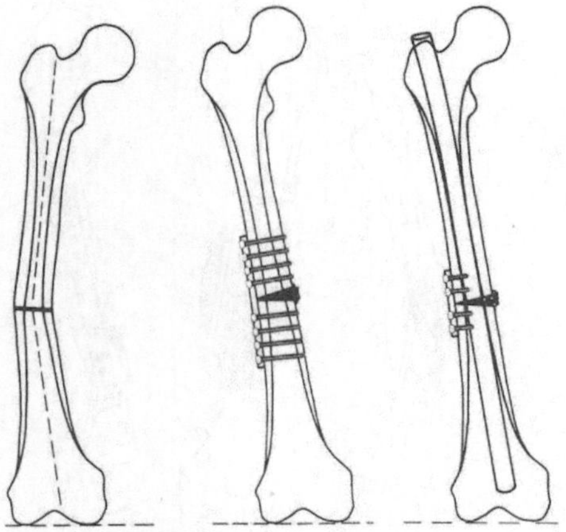

Fig. 2. Transverse open wedge osteotomy

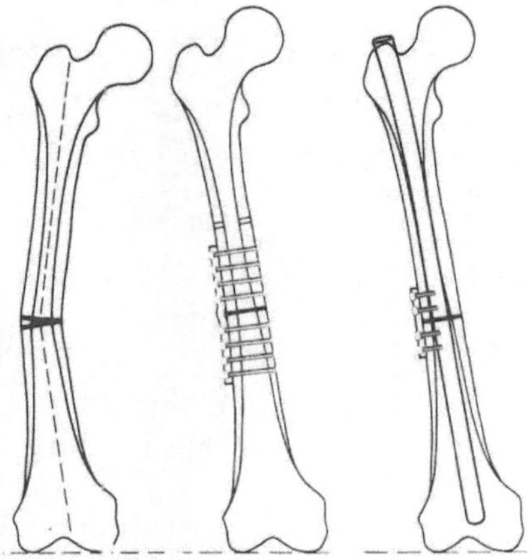

Fig. 3. Transverse closed wedge osteotomy

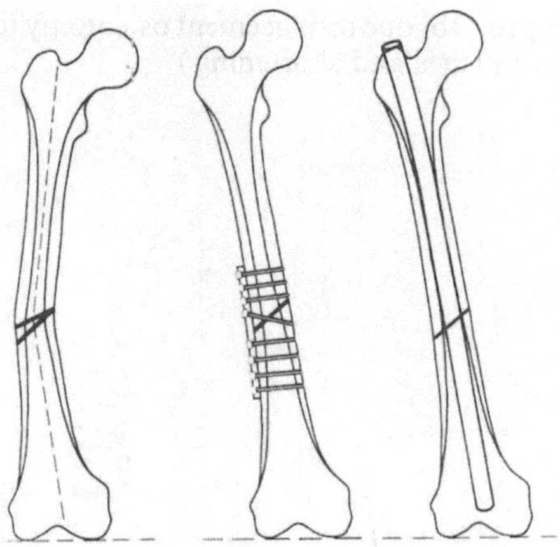

Fig. 4. Oblique closed wedge osteotomy

Deformities of the femoral shaft are frequently accompanied by shortening. The oblique displacement osteotomy makes it possible to correct this shortening while preserving apposition of the bone ends. Concurrent wedge resections may be used to correct axial and rotational alignment and are particularly useful if a massive callus is present at the site of the deformity. The long, oblique osteotomies are performed in the sagittal or the frontal plane, depending on the nature of the deformity.

These osteotomies are easily stabilized with lag screws and a neutralization plate. Resected bone wedges can be securely fixed in existing defects to serve as grafts. Usually, healing between the compressed osteotomy surfaces is swift (Figs. 5 and 6).

Another technique for restoring length equality is the step-out displacement osteotomy. It is especially suited for malunions with overlapping and shortening. With proper placement of the osteotomy planes, angulation can also be corrected (Fig. 7).

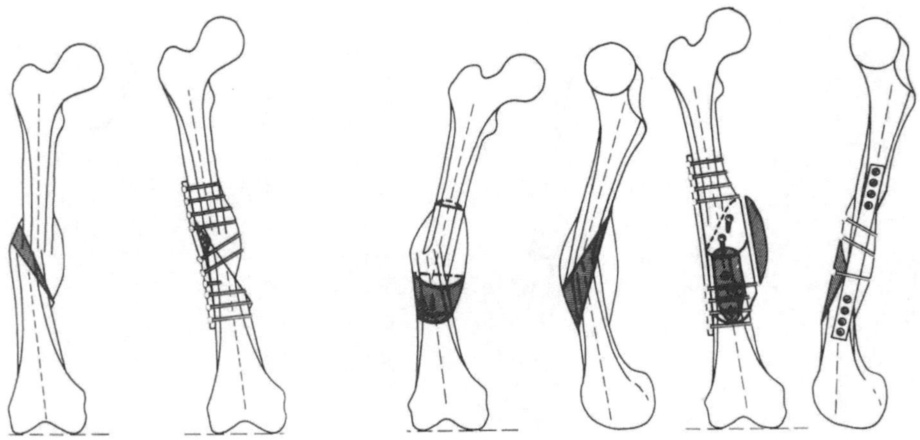

Fig. 5 **Fig. 6**

Fig. 5. Oblique displacement osteotomy to correct a double deformity (angulation and shortening)

Fig. 6. Oblique displacement osteotomy to correct a complex deformity (angulation in two planes and shortening)

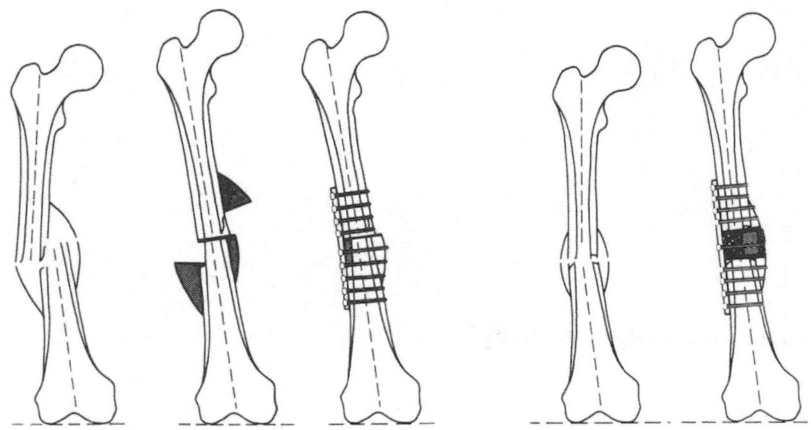

Fig. 7 **Fig. 8**

Fig. 7. Step-cut displacement osteotomy to correct shortening and angulation

Fig. 8. Lengthening osteotomy. The gap is bridged with a plate, a block of corticocancellous bone is interposed to buttress the fragments, and the defect is packed with cancellous bone

Lengthening osteotomies should be used sparingly due to their protracted healing time. Their main indication is in limb shortening caused by axial impaction in cases where the bone has a normal cross-section.

The bone may be lengthened up to 4 cm in one stage [8]. If greater lengthening is needed, it should be effected in multiple stages.

A plate bridging the lengthening defect is subjected to high bending loads. These loads can be reduced by interposing a block of corticocancellous bone on the compression side of the bone to serve as a buttress. Extensive cancellous bone grafting is also necessary to restore continuity across the defect (Fig. 8).

Applied Corrective and Stabilizing Procedures

In the 25 cases reviewed, a simple transverse osteotomy was performed in 6. There were for derotation, and three were for correction of angulation. Five patients had an oblique displacement osteotomy, three with a concurrent wedge resection to correct angular deformity. The step-cut displacement osteotomy was performed in two patients. A total of six lengthening osteotomies were carried out – four in one stage and two in multiple stages.

Sixteen of the osteotomies were stabilized by plate osteosynthesis, seven by a combination of intramedullary fixation and plate osteosynthesis, and two by intramedullary fixation alone. Figure 9 (see pp. 124 and 125) illustrates the correction of a complex midshaft deformity.

Complications

A total of five significant complications developed in four patients. All remaining osteotomies healed uneventfully.

In a one-stage lengthening of 3 cm with concurrent axial realignment, ischemia of the leg was noted postoperatively. Circulation was restored by shortening the defect to 1.5 cm and freeing the blood vessel from surrounding scar tissue.

Plate loosening occurred in one closed wedge osteotomy, and the fixation had to be revised.

One plate used to fix a one-stage lengthening became bent and had to be replaced.

Another plate became bent during the course of a multistage lengthening. During revision of the fixation, new cancellous bone grafts were applied. Later, as the defect was consolidating, the plate fractured, and another revison had to be carried out.

Summary

One of the most rewarding tasks in reconstructive surgery is the correction of limb deformities in yound adults. Through optimum planning and perfect techniques of osteotomy and internal fixation, it is possible to perform the correction at the site of the deformity and, by restoring bony anatomy, lay the groundwork for the recovery of full functional capacity in the limb.

The femoral shaft poses a special challenge due to the shortening that often accompanies axial deformities in that region.

The displacement osteotomy offers a powerful means of correcting shortening and angulation while preserving contact between the bone ends.

In lengthening osteotomies, typical complications such as plate bending and plate fracture can be largely avoided by inserting a compression-resistant bone graft into the defect.

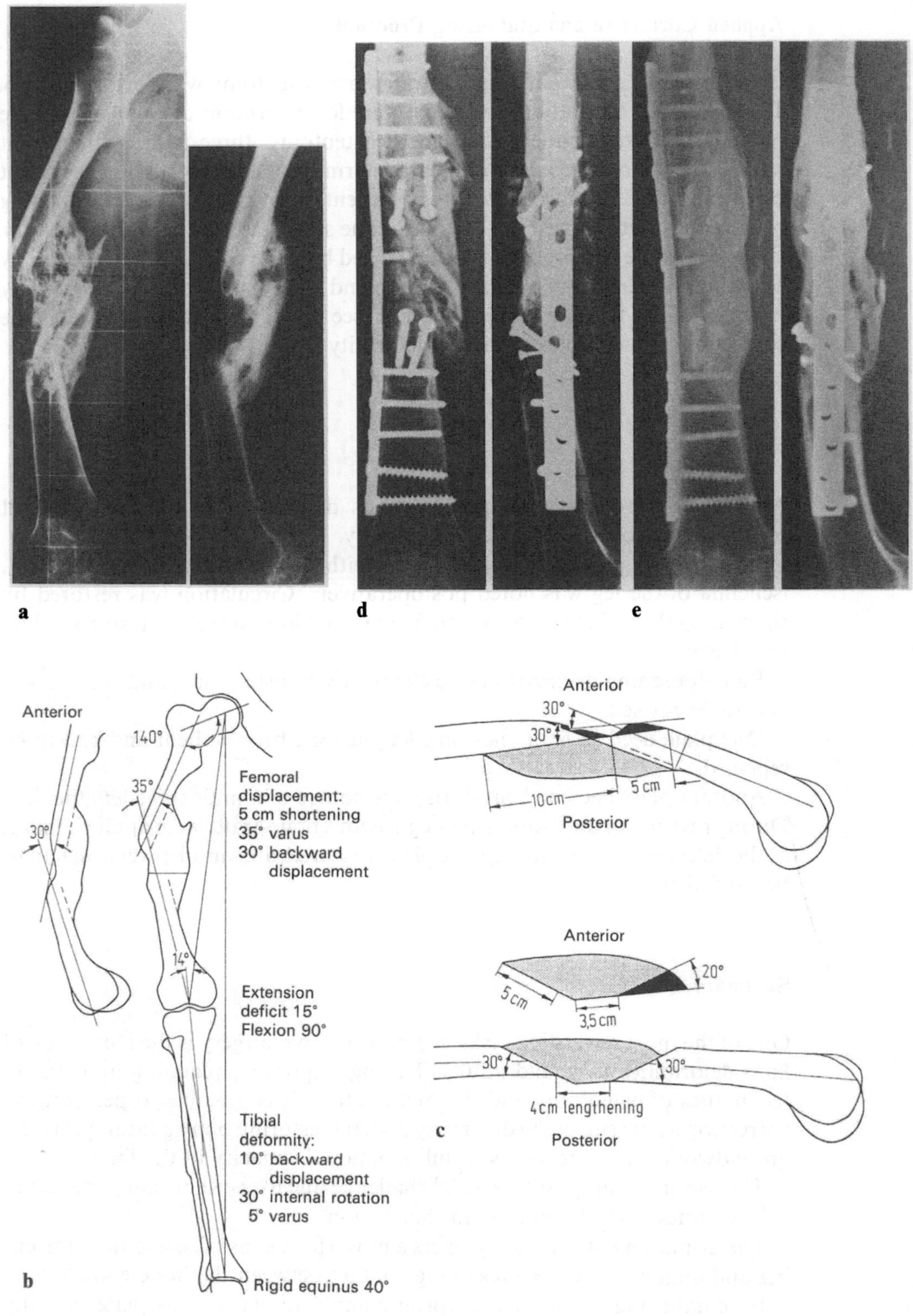
a
d
e
Anterior
140°
35°
30°
Femoral
displacement:
5 cm shortening
35° varus
30° backward
displacement
14°
Extension
deficit 15°
Flexion 90°
Tibial
deformity:
10° backward
displacement
30° internal rotation
5° varus
b
Rigid equinus 40°
Anterior
30°
30°
5 cm
10 cm
Posterior
Anterior
20°
5 cm
3,5 cm
30°
30°
4 cm lengthening
c
Posterior

Fig. 9a–e

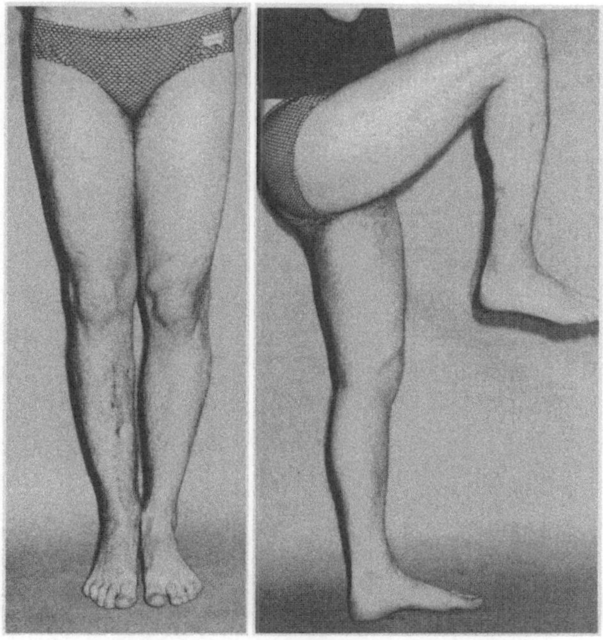

f

Fig. 9 a–f. Correction of a complex deformity of the right femur 18 months after fracture. **a** Preoperative roentgenogram of the malunited femoral fracture (35° varus, 30° backward displacement, 5 cm shortening). **b** preoperative drawing of the femur and tibia. There were coexisting tibial deformities secondary to a noncomitant tibial fracture (30° internal rotation, 10° backward displacement, 5° varus). There was also a fixed 40° equinus deformity and severely limited motion in the right knee. **c** Drawings showing the correction of the femoral deformity and the osteotomy planes; after angulation is corrected and the bone is lengthened 4 cm, the resected callus is used to bridge the defect. **d** Postoperative roentgenograms. In the same operation the tibial deformities were corrected and the Achilles tendon was lengthened by Z-plasty; then an external frame was applied for gradual correction of the equinus deformity. **e** Roentgenologic status 18 months after surgery; there is complete integration of the graft. **f** Appearance and function of the limb 18 months after surgery

References

1. Bragard K (1932) Das Genu valgum. Z Orthop Chir [Suppl] 57
2. Bouillet R, Gaver van P (1961) Arthrose du genou. Acta Orthop Belg 27:5
3. Debrunner AM, Seewald K (1964) Die Belastung des Kniegelenkes in der Frontalebene. Z Orthop 98:508
4. Ecke H, Neubert C, Neeb W (1980) Analyse der Behandlungsergebnisse von 1127 Patienten mit Oberschenkelfrakturen aus der Bundesrepublik Deutschland und der Schweiz. Unfallchirurgie 6:38
5. Gotzen L, Haas N, Strohfeld G (1981) Zur Biomechanik der Plattenosteosynthese. Unfallheilkunde 84:439
6. Lanz v T, Wachsmuth W (1972) Praktische Anatomie, Bd I/4, Bein und Statik. Springer, Berlin Heidelberg New York
7. Tscherne H, Gotzen L (1979) Posttraumatische Fehlstellungen. Chirurgie der Gegenwart, Bd IVa. Unfallchirurgie. Urban & Schwarzenberg, München Wien Baltimore
8. Wagner H (1972) Technik und Indikation der operativen Verkürzung und Verlängerung von Oberschenkel und Unterschenkel. Orthopäde 1:59

Corrective Osteotomies of the Tibial Shaft

G. Hörster

Introduction

Malunited fractures of the tibial shaft place unphysiologic loads on adjacent joints and, beyond a certain magnitude, should be regarded as preosteoarthritic and treated accordingly [7]. It is the alteration of *functional loads* on the joints that has the greatest pathophysiologic significance.

In selecting patients for corrective surgery of the tibia and in formulating a plan of operation, it is important to consider the peculiar topographical features of the bones and soft tissues of that region. In the present article we shall give special attention to the details of preoperative planning (site, type and stabilization of the osteotomy), beginning with an examination of the pathophysiologic aspects of joint loading in the presence of significant tibial shaft deformity. We shall limit our attention to deformities in the frontal plane that have a high degree of clinical significance.

Physiologic Aspects of Knee and Ankle Joint Loading

A complete load analysis is not yet possible, for studies in the gait laboratory are not yet able to provide complete functional data on knee and ankle joint loads [12]. Drawing on the work of Braune [2], Debrunner [3], Eberhard (quoted in Debrunner [3]), Fischer [6] and Pauwels [18], we have constructed a two-dimensional model which highlights some details of the stance phase of gait (Fig. 1). This model is a useful source of information on knee and ankle loads during gait.

The following assumptions are made in our necessarily simplified model:

a) Femoral length is 50 cm, tibial length is 40 cm.
b) The pelvis is tilted 5° toward the supporting side.
c) The supporting surface of the weight-bearing leg is at the base of a perpendicular dropped from the center of gravity in the symmetrical two-legged stance.
d) The weight-bearing axis from the partial center of gravity S5 is inclined 3° in a medial-to-lateral, cranial-to-caudal direction.

When considering the loads on the leg joints, it is important to understand that the weight-bearing axis does not traverse the joint centers during gait. As a result, the body weight exerts bending moments on the different joints through lever arms of varying length. Even the ankle joint is affected, because the equilibrium that is established during gait is dynamic, and the supporting

Corrective Osteotomies of the Lower Extremity
Edited by G. Hierholzer, K. H. Müller

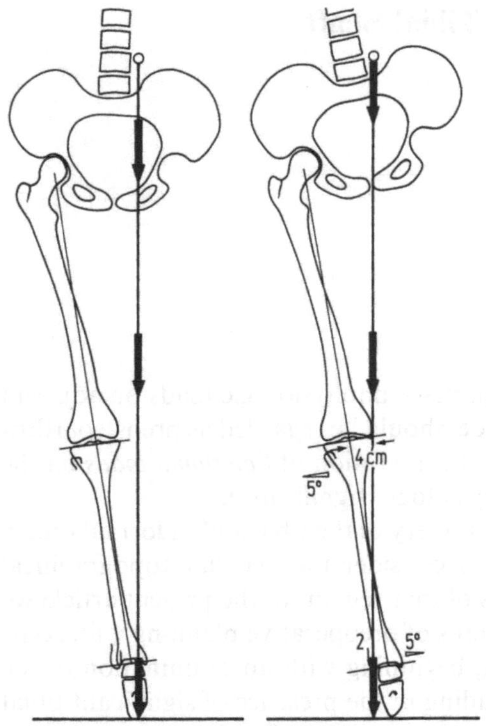

Fig. 1 a,b. Model drawings showing the position of the joints in relation to the weight-bearing axis. **a** Static equilibrium during one-legged stance; **b** dynamic equilibrium in the stance phase of gait

surface of the weight-bearing foot does not necessarily coincide with the base of the weight-bearing axis. The inclination of this axis results from a combination of the perpendicular dropped from S5 and a small transverse force directed toward the weight-bearing side that is produced by the alternation of supporting sides during gait (Eberhard et al. 1947, quoted in Debrunner [3]). Its origin lies at the partial center of gravity S5 (center of gravity of the body minus the supporting leg), with S5 being shifted toward the midline during gait by a slight pelvic tilt toward the supporting side. Pauwels notes that the changes in the length of the lever arm of the body weight during the different phase of gait are not significant as far as the hip joint is concerned, so that changes in the position of S5 may be disregarded [18]. The distance of the weight-bearing axis from the center of the knee joint is approximately 4 cm, and its distance from the center of the ankle joint is approximately 2 cm. Both joints are subjected to roughly the same body weight in the weight-bearing phase. (In theory, the partial weights of the limb would have to be subtracted in a separate consideration of the knee and ankle joints.)

The eccentric position of the knee and ankle joints gives rise to bending moments that must be counteracted by the muscles and ligaments. This is necessary in order for compressive forces to act on the joints [14]. Because the knee joint is not guided by bony structures, the body weight that acts on the knee joint through a substantial lever arm poses a serious threat to the medial compartment of the knee (Eberhard at al. 1947, quoted in Debrunner [3])

[11]. The ankle joint, on the other hand, is loaded most heavily in its lateral portion. Because it is guided by bony structures, and because its center is nearer the weight-bearing axis than that of the knee, it is less susceptible to decompensation [24].

From our description of the position of the supporting surface of the foot and from the anatomy of the lower extremity, we find that the mechanical axis of the leg (line connecting the centers of the hip, knee and ankle joints) is inclined 5° in a proximal-to-distal, lateral-to-medial direction [11]. With perfect axial relationships, the mechanical axis will coincide with the resultant load on the knee. But deviation of the mechanical axis from the center of the knee signifies only a *qualitative* alteration of knee loading. Given the eccentricity of the knee joint with respect to the weight-bearing axis, the deviation of the mechanical axis cannot be taken as a *quantitative* measure of knee loads.

The 5° slope of the mechanical axis results in a 2° varus inclination of the knee baseline and talar baseline in the stance phase of gait. As a result, slight pronation of the subtalar joint is necessary to achieve a plantigrade landing of the foot. The knee baseline and talar baseline from a 5° angle with the weight-bearing axis, which causes physiologic shear forces to act on the knee and ankle joints during gait [3].

Loading of the Knee and Ankle Joint in the Presence of Diaphyseal Varus and Valgus Deformity

With the help of our model, we are able to depict simple and complex axial deformities, recognize alterations of joint loads, and formulate specific plans of treatment (cf. [5]).

Since joint loads cannot be analyzed in quantitative terms, considerable importance is placed on two measurable, variable quantities:

1. The distance of the weight-bearing axis from the center of the knee or ankle joint. This provides a measure of the change in the rotational moment of the body weight.
2. The degree of obliquity of the knee baseline and talar baseline and the associated change in shear forces. Because the deformities of interest are located between the knee and ankle, they result in fundamentally different inclinations of the knee and ankle joint with respect to the weight-bearing axis.

Measurements for different deformities are comparable only on the condition that the position of the partial center of gravity S5, the center of the femoral head, and the supporting surface of the foot remain constant. This means that the patient must abduct the hip slightly in a varus deformity and abduct it in a valgus deformity. Only in this way can the foot land centrally during the stance phase of gait (Figs. 2 and 3).

In the interest of reproducibility, we shall assume that we are dealing with a 10° deformity located precisely at the center of the tibial shaft.

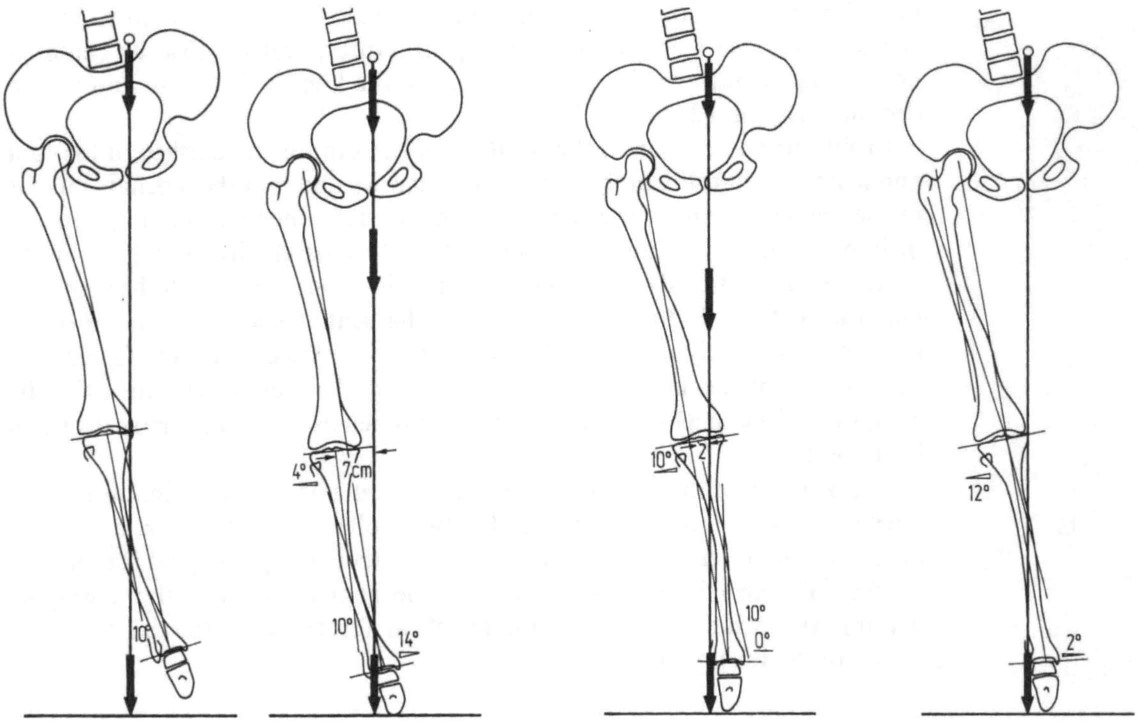

Fig. 2 a **b** **Fig. 3** **Fig. 4**

Fig. 2 a,b. Loads on the knee and ankle with a diaphyseal varus of 10°. **a** Without compensatory hip abduction; **b** in the stance phase of gait

Fig. 3. Loads on the knee and ankle with a diaphyseal valgus of 10° in the stance phase of gait

Fig. 4. Femoral and tibial deformities that are equal in magnitude but opposite in direction center the mechanical axis but cause unphysiologic joint obliquity

Varus Deformity (Fig. 2):

Varus deformity of the shaft increases the distance of the weight-bearing axis from the center of the knee joint by more than 50% relative to the normal limb. The inclination of the knee baseline is virtually unchanged. In the ankle joint, the weight-bearing axis is moved closer to the joint center, while the varus inclination of the talar baseline reaches 14°.

Valgus Deformity (Fig. 3):

Valgus deformity of the shaft moves the weight-bearing axis much closer to the center of the knee joint while increasing the inclination of the knee baseline to 10°. It increases the distance of the weight-bearing axis from the center of the ankle joint by 50% and rotates the talar baseline perpendicular to the axis.

These facts explain why the loads on the knee and ankle differ so greatly for equal degrees of varus and valgus deformity. It is clear that equivalent medial and lateral shifts of the mechanical axis from the center of the knee will have very different effects on joint loads, as Bragard and Kostuik have demonstrated [1,10]. The magnitude of the load is critically influenced by the change in the rotational moment of the body weight associated with lever arms of different lengths. The observed susceptibility of the medial compartment of the knee to degenerative change in patients with varus deformity is explained by the tendency of the muscles and ligaments to decompensate in the face of a significant increase in the length of the lever arm. With a valgus deformity, our models indicate that the knee joint would be likely to decompensate only if the weight-bearing axis were to cross the center of the knee, because the medial part of the joint lacks the intrinsic compensatory structures of the lateral side. Thus, a diaphyseal valgus of 10° does not subject the knee joint to potentially damaging bending loads.

A simple displacement of the fragments without varus or valgus angulation also shifts the mechanical axis relative to the knee, but the magnitude of the shift does not depend on the site of the deformity. Accordingly, the frequency and severity of osteoarthritis in neighboring joints will depend directly on the amount of displacement that occurs [24]. Because the supporting surface of the foot is only a short distance from the center of the ankle joint, different deformities produce only slight changes in the length of the lever arm for this joint. Thus, the association of diaphyseal deformity with degenerative disease of the ankle joint postulated by Rosemeyer appears to be unlikely [19].

Just as the described change in the rotational moment of the body weight in varus and valgus deformities results in different loads on the joints, the inclinations of the knee baseline and talar baseline also have different consequences. Increased obliquity of the joints relative to the weight-bearing axis has the effect of increasing shear forces on the joints. The main danger of these forces is that they act in the same direction as the bending loads exerted by body weight, and so they exacerbate the stresses imposed on a localized region of the joint. With a varus deformity of the tibia, the lateral compartment of the ankle is at particular risk for damage to its stabilizing structures, especially the syndesmosis.

Besides the pathologic shear forces mentioned above, excessive obliquity of the talar baseline due to varus deformity also compromises the ability of the subtalar joint to maintain a plantigrade gait through pronation. With a diaphyseal varus of 10°, this compensatory ability is already lost. In principle, we feel that this is the prime indication for corrective osteotomy in patients with varus deformities of the distal half of the tibia.

When we consider the position of the weight-bearing axis on the one hand and the inclinations of the knee and talar baselines on the other, we find that concomitant deformities of the femur and tibia that are equal in magnitude but opposite in direction do tend to center the mechanical axis, but they do not eliminate unphysiologic shear forces [14,16] (Fig. 4). This pathologic inclination of the joint line, which is especially pronounced in the knee, can in itself justify corrective surgery for deformities in excess of 10°.

Guidelines for Preoperative Planning

Whole-leg roentgenograms of the affected and unaffected sides are essential for determining the degree of the deformity and planning its correction. The true extent of diaphyseal deformities is best appreciated with the patient standing. It does not matter whether the patient bears weight on the injured leg or both legs, because the spatial relations of the limb axes to the center of body gravity are of no relevance. Whole-leg films can sometimes be dispensed with in deformities involving the distal third of the tibia, in which case the relative inclination of the talar baseline is the decisive factor in patient selection.

Tracings are made from the roentgenograms of both limbs, and the relevant axes, axial intersections and joint baselines are indicated [8,9,12,17]. By superimposing the two tracings, one can plan a theoretically ideal realignment of the extremity. When local clinical findings are known, various ojptions may be considered with regard to the site, type and stabilization of the osteotomy.

Rotational deformities of the tibia are manifested roentgenologically by an increased inclination of the talar baseline, regardless of coexisting deformity in the frontal plane. A tibial malunion with external rotation produces an inclination in the valgus direction, while a malunion with internal rotation produces a varus inclination. This knowledge is necessary in order to avoid planning errors and to avoid the attempt to correct, say, an external rotation deformity (with obliquity of the talar baseline) by varus repositioning. While such an operation would appear to restore parallel alignment of the knee and ankle joints on x-rays, it would actually superimpose a varus deformity on the preexisting rotational deformity.

Site of the Correction

While knowledge of the relative positions of the joint centers and weight-bearing axis is important in assessing the need for surgery, preoperative planning must necessarily be guided by the position of the mechanical axis. Only when the mechanical axis is centered in the knee, and the knee and talar baselines are inclined 3° relative to the mechanical axis, can one be certain that a physiologic weight-bearing alignment has been restored.

With varus deformity of the knee joint, an overcorrection can be made to relieve postoperative stresses on the damaged portions of the joint. This should be included in the plan of operation [15,21]. Overcorrection of a valgus deformity should be avoided.

Ideally, a *simple* diaphyseal deformity is corrected by an open- or closed-wedge osteotomy performed at the level of intersection of the partial tibial axes. This intersection defines the level of the deformity. Details of planning are described by Oest, taking a high tibial osteotomy as an example [16]. The steps are as follows:

1. Define the level of the deformity as the level of the osteotomy.
2. Draw the proximal segment of the mechanical axis from the center of the femoral head through the center of the knee joint to the osteotomy.
3. Draw a line from the center of the ankle joint to the intersection of the osteotomy with the proximal segment of the mechanical axis.

The angle enclosed by the partial axes equals the angle of correction. If the steps above are carefully followed, this angle should be identical to the angle of the deformity (Fig. 5).

If the axial intersection does not coincide with the level of the fracture visible on roentgenograms, it may be concluded that a *combined* deformity exists. The fracture has undergone secondary lateral or medial displacement during healing, usually with a varus or valgus component predominating both visually and functionally. This type of deformity is also corrected by the method of Oest, i.e., at the level of the axial intersection on preoperative drawings. The advantage of this method is that the secondary displacement may be disregarded during planning. A discrepancy between the site of the deformity and the axial intersection is often advantageous in the lower leg, as it allows the osteotomy to be performed in an area with better osseous and soft-tissues conditions. If the site of the axial intersection is disregarded and the osteotomy is done at the level of the deformity, it will be necessary to correct both the angulation and the displacement in order to center the mechanical axis.

The coexistence of two deformities also has an important bearing on patient selection. This is because the joint load depends both on the magnitude of the deformity and on the location of the axial intersection. Medial displacement of the distal fragment impairs the biomechanics of the knee joint in the presence of a coexisting varus deformity. For example, a diaphyseal varus deformity of 10° coexisting with a medial displacement of the distal fragment by the diameter of the shaft is equivalent to a varus deformity of equal magnitude located in the upper tibia (Fig. 6).

When dealing with malunited fractures of the tibial shaft, local conditions frequently make it necessary to perform the osteotomy in the metaphysis. It should be noted, however, that the farther the osteotomy is from the axial intersection, the more difficult it is to center the mechanical axis and also obtain a physiologic position of the joint baselines [23]. Oest points out that a deviation of the level of the osteotomy from the axial intersection is negligible only if it is small [16]. As the osteotomy is moved proximally from the axial intersection, the angle of correction becomes smaller while the obliquity of the talar baseline increases. In our example of a 10° diaphyseal varus deformity, the planing of a proximal metaphyseal osteotomy by the method of Oest leads to a correction angle of 6°. This centers the mechanical axis in the knee, but there persists a 9° inclination of the talar baseline (Fig. 7). This approaches the limit of compensatory pronation in the subtalar joint. An operation on the distal tibia cannot be planned using this method, because the intersecton of the level of the osteotomy and proximal mechanical axis lies outside the bone.

If the angle of correction in the metaphyseal osteotomy equals the angle of the deformity, parallel alignment of the knee baseline and talar baseline will be restored. The resulting shift of the mechanical axis in the knee joint is then corrected by displacing the osteotomy surfaces reltive to each other [9,13]. Generally this involves some degree of compromise, for a diaphyseal deformity of 10° would require displacement of the metaphyseal osteotomy surfaces by more than half the diameter of the shaft in order to center the mechanical axis. This type of osteotomy can be done in either the proximal or distal tibial metaphysis; the former operation causes a lateral shift of the mechanical axis relative to the knee, while the latter causes a medial shift

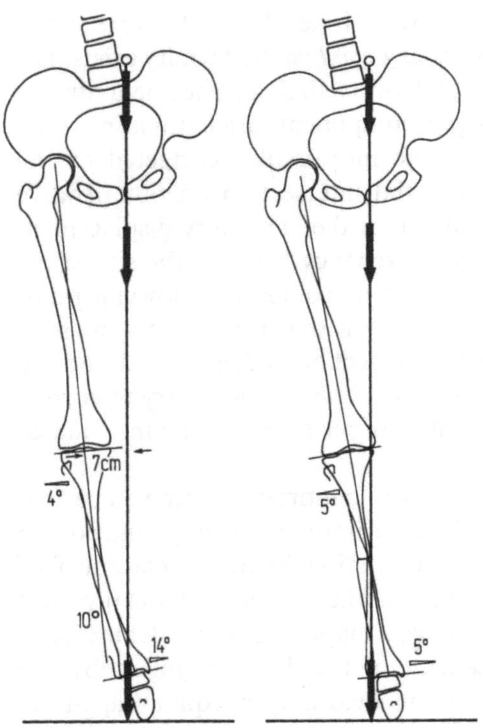

Fig. 5a **b**

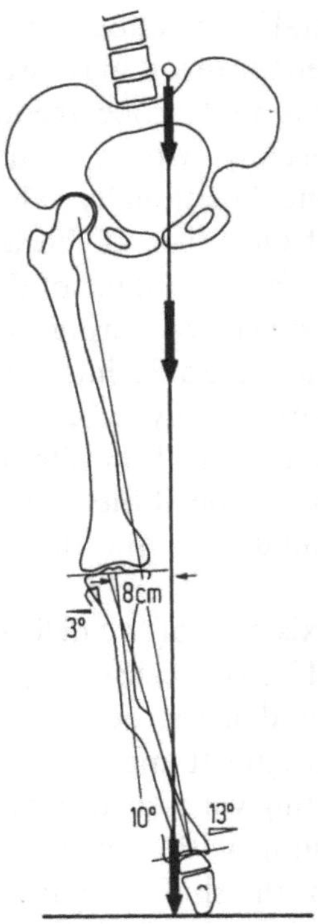

Fig. 6

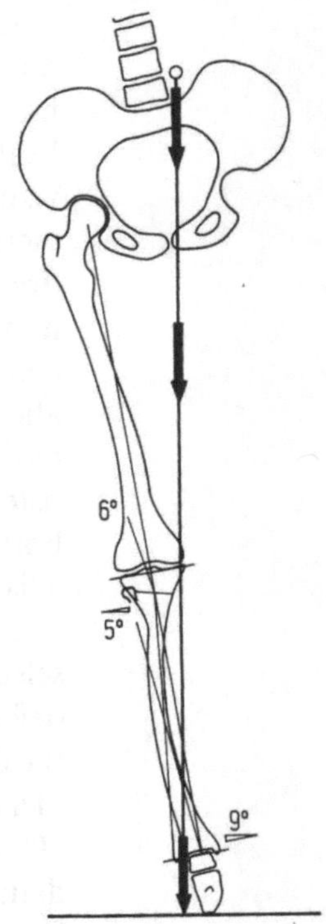

Fig. 7

Fig. 5 a,b. Transverse closed wedge osteotomy to correct a diaphyseal varus of 10°. **a** Before the correction; **b** after the correction

Fig. 6. The combination of diaphyseal varus and medial displacement of the distal fragment leads to a proximal migration of the axial intersection and thus to a deterioration of the biomechanics of the knee

Fig. 7. The proximal metaphyseal correction of a 10° diaphyseal varus deformity (by the method of Oest) leads to a 6° angle of correction with an abnormal 9° inclination of the talar baseline to the weight-bearing axis

(Figs. 8 and 9). With a diaphyseal varus deformity, the proximal metaphyseal osteotomy shifts the mechanical axis into the lateral compartment of the joint, and so that operation would be preferred. A valgus deformity in the same location should be corrected with a distal osteotomy. If at all possible, the mechanical axis should not pass medial to the center of the knee joint following surgery. For biomechanical reasons we do not agree with Janssen's statement that distal metaphyseal osteotomies are generally appropriate for deformities of the shaft [9].

Types of Osteotomy

As a rule, closed wedge osteotomies are used to correct posttraumatic diaphyseal deformities. The tibial shaft is not a favorable site for open wedge procedures. Transverse osteotomies of the diaphysis carry a risk of delayed union, especially when they are fixed with an internal plate. Healing is assisted in such cases by the concurrent application of a medial cancellous bone graft [23].

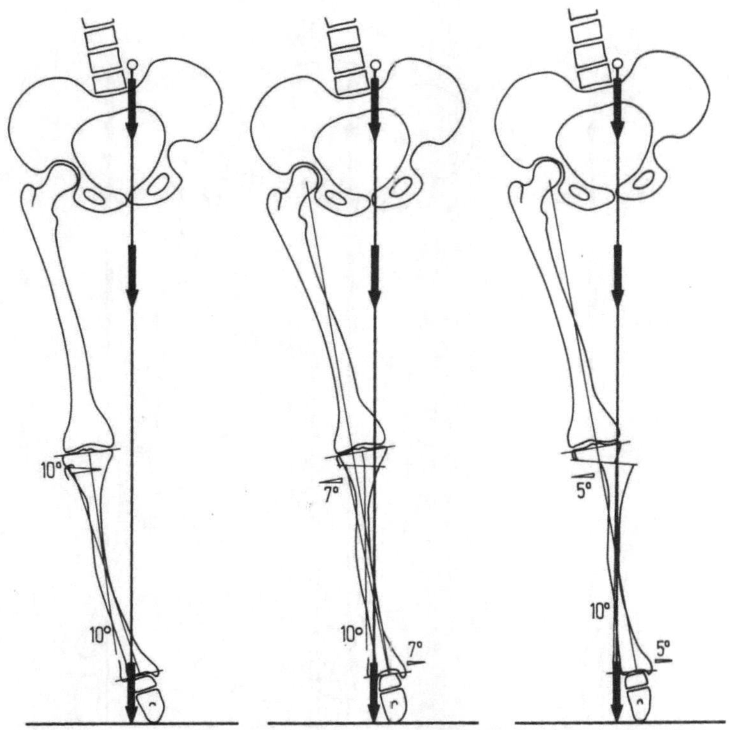

Fig. 8 a–c. Proximal metaphyseal correction of a 10° diaphyseal varus deformity. **a** Before correction; the angle of correction equals the angle of the deformity. **b** This correction shifts the mechanical axis lateral to the center of the knee joint. **c** Mechanical axis and joint obliquity are normalized by lateral displacement of the proximal fragment

The risk of delayed union can also be reduced by using oblique osteotomy surfaces to increase the area of interfragmental contact. Step-cut osteotomies may also be employed [23]. An important advantage of the oblique diaphyseal osteotomy is that lag screws may be inserted across the osteotomy to increase interfragmental compression and enhance stability. Another advantage is that the osteotomy surfaces can be displaced relative to each other along the oblique plane to shorten or lengthen the extremity. This is considered during preoperative planning.

Accurate centering of the mechanical axis depends both on the amount of angular correction achieved and on the level of the center of rotaton of the osteotomy (i.e., the point where the osteotomy surfaces intersect). The closer the osteotomy center of rotation is to the point of axial intersection, the more accurately the mechanical axis will be centered in the knee. For a given distance of the center of rotation from the axial intersection, the orientation of the osteotomy has no effect on the biomechanical result, only on the area of the apposed bone surfaces (Figs. 5 and 10). Also, it does not matter whether the oblique osteotomy is carried out proximal or distal of the axial intersection. If possible, the correction should be planned suct that displacement of the

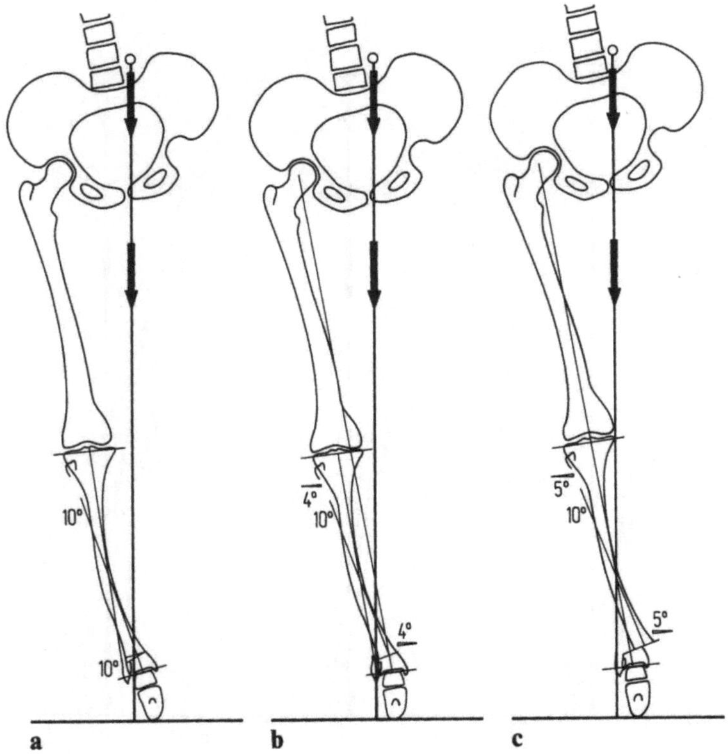

Fig. 9

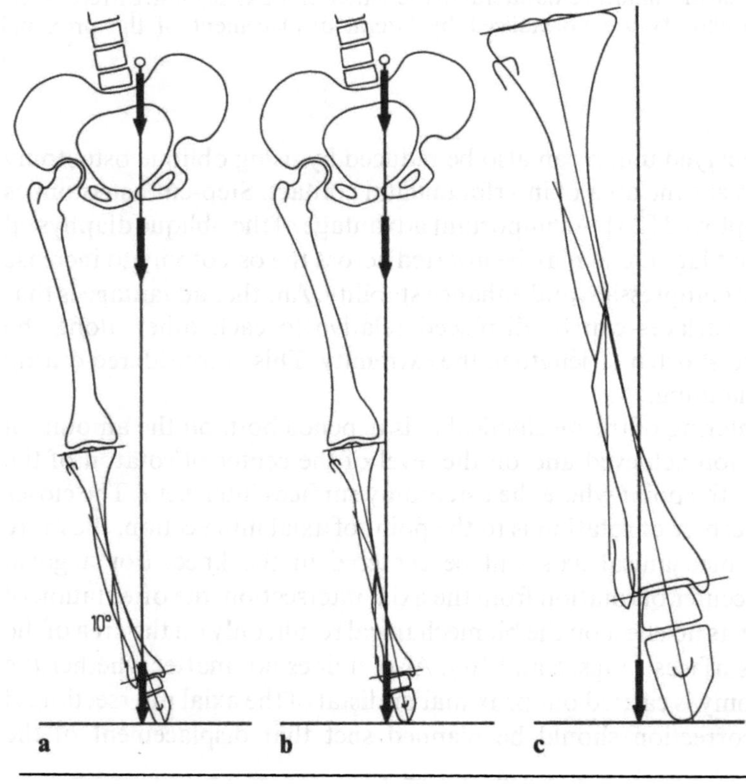

Fig. 10

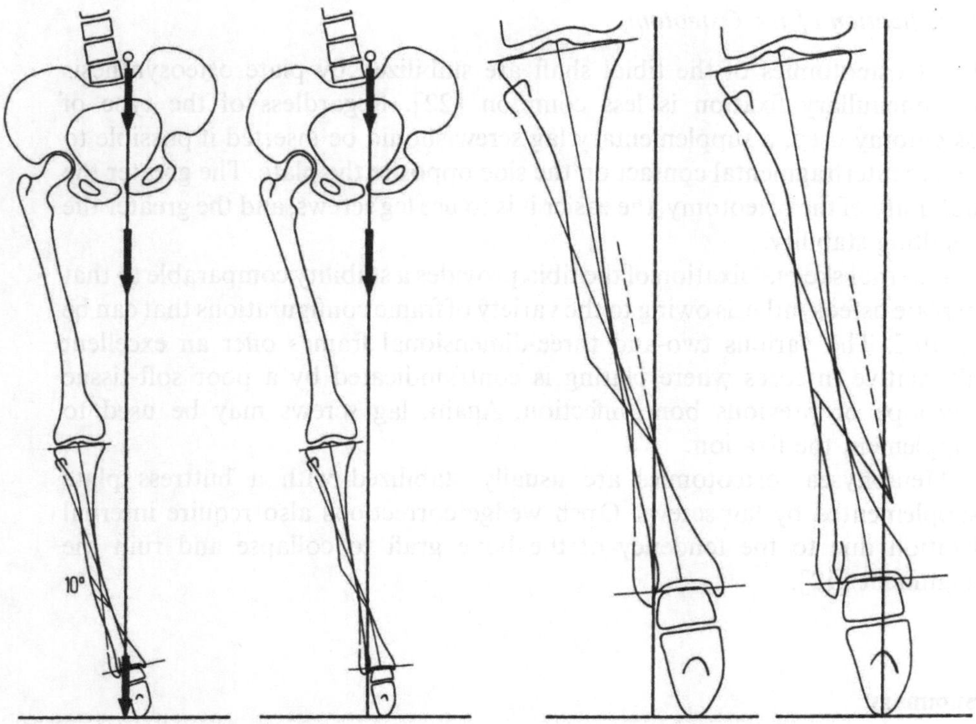

Fig. 11 a – d. Oblique closed wedge diaphyseal osteotomy to correct a varus deformity of 10°. **a** Before correction; the proximal part of the base of the wedge is at the level of the axial intersection. **b** After correction; the correction produces a medialization of the distal fragment with a corresponding shift of the mechanical axis. **c** Detailed view of the osteotomy site. **d** Detailed view of the osteotomy site after the mechanical axis has been centered by displacement of the osteotomy surfaces; note the significant shortening that results

fragments along the osteotomy plane will center the mechanical axis and also equalize the limb lengths (Fig. 11).

In the metaphysis, open wedge osteotomies using corticocancellous grafts may be appropriate depending on the age of the patient. These procedures are also useful for correcting length discrepancy. The large area of interfragmental contact obviates the need for an oblique osteotomy.

Fig. 9 a – c. Distal metaphyseal correction of a 10° diaphyseal varus deformity. **a** Before correction; the angle of correction equals the angle of the deformity. **b** This correction shifts the mechanical axis medial to the center of the knee joint. **c** Mechanical axis and joint obliquity are normalized by medial displacement of the proximal fragment

Fig. 10 a – c. Oblique diaphyseal osteotomy to correct a varus deformity of 10°. The level of the center of rotation coincides with the axial intersection. **a** Before correction. **b** After correction; the mechanical axis is centered, and joint obliquity is normal. **c** Detailed view of the osteotomy site

Stabilization of the Osteotomy

Most osteotomies of the tibial shaft are stabilized by plate osteosynthesis intramedullary fixation is less common [22]. Regardless of the type of osteotomy used, a supplementary lag screw should be inserted if possible to secure interfragmental contact on the side opposite the plate. The greater the obliquity of the osteotomy, the easier it is to use leg screws, and the greater the resulting stability.

External skeletal fixation of the tibia provides a stability comparable to that of plate osteosynthesis owing to the variety of frame configurations that can be created. The various two-and three-dimensional frames offer an excellent alternative in cases where plating is contraindicated by a poor soft-tissue envelope or previous bone infection. Again, lag screws may be used to supplement the fixation.

Metaphyseal osteotomies are usually stabilized with a buttress plate supplemented by lag screws. Open wedge corrections also require internal fixation due to the tendency of the bone graft to collapse and ruin the alignment [12].

Summary

The principles of corrective osteotomies for tibial shaft deformities in the frontal plane are described. A biologically and biomechanically optimum correction relies on detailed preoperative planning based on drawings of the affected and unaffected sides. Patient selection requires a knowledge of the functional pathophysiology of the knee and ankle joints. In a simplified two-dimensional model, it is shown how a diaphyseal varus deformity of 10° clearly justifies operative correction. An equivalent valgus deformity apparently poses no significant threat to neighboring joints from a biomechanical standpoint. Finally, details of operative technique are described, pointing out the advantages and disadvantages of particular sites and types of osteotomy. Theoretical considerations are valuable only when clinical and roentgenologic findings are taken into account.

References

1. Bragard K (1932) Das genu valgum. Z Orthop Chir [Suppl] 57
2. Braune W, Fischer O (1895) Der Gang des Menschen. I. Teil: Versuche am unbelasteten und belasteten Menschen. Abhandl K S Ges Wissensch 21/4:152
3. Debrunner AM, Seewald K (1964) Die Belastung des Kniegelenkes in der Frontalebene. Z Orthop 98: 508
5. Endler F (1974) Biomechanische Probleme bei kombinierten Achsenfehlern der unteren Extremitäten. Orthop Prax 7/10:423
6. Fischer O (1899) Der Gang des Menschen. II Teil: Die Bewegung des Gesamtschwerpunktes und die äußeren Kräfte. Abhandl K S Ges Wissensch 25/1:3

7. Hackenbroch M (1957) Degenerative Gelenkerkrankungen. In: Hohmann G, Hackenbroch M, Lindemann K (Hrsg) Thieme, Stuttgart (Handbuch der Orthopädie, Bd I)
8. Hippe P (1976) Die Indikation zur Korrektur diaphysärer Achsenfehler der unteren Extremität. Orthop Prax 3/12:299
9. Janssen G, Dietschi C (1974) Die supramalleoläre Korrekturosteotomie nach Unterschenkelfrakturen. Z Orthop 112:444
10. Kostuik JP, Schmidt O, Harries WR, Woldridge C (1975) A study of weight transmission through the knee joint with applied varus and valgus loads. Clin Orthop 108:95
11. Lang J, Wachsmuth W (1972) Praktische Anatomie, Bd I/4. Bein und Statik. Springer, Berlin Heidelberg New York
12. Limmer L, König G, Leitz G (1977) Die Individualität der Belastungsmuster des menschlichen Ganges. Z Orthop 115:321
13. Müller KH, Bieberach M (1977) Korrekturosteotomien und ihre Ergebnisse bei kniegelenknahen posttraumatischen Fehlstellungen. Unfallheilkunde 80:359
14. Müller ME (1967) Posttraumatische Achsenfehlstellungen an den unteren Extremitäten. Huber, Bern Stuttgart
15. Noesberger B (1976) Osteotomien im Kniebereich. Orthop Prax 2/12:168
16. Oest O (1973) Röntgenologische Beinachsenbestimmung. Z Orthop 111:497
17. Oest O, Sieberg HJ (1971) Die Röntgenganzaufnahme der unteren Extremitäten. Z Orthop 109:54
18. Pauwels F (1965) Gesammelte Abhandlungen zur funktionellen Anatomie des Bewegungsapparates. Springer, Heidelberg Berlin New York
19. Rosemeyer B, Pförringer W (1979) Posttraumatische Unterschenkelfehlstellungen. Münch Med Wochenscher 121:1251
20. Tjörnstrand B, Egund N, Hagstedt B, Lindstrand A (1981) Tibial osteotomy in medial gonarthrosis. Arch Orthop Trauma Surg 99:83
21. Tscherne H, Gotzen L (1978) Posttraumatische Fehlstellungen. Chir Ggw 4a:52
22. Wagner H (1977) Prinzipien der Korrekturosteotomie am Bein. Orthopäde 6:145
23. Weber BG (1966) Verletzungen des oberen Sprunggelenkes. Aktuel Probl Chir 3
24. Ziernhöld G, Beck E (1977) Einfluß der Seitenverschiebung geheilter Unterschenkelbrüche auf das Knie- und Sprunggelenk. Unfallchirurgie 3:191

The Displacement Osteotomy as a Correction Principle

H. Wagner

The principle of the displacement osteotomy offers a valuable alternative to the classic closed wedge osteotomy and effectively augments our capabilities for the surgical treatment of posttraumatic deformities. With the displacement osteotomy it is possible to align the fragments with the mechanical axis of the joints while simultaneously correcting angular deformity. This restores a physiologic weight-bearing alignment and transforms bending forces into compressive forces, which are favorable for bone consolidation. The displacement osteotomy does not require the resection of a bone wedge, and axial correction is effected by aligning and then impacting the osteotomy fragments. This produces a good primary stability and provides a secure foundation for internal fixation. The osteotomy can also be used to lengthen an entire bone or a portion of it, such as the femoral neck in a double intertrochanteric osteotomy.

The classic procedure for correcting a posttraumatic axial deformity is the closed wedge osteotomy, in which a wedge of bone is resected from the apex of the deformity, the osteotomy surfaces are apposed in the desired alignment, and the osteotomy is stabilized by internal fixation or an external frame (ASIF Manual 1977 [1]) (Fig. 1).

However, the closed wedge osteotomy has several disadvantages, which are most apparent in cases of very severe angular deformity or when there is extensive bowing involving a long segment of bone (Figs. 12 and 13). In these cases the closed wedge osteotomy will correct the angular deformity, but the longitudinal axis of the shaft will be displaced relative to the mechanical axis of the neighboring joints (Fig. 1 b). This places a bending stress on the osteotomy and leads to asymmetric joint loading and an esthetically poor result [2].

The supracondylar femoral osteotomy illustrates these problems particularly well (Fig. 1): Resection of the bone wedge and closure of the osteotomy produces an undesired lateralization of the proximal fragment on the femoral condyle. Of course the proximal fragment can then be displaced medially to center it over the condyle, but this reveals yet another disadvantage of the closed wedge osteotomy: The correction of severe axial deformities requiring a large wedge resection results in proximal and distal osteotomy surfaces that differ markedly in cross-section. As a result, the thinner proximal fragment rests upon the larger and entirely cancellous surface of the distal fragment and may sink into it if the cancellous bone is soft.

These problems are easily solved by the displacement osteotomy (Figs. 2–4). First the shaft is transversely osteotomized. Then the distal fragment is

Corrective Osteotomies of the Lower Extremity
Edited by G. Hierholzer, K. H. Müller

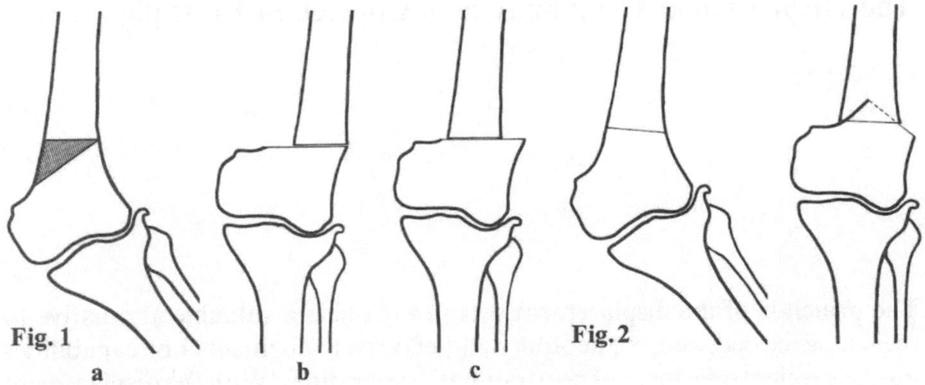

Fig. 1. a Supracondylar closed wedge osteotomy of the femur to correct severe valgus deformity. **b** Closure of the osteotomy at the lateral apex results in lateralization of the proximal fragment. **c** Medial displacement of the proximal fragment aligns it with the mechanical axis of the joint, but due to the size discrepancy of the osteotomy surfaces, the proximal fragment rests upon the (soft) cancellous surface of the distal fragment

Fig. 2. Supracondylar displacement osteotomy of the femur for severe valgus deformity. Following the transverse osteotomy, the proximal fragment is concurrently aligned and medialized. The medial edge of the distal fragment is impacted into the medullary canal of the proximal fragment. Overlapping of the cortices on the medial side ensures good primary stability and provides an effective medial buttress for internal fixation

displaced toward the concave side of the axial deformity until the deformity is corrected. Finally the edge of the distal fragment on the original convex side of the deformity is impacted into the modullary canal of the proximal fragment to create a wedging effect. The distal fragment is displaced laterally for correction of a valgus deformity, medially for a varus deformity, and posteriorly for a flexion deformity. Besides realigning the fragments with the mechanical axis of the limb, the displacement osteotomy also provides excellent stability. The impaction of the fragments and interlocking of the cortices creates a solid buttress for the osteotomy and a good foundation for internal fixation. Because supracondylar femoral osteotomies are most commonly performed in the geriatric age group, the question of primary stability is an important one – for the cancellous bone of the distal femoral metaphysis, is always atrophic, and elderly patients often have difficulty mastering partial weight bearing on crutches.

The distal fragment of the displacement osteotomy projects beyond the bony silhouette on the concave side of the original deformity. Depending on the amount of the correction, this may create a sharp "step" that jeopardizes soft tissues and therefore must be smoothed. This is especially important following the correction of a flexion deformity of the knee by a supracondylar anterior displacement osteotomy, which may leave a dangerous bony spike among the large blood vessels in the popliteal plane (Fig. 10).

In axial corrections of the upper tibia, basically the same phenomena are encounted as in a supracondylar femoral osteotomy (Fig. 5). Again, the displacement osteotomy can provide a more favorable orientation of the fragments and good primary stability in cases where angular deformity is

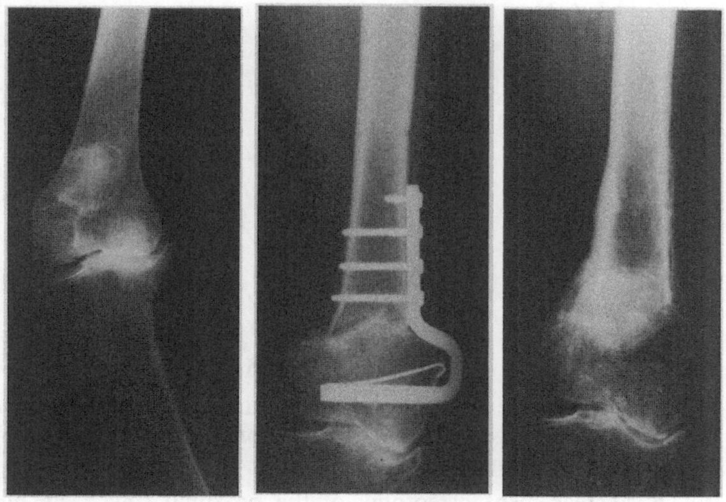

a b c

Fig. 3 a – c. Example of a supracondylar displacement osteotomy of the femur. **a** Severe, unstable osteoarthritis of the knee with valgus deformity in woman 66 years of age. **b** Supracondylar displacement osteotomy. (The lateral epicondyle was transposed proximally to advance the lateral collateral ligament and is fixed with a Kirschner wire.) **c** Three years after the supracondylar displacement osteotomy

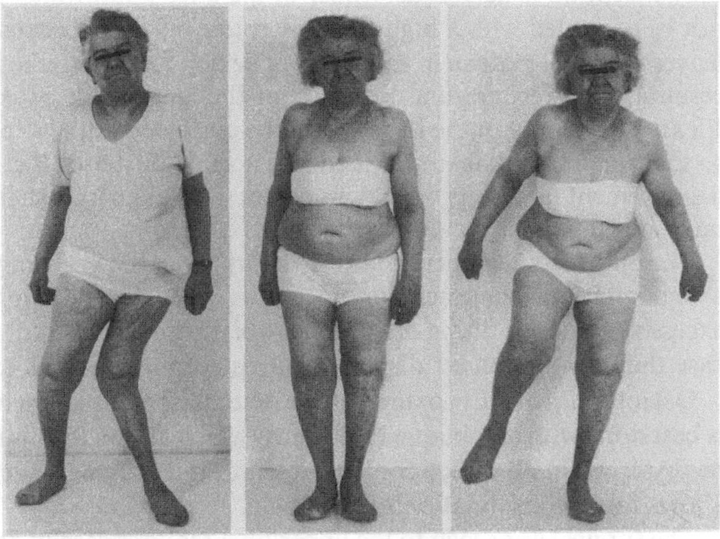

a b

Fig. 4 a,b. Supracondylar femoral displacement osteotomy for severe, unstable valgus osteoarthritis of the knee in woman 66 years of age (same patient as in Fig. 3). **a** Status fefore surgery; the left leg is unable to bear weight. **b** Status 5 years after surgery

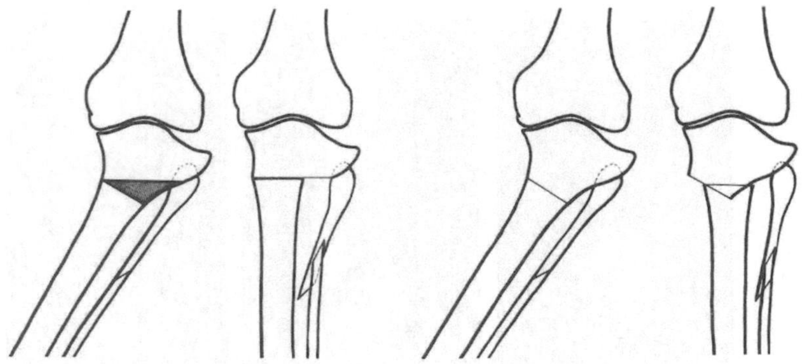

Fig. 5 Fig. 6

Fig. 5. Closed wedge osteotomy of the proximal tibia. With severe angular deformity, the resection of a large wedge creates osteotomy surfaces of unequal size and poor axial alignment of the fragments

Fig. 6. Displacement osteotomy of the proximal tibia. The bone is transversely osteotomized, and the distal fragment is aligned and moved laterally into the mechanical axis of the joint. The proximal fragment is impacted into the medullary canal of the distal fragment

severe (Fig. 6). Correction is effected by displacing the distal fragment toward the convex side of the original deformity and impacting the convex edge of the proximal fragment into the distal medullary cavity. Anatomic conditions make the displacement osteotomy thechnically more difficult in the upper tibia than in the distal femur, and displacement of the fragments is limited by the relatively thin anterior soft-tissue envelope. Nevertheless, even very severe angular deformities can be corrected in the proximal tibia (Figs. 7 and 8). The only exception is flexion deformity of the knee joint, which generally should not be corrected with a high tibial osteotomy. This is because the osteotomy leaves the tibial plateau in a position of flexion relative to the femoral condyle, resulting in a recurvatum deformity at the level of the osteotomy (Fig. 9). Flexion deformity of the knee should be corrected at the supracondylar level so that the tibial plateau will retain its normal posterior tilt, and the anterior displacement of the proximal fragment will align the shaft axes with the mechanical axis of the limb (Fig. 10).

The only instance where a flexion deformity of the knee may be treated with a high tibial displacement osteotomy is when the deformity is caused by excessive posterior tilting of the upper tibial articular surface (Fig. 11). In this case the intratuburcular displacement osteotomy gives an ideal correction.

Osteotomies of the proximal tibia also require transection of the fibula. This is best done with an oblique osteotomy, which allows the fibular fragments to be displaced in all directions yet preserves interfragmental contact and thus allows rapid consolidation of the fibula.

The surgical approach to the upper tibia requires careful detachment of the intervening anterior muscles. After the osteotomy is completed, the origins of the muscles are reattached, and the fascia is closed without tension. Under no circumstances should a tight fascial suture be allowed to put pressure on the

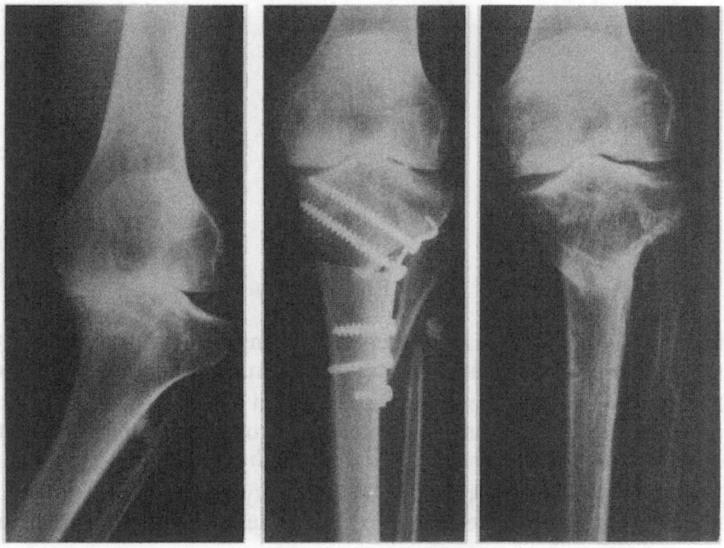

a b c

Fig. 7 a–c. Example of a displacement osteotomy of the proximal tibia. **a** Severe, unstable osteoarthritis of the knee with varus deformity in man 54 years of age. **b** High tibial displacement osteotomy. **c** Three years after surgery

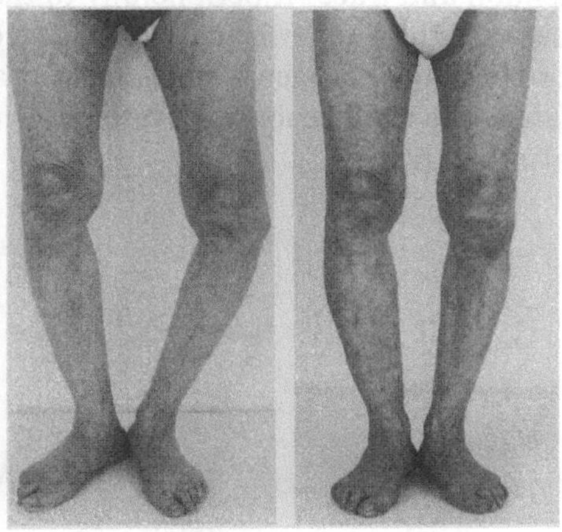

a b

Fig. 8. a Severe, unstable varus osteoarthritis of the knee in 54-year-old man (same patient as in Fig. 7); the affected leg is unable to bear weight. **b** Status 3 years after high tibial displacement osteotomy

anterior compartment; otherwise an anterior compartment syndrome could result and cause irreversible harm. In doubtful cases the fascia should be left open; closure may be possible later when the internal fixation material is removed.

Care should also be taken to avoid fascial tension over the peroneal nerve. The correction of a valgus deformity invariably places tension on lateral fascial tissues. This tension can lead to ischemic nerve injury by compressing the blood vessels of the peroneal nerve. Peroneal nerve palsy following the correction of a valgus deformity is not caused by stretching of the nerve, as is often claimed, but is the result of pressure from tight fascia. Thus, when

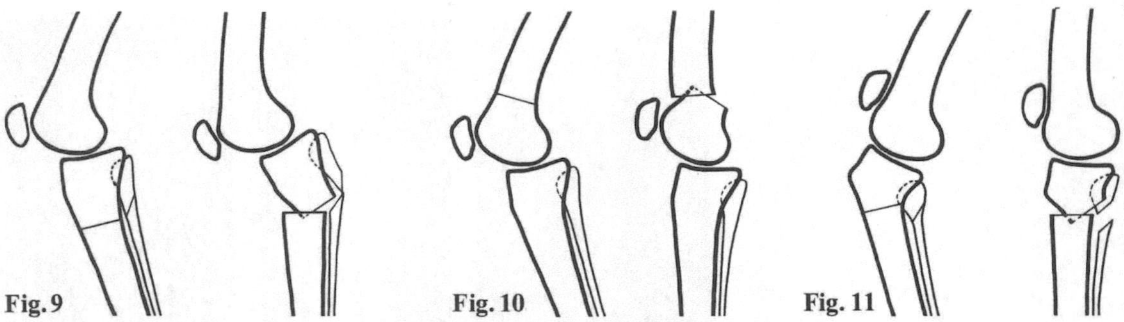

Fig. 9. The high tibial displacement osteotomy is not appropriate for the correction of a flexion deformity of the knee, because it leaves the tibial plateau in a position of lexion, creating a recurvatum deformity
Fig. 10. When a supracondylar displacement osteotomy of the femur is used to correct flexion deformity of the knee, the anterior displacement of the proximal fragment moves the diaphyses into the mechanical axis of the joints and restores a favorable weight-bearing alignment
Fig. 11. Only when the knee flexion deformity is caused by an angulation of the proximal tibia can the high tibial displacement osteotomy create an ideal weight-bearing alignment

correcting a valgus deformity, the surgeon should always make a point of splitting the fascia over the peroneal nerve. From the lateral approach the surgeon locates the peroneal nerve at its site of emergence behind the biceps tendon and traces it peripherally to the origin of the first muscular branches distal to the fibular head, splitting the overlying fascia as he proceeds. At the origin of the peroneus longus muscle, a narrow, sharp-edged, curved strip of fascia often will be found covering the nerve. It is recommended that this strip also be divided.

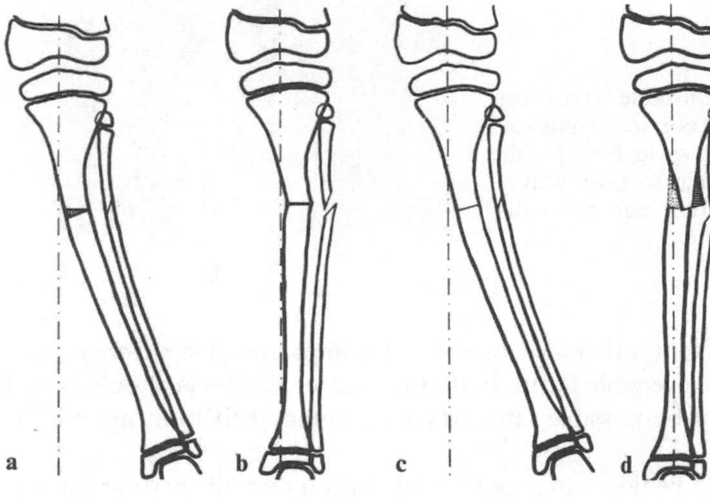

Fig. 12. a,b When there is a general bowing of the shaft of a long bone, a closed wedge osteotomy will leave the fragments outside the mechanical axis. **c,d** By contrast, the displacement osteotomy aligns the fragments with the mechanical axis of the joints. To smooth the bone surface and facilitate internal fixation, the projecting edge created by the displacement is tangentially resected and **d** is inserted into the "step" on the opposite side

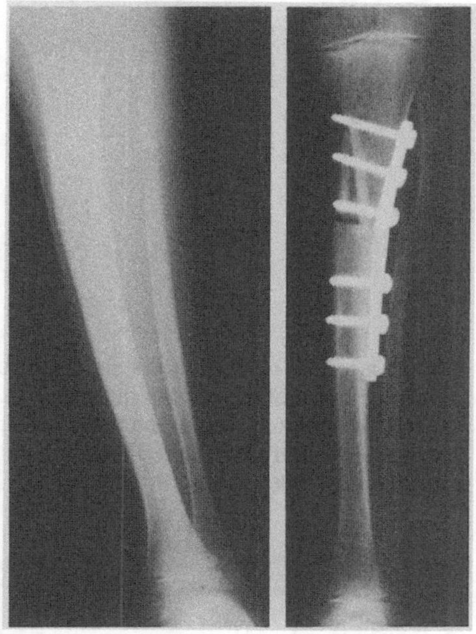

Fig. 13. Roentgenographic example of a diaphyseal displacement osteotomy (of the type shown in Fig. 12 c,d). The laterally projecting edge of the proximal fragment was tangentially resected and interposed as a graft on the opposite side

The displacement osteotomy is very well suited for the correction of deformities in which there is a more or less generalized bowing of the shaft (Figs. 12 and 13). An ideal correction by wedge resection in such cases would require that multiple osteotomies be performed at various levels of the bone. The displacement osteotomy can restore axial alignment and center the mechanical axis, all on a single osteotomy plane.

The displacement osteotomy is especially useful in cases where lateral or medial displacement of a short peripheral fragment is desired, but even a large wedge resection would not provide sufficient medialization or lateralization of the small fragment.

An excellent example of this application is the calcanean displacement osteotomy for valgus deformity of the hindfoot (Figs. 14–17).

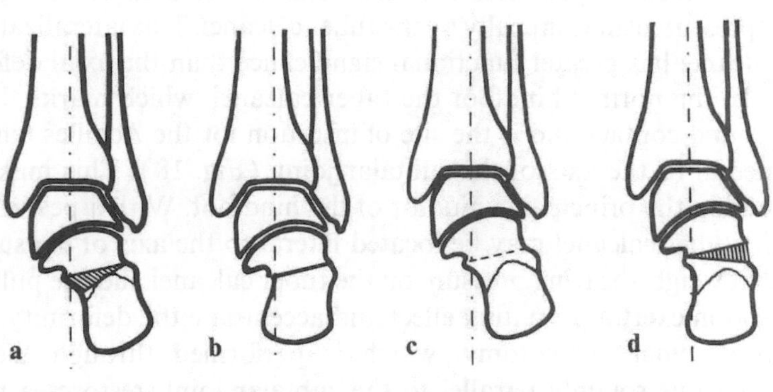

Fig. 14 a–d. The closed wedge osteotomy **a,b** and the open wedge osteotomy of the calcaneus **c,d** have relatively little medializing effect on the tuber calcanei, even with a large wedge resection, because of the short peripheral fragment

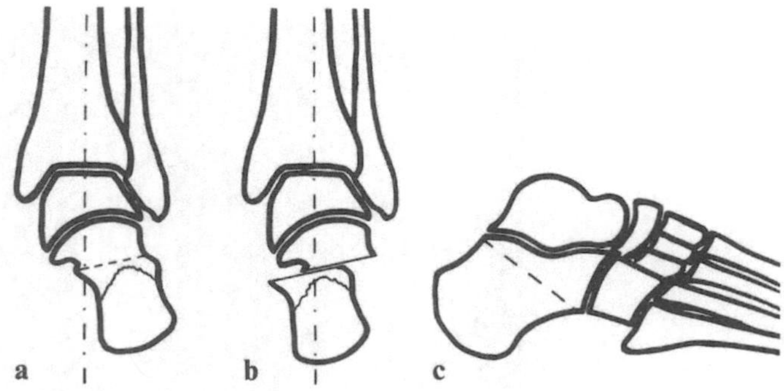

Fig. 15 a,b. The calcanean displacement osteotomy does not significantly change the axial alignment of the peripheral fragment. Its beneficial effect on function derives from the medial displacement of the tuber calcanei. c The line of the osteotomy extends from the posterior margin of the subtalar joint to the inferior margin of the calcaneocuboid joint, leaving both joints intact

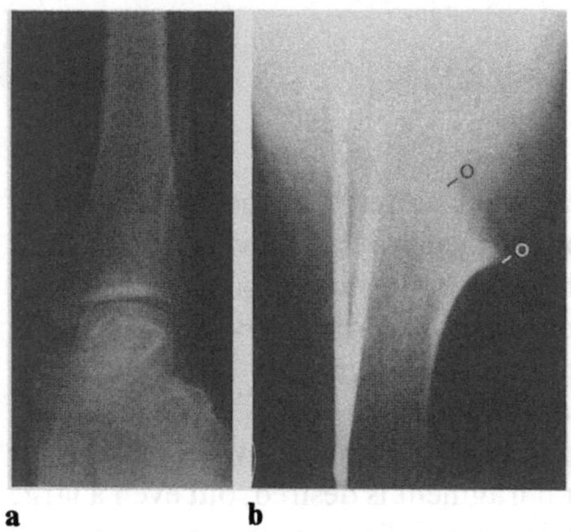

Fig. 16 a,b. Example of a calcanean displacement osteotomy. **a** Very severe valgus deformity of the hindfoot associated with dysplasia of the ankle joint and fibular hypoplasia with absence of the lateral malleolus in girl 15 years of age. **b** The extent of the displacement is indicated by the edges of the osteotomy ("O") in this axial view

In this deformity, which may present as a congenital, functional or posttraumatic pes valgus, two interrelated problems exist, both of which require correction. First, there is a valgus deformity of the calcaneus; second, this deformity produces a lateral shift in the area of heel-ground contact, represented anatomically by the tuber calcanei. This lateralization of the tuber calcanei has greater functional significance than the axial deformity as such.

In the normal hindfoot the tuber calcanei, which marks the area of heel-ground contact and is the site of insertion for the Achilles tendon, is located medial to the axis of the subtalar joint (Fig. 18). This makes the Achilles tendon the principal supinator of the hindfoot. With a pes valgus deformity, the tuber calcanei may be located lateral to the axis of the subtalar joint, so that weight-bearing pressure on the tuber calcanei and the pull of the Achilles tendon exert a pronating effect and accentuate the deformity. The calcanean displacement osteotomy, which is performed through the body of the calcaneus roughly parallel to the subtalar joint, restores a normal weight-bearing alignment through medial displacement of the tuber calcanei. The large cancellous surfaces of the osteotomy permit early partial weight-bearing

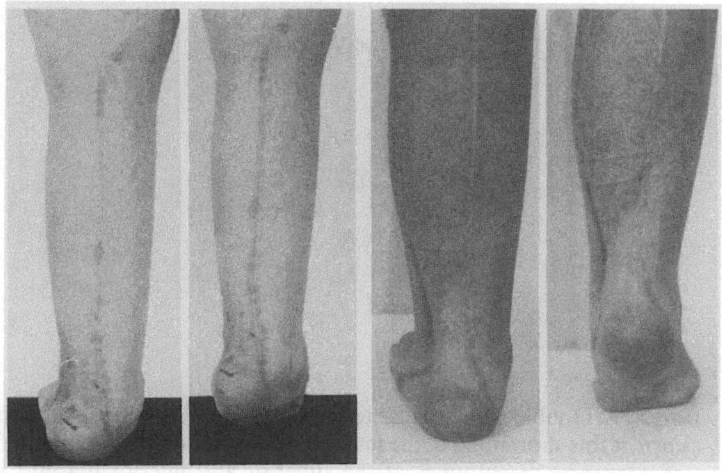

Fig. 17 a,b. Displacement osteotomy of the left calcaneus in girl 15 years of age (same case as in Fig. 16). **a** Before surgery the severe valgus deformity of the hindfoot and abducted position of the forefoot are evident in the plantigrade stance and flat toe stance. (The long cutaneous scar is from a fascial revision with lengthening of the Achilles tendon due to excessive equinovalgus contracture.) **b** Nineteen months after calcanean displacement osteotomy the heel is in the neutral position in plantigrade stance and shows slight supination in flat toe stance, while the forefoot assumes an adducted position and the longitudinal plantar arch is well raised

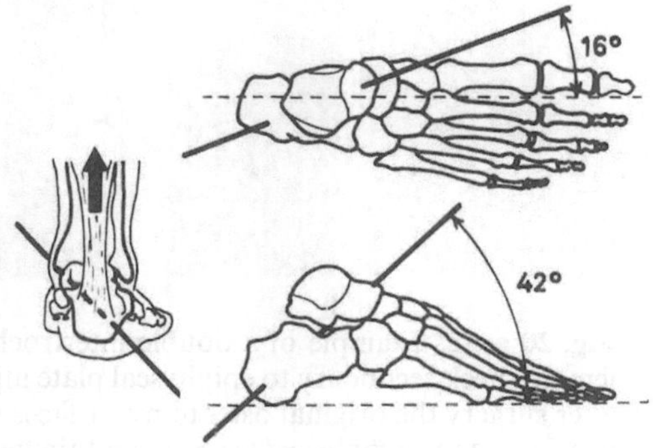

Fig. 18. Axis of the subtalar joint. The tuber calcanei, with the insertion of the Achilles tendon, is located medial to this axis, so that both the heel strike and the pull of the Achilles tendon produce a supinating effect

and rapid union. The efficacy of the displacement osteotomy is most evident in cases where the valgus deformity results from a congenital or acquired loss of the lateral malleolus with extreme instaility (Figs. 16 and 17). Although valgus deformity is the most common indication for the calcanean displacement osteotomy, a supination deformity of the hindfoot is also correctable by lateral displacement of the tuber calcanei.

Finally, the principle of the displacement osteotomy is useful in cases where severe deformity has altered the proportions of the individual parts of a bone. It is particularly useful in diacondylar or intertrochanteric corrections. A good example is the double intertrochanteric osteotomy. When severe shortening of the femoral neck has developed secondary to epiphyseal plate injury, this procedure can lengthen the femoral neck by displacement of the fragments (Figs. 19 and 20). By making one osteotomy at the superior margin of the

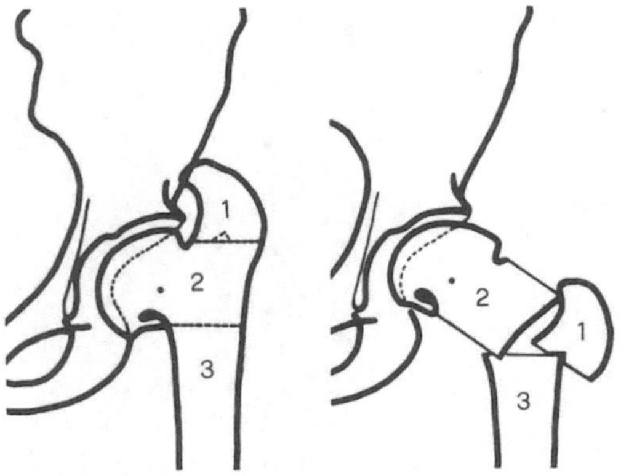

Fig. 19. Double intertrochanteric osteotomy. Only a displacement osteotomy can correct this shortening of the femoral neck secondary to epiphyseal plate injury. A pair of transverse osteotomies at the superior and inferior margins of the femoral neck divide the upper femur into three fragments, which can be independently displaced. The diaphysis and greater trochanter are displaced laterally to lengthen the femoral neck. The femur as a whole is lengthened by positioning the femoral neck segment in valgus

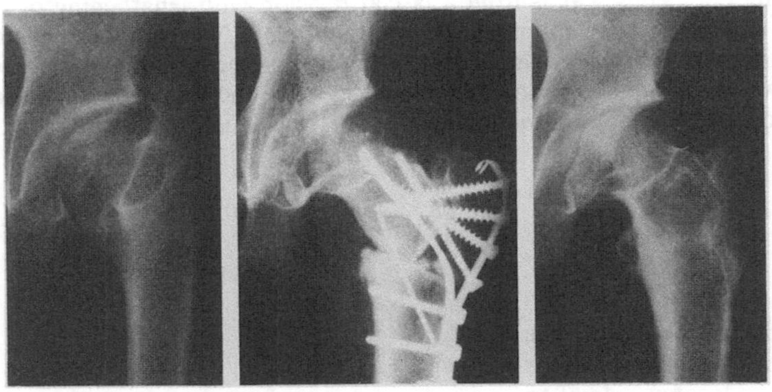

a **b** **c**

Fig. 20 a–c. Example of a double intertrochanteric osteotomy. **a** Shortening of the femoral neck secondary to epiphyseal plate injury in boy 16 years of age. **b** Eight weeks after surgery the original osteotomy surfaces are still clearly visible. The tension-band fixation was accomplished using a semitubular hook plate [2]. Kirschner wires stabilize the fragments against lateral displacement. **c** 18 Months after the double intertrochanteric osteotomy, bone remodeling has obliterated the osteotomy lines, and the proximal femur shows an essentially normal configuration

femoral neck segment and another at the inferior margin, the proximal end of the femur is divided into three fragments which can be independently displaced to lengthen the femoral neck and the femur as a whole.

References

1. Müller ME, Allgöwer M, Schneider R, Willenegger H (1977) Manual der Osteosynthese, 2. Auflage. Springer, Berlin Heidelberg New York
2. Wagner H (1977) Prinzipien der Korrekturosteotomie am Bein. Orthopäde 6:145–177

Lengthening and Shortening Osteotomies of the Diaphyses

I. Scheuer and A. Lies

Besides their cosmetic effect, leg length discrepancies have profound functional significance with regard to their effect on gait. Leg length discrepancies of 1 cm or less are easily compensated for and tolerated. But discrepancies of only 2–3 cm lead to postural changes, abnormalities of gait, and pain referrable to unphysiologic loads on the lower limb joints and especially on the spine, which must compensate for the pelvic obliquity during gait. Apparent or "functional" inequalities of leg length resulting from a flexion contracture of the knee or other causes must be distinguished from true posttraumatic leg length discrepancies, which are dealt with in the present article.

Leg length discrepancies may be treated conservatively by the use of orthopedic appliances or they may be corrected surgically. First it must be determined whether orthopedic care is adequate. Discrepancies of 3 cm or less are easily managed by applying elevation to the sole and heel of an ordinary shoe, possibly combined with a special insole [12]. However, this makes for a heavy and "fat looking" shoe that renders the short limb all the more conspicuous to the casual observer. Young women in particular are often willing to tolerate a significant inequality of limb length, and it is remarkable how well some women are able to affect a reasonably normal gait even with a discrepancy of 4–6 cm (Fig. 1).

In patients 40 years of age or older, the metaphysis is the preferred site for the surgical correction of severe leg length discrepancies. An osteotomy of the proximal femur, for example, tends to heal much more readily than an osteotomy of the diaphysis.

The first successful "aperiosteal lengthening of short femora in dwarfs" was described by Bier [4] at the German Surgeons' Congress of 1922. Several years later Abbott [1] reported on the operative lengthening of the tibia and fibula. In Bier's technique the femur was transversely osteotomized, and continuous longitudinal traction was applied to the limb. In young patients he observed excellent osseous bridging of the gradually elongating gap between the fragments. Some years later this principle was adopted by Anderson [2].

Numerous lengthening devices have been developed that permit application of a continuous external distraction to the osteotomized limb [7,9,11,13]. Basically these devices represent modifications of the external skeletal fixation frame. Wagner [14,15] modified the lengthening apparatus of Anderson and developed his own technique of diaphyseal lengthening that combines continuous distraction with the use of special fixation plates that bridge the gap between the fragments (Fig. 2).

Corrective Osteotomies of the Lower Extremity
Edited by G. Hierholzer, K. H. Müller

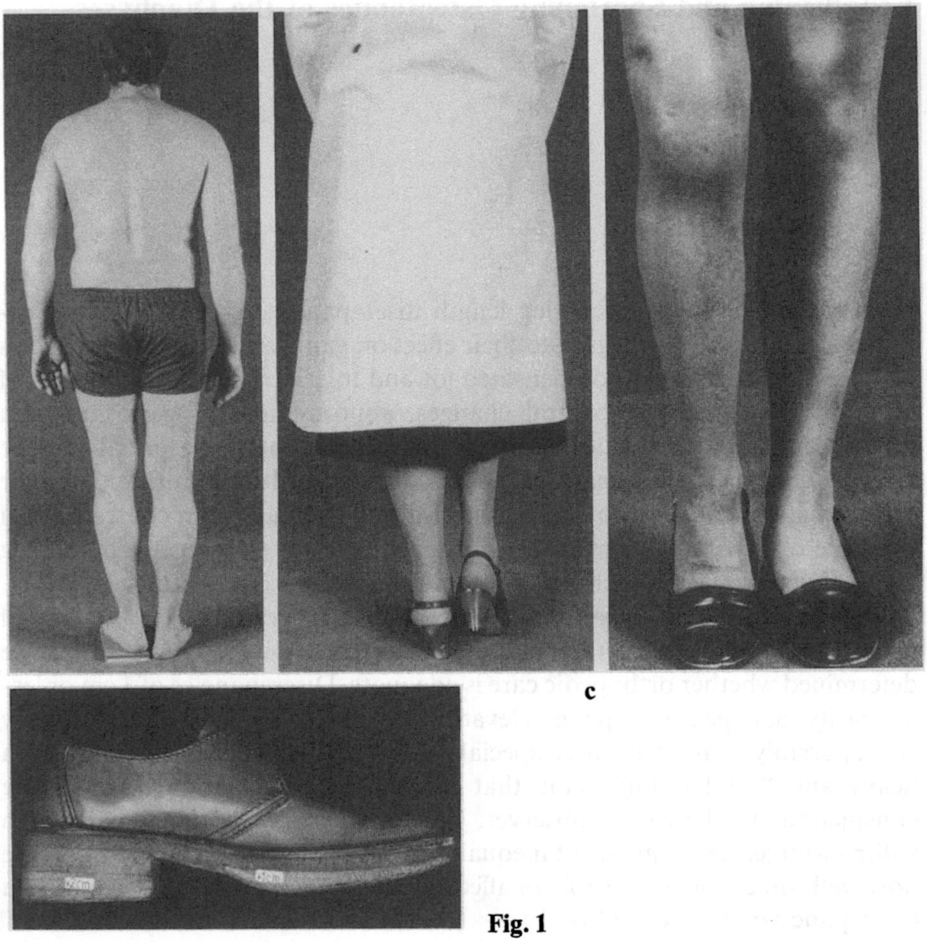

a d c b Fig. 1

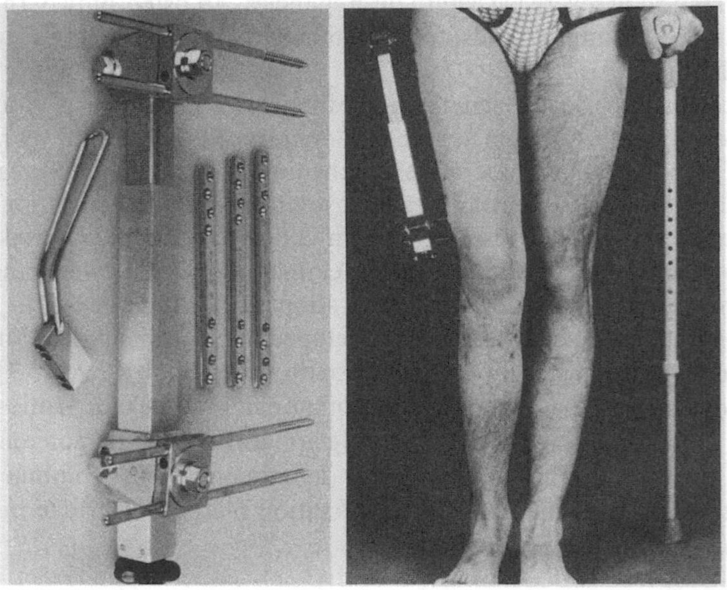

a b Fig. 2

Other types of lengthening devices have also been developed. One is a telescoping rod that fits within the intramedullary cavity of the diaphysis [3]. Gotz and Schellmann [6] designed an intramedullary rod equipped with an hydraulic cylinder that produced continuous distraction under the control of an external transducer. This technique did not gain wide acceptance, however. Witt and Jäger [17,18] have developed a fully implantable distraction device that effects continuous lengthening via a motor-driven angled-blade plate with sliding rails, a transmitter, and a receiver. This system is presently undergoing clinical trials.

Types of Osteotomy

Various types of osteotomy are known. Transverse, oblique and step-cut osteotomies may be used in the diaphyseal region. Each of these osteotomies has its risks and advantages. The transverse osteotomy is the easiest to perform, but it is relatively unstable and susceptible to varus, valgus and rotational malalignment. The oblique diaphyseal osteotomy is less prone to secondary loss of correction, because it provides better contact between the fragments. The step-cut osteotomy is the most difficult technically, but it ensures good bony contact and virtually eliminates the possibility of secondary angulation or rotation of the fragments. Numerous operative methods have been described. Lange [8], for example, osteotomized the femur with a stepped cut, stabilized it with a medullary nail, and applied traction until the desired limb length was obtained. Combined procedures are possible by excising a bone segment from the diaphysis of the longer limb and interposing it between the osteotomized bone ends of the shorter limb [10]. In femoral operations this can provide up to 7 cm of overall length correction. The disadvantage of this technique is that it requires shortening of the healthy leg, both legs must be operated on at once, and the patient is left with a duplication of the deformity.

Evaluation and Indications for Surgical Correction of Leg Length

It is known that a metaphyseal osteotomy heals more rapidly than a diaphyseal osteotomy. However, when there is significant posttraumatic angulation and shortening of the shaft, the diaphyseal lengthening osteotomy is preferred over the metaphyseal operation, because it avoids a statically

Fig. 1. a The board method of detecting leg length discrepancy. **b** Corrective shoe with elevation of sole and heel. **c,d** Woman with 7-cm leg length discrepancy after osteomyelitis of the upper tibia in childhood. The woman, now 48, refuses orthopedic aids, wears an ordinary shoe, and has a reasonably normal-appearing gait

Fig. 2. a The lengthening apparatus of Wagner and the Special plates used for internal fixation of the lengthened bone. **b** The distraction apparatus applied to the femur

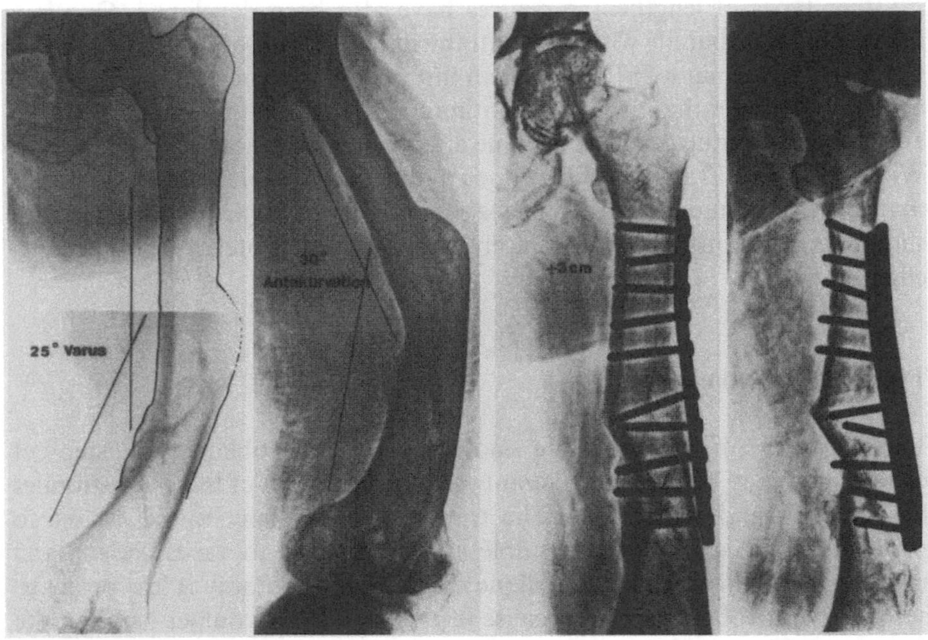

a **b**

Fig. 3. a Conservatively treated femoral shaft fracture that healed with severe shortening, varus and backward displacement in woman 72 years of age. **b** The straightening osteotomy corrected the angular deformity and also lengthened the femoral shaft by 3 cm

unfavorable S-shaped bowing of the femur while affording a length gain of 4–6 cm or more.

Whenever a leg length discrepancy is detected, a search should be made for associated deformities such as valgus or varus bowing of the shaft or rotational malalignment (Fig. 3). The complex deformity thus identified must be treated accordingly. Wagner [14] states that, as a general rule, leg length discrepancies should be treated surgically only if the coexisting deformities can also be corrected, the objective being to free the patient from reliance on orthopedic aids. If this is not possible, then both the length discrepancy and associted deformities should be corrected with orthopedic aids.

Clinically, leg length discrepancies are measured by placing a board under the foot and checking pelvic obliquity with a level. When the pelvis is horizontal, the thickness of the board equals the length discrepancy. Whole-leg roentgenograms in the standing, weight-bearing posture provide additional information on length discrepancy when magnification factors are taken into account. The exact site of the deformity can be identified on these films. Computed tomograms are helpful in disclosing occult rotational deformities of the femur or tibia.

When a posttraumatic leg length discrepancy of more than 4 cm is present in an adult, or more than 2 cm in a child, a decision must be made whether to lengthen the affected limb, shorten the unaffected limb, or perform both operations in either one or two stages. Numerous factors will determine

Table 1

Decision between lengthening and shortening depends on

A. General factors	B. Special factors
▶ Age of patient	▶ Fracture type
▶ Body height	▶ Progress of fracture healing
▶ Body proportions	▶ Soft tissues
▶ Anticipated effect on gait	▶ Scars
▶ Cosmetic result	▶ Number of prior operations
▶ Psychological aspects	▶ Local infections
	▶ Associated deformities

whether a lengthening operation or a shortening operation is most appropriate for a given patient. The healing potential of an osteotomy, especially in diaphyseal lengthening, decreases rapidly with advancing age, despite the use of adjunctive measures such as cancellous bone grafting. Thus, continuous leg lengthening should be completed before the end of the growth period if possible, and this operation should rarely be attempted in adults due to the risks that are involved.

Body height is another factor to be considered, and the safer shortening operation would be preferred in tall patients where preservation of height is not critical. In short patients, a lengthening operation would be the more reasonable option. Other considerations are body proportions, gait pattern, and the anticipated cosmetic result (Table 1). The operation of choice will also depend on local conditions, including the status of the soft tissues and the blood flow in the operative area. The number of prior operations and the amount and quality of scar tissue should also be taken into account. Multiple prior operations on the limb, a previous open fracture or previous local infection would make further surgery on the limb inadvisable, and equalization of leg lengths would be best accomplished by surgical shortening of the healthy limb (Fig. 4).

Leg Lengthening

When there is severe angular deformity of a diaphysis, up to 2–3 cm of length increase can be obtained with a straightening osteotomy. On the other hand, leg lengthening by osteotomy and distraction makes it possible to correct even greater length discrepancies with a high degree of accuracy. This operation may be performed in one or more stages. Continuous distraction often is applied over a period of weeks, using a rate of elongation of no more than 1.5 mm per day. After the desired distraction has been obtained, a second operation is performed in which the fragments are fixed internally with a plate. The distraction apparatus may then be removed.

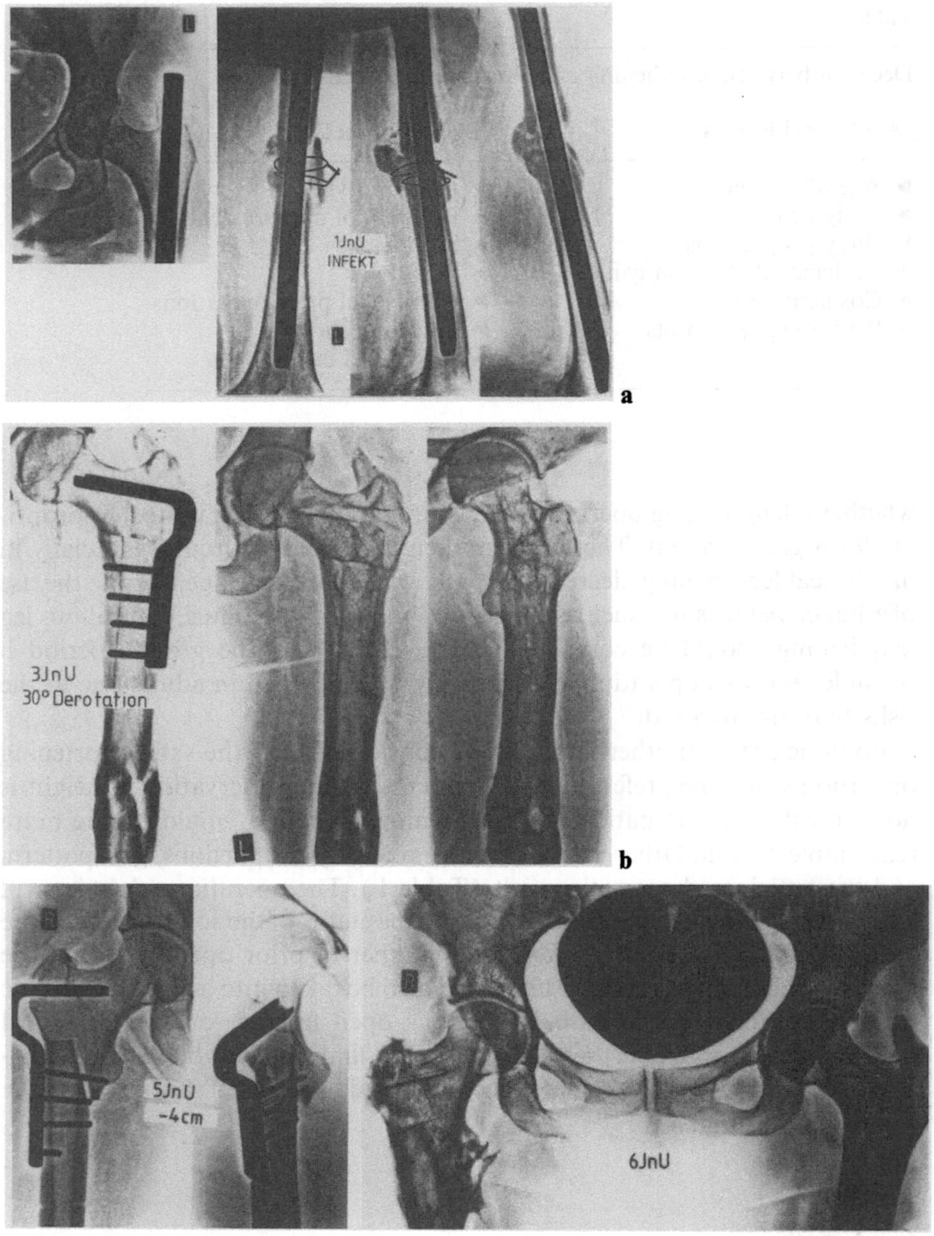

a b c d

Fig. 4. a Medullary nailing and cerclage of this femoral fracture with comminution of a 22-year-old woman was followed by infection and then finally by union with 4 cm of shortening and 30° of external rotation. **b** After the infection cleared, an intertrochanteric derotation osteotomy was performed away from the focus of infection. **c** Two years later a 4-cm shortening osteotomy was performed on the unaffected leg. **d** Result 6 years after the fracture

Table 2. Posttraumatic leg Shortening

Type I.	Deformities *without* bone loss	
	Lengthening favorable:	▶ Angulation ▶ Overlap
Type II.	Deformities *with* bone loss	
	Lengthening favorable: up to age 20	▶ After epiphyseal plate injury
	Difficult: up to age 40	▶ Collapsed bone fragments
	Very difficult: after age 40	▶ Osteomyelitis with bone loss

Two types of posttraumatic leg shortening are recognized (Table 2):

Type I leg shortening results from deformities without bone loss and is caused entirely by severe angulation or by overriding of the fragments. In these cases lengthening is effected by means of an oblique or step-cut osteotomy. The prospect for healing is good even in elderly patients, because the osteotomy can be designed to maintain secure interfragmental contact after lengthening. We always plate these osteotomies, because medullary nailing does not give sufficient rotational stability, especially in the femur (Fig. 5).

Type II leg shortening results from diaphyseal deformities that are associated with bone loss. The cause of the longitudinal defect is the premature traumatic closure of an epiphyseal plate, the collapse of a bone fragment, or osteomyelitis with bone loss. In adults this type of shortening, the defect produced by lengthening should always be grafted with cancellous bone. Owing to the presence of the lengthening defect and the absence of a bony buttress, union is slow and the prognosis uncertain. This contrasts with skeletally immature patients, who tend to recover well. With increasing age, the rate of complications such as bowing, fracture healing disturbances, and persistent bony defects rapidly increases (Fig. 6).

Shortening and lengthening operations on the tibia are technically more difficult than on the femur, where conditions are more favorable owing to the thickness and mobility of the soft tissue envelope. The soft-tissue status of the lower leg greatly limits the indications for surgery and the amount of lengthening that can be obtained. Nevertheless, there may be cases in which severe shortening of the tibia relative to the femur causes a gait disturbance sufficient to justify a lengthening osteotomy of the tibia.

Diaphyseal limb lengthening in one or more stages may be performed early during the first weeks after a fracture is sustained, or it may be done as a late procedure following the malunion of a fracture [Table 3].

The length increases indicated here, which are arranged by fracture type and location, represent the approximate lengthenings that can be obtained based on available experience. Even with a femoral fracture that is healing with deformity, a one-stage lengthening in excess of 6 cm is not advised due to the

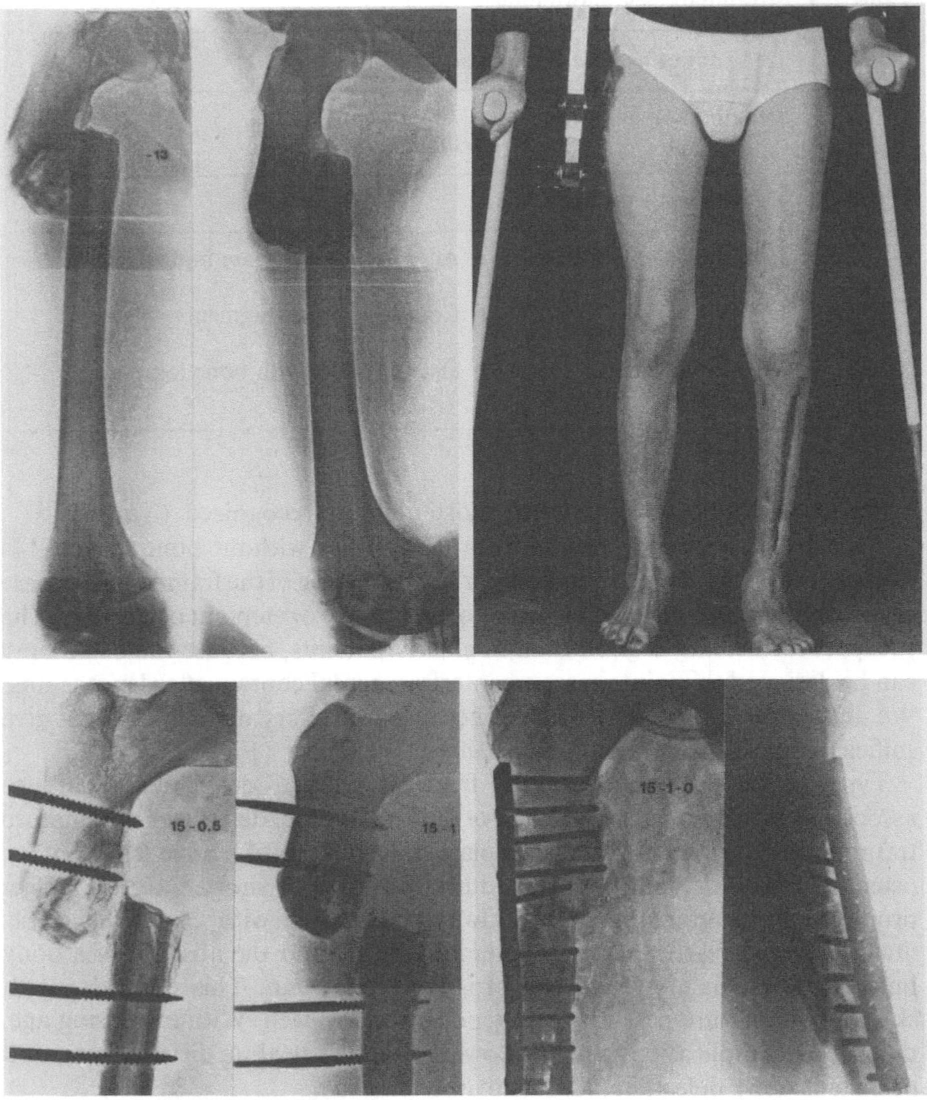

a c b d

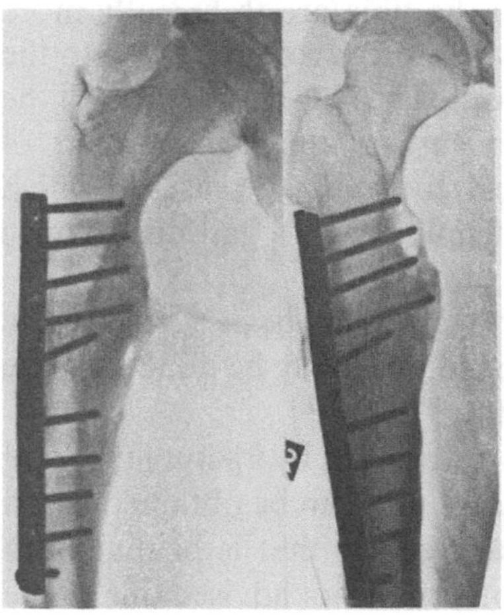

e

Fig. 5 a – e. Example of a type I posttraumatic leg shortening. **a** A femoral fracture in a 17-year-old man with multiple injuries healed with significant overriding of the fragments and 10 cm of shortening (13 months after injury). **b, c** The area of the malunion was osteotomized, and continuous distraction was applied. **d** After lengthening was completed, the bone was fixed with a compression plate. The picture of a resolved tibialis anterior syndrome following an open tibial fracture is evident in the left leg. **e** Bony consolidation 2 years after plating. The leg shows unrestricted joint function, good axial alignment, and 1.5 cm of residual shortening

Table 3. Diaphyseal Leg Lengthening

Early (healing fracture ≃ 8 wks)				Late (malunited fracture)		
A. One stage	Safe	Borderline	Not advised	Safe	Borderline	Not advised
Femur:	4 cm	6 cm	>6 cm	4 cm	–	>4 cm
Tibia:	2 cm	4 cm	>4 cm	2 cm	3 cm (tibialis anterior syndrome)	>4 cm
B. Multistage (continuous)						
Femur:	4–6 cm	?	?	6 cm	8 cm (knee function!)	?
Tibia:	4 cm	?	?	3 cm	4 cm ● ankle function ● tenotomy	?

danger of excessive soft-tissue scarring, muscle contractures and peripheral nerve complications. The tibia should not be lengthened more than 4 cm at one time following a recent fracture. Tibial lengthening significantly increases soft-tissue pressure in the muscle compartments of the lower leg and may cause severe neurovascular complications that are manifested clinically as a compartment syndrome.

Multistage or continuous leg lengthening following the established malunion of a fracture can accurately restore limb length in young patients. Length increases up to 6 cm can be safely achieved in the femur. In posttraumatic diaphyseal leg lengthening, soft-tissue conditions limit the amound of increase that can be obtained. Bands of scar tissue that interfere with the lengthening should be incised or divided. At least a temporary limitation of knee flexion may be expected to occur when femoral lengthening exceeds 8 cm. In the tibia, a length increase of only 4 cm leads to functional disturbances of the ankle joint. If an equinus deformity develops, secondary procedures such as an Achilles tenotomy will be required.

Complications about the osteotomy site become more frequent and severe as the length of the defect increases. This even applies to continuous distraction with the Wagner apparatus, especially in adults. The greater the amount of lengthening, the more tedious and time-consuming is the course of treatment, for bony bridging of the gap between the fragments is a very slow process that sometimes necessitates multiple cancellous bone grafts. Despite the subsequent application of lengthening plates in various positions (posterior, lateral, or even anterior), secondary medial or anterior displacement of the femur cannot always be avoided [5,16]. Plate fractures and dislodgments are common (Fig. 6). Before such a procedure is undertaken, the patient should be informed about these potential complications and about the prolonged course of treatment, which may span a period of months or even years. Unlike Wagner, we almost always observe a low-grade soft-tissue

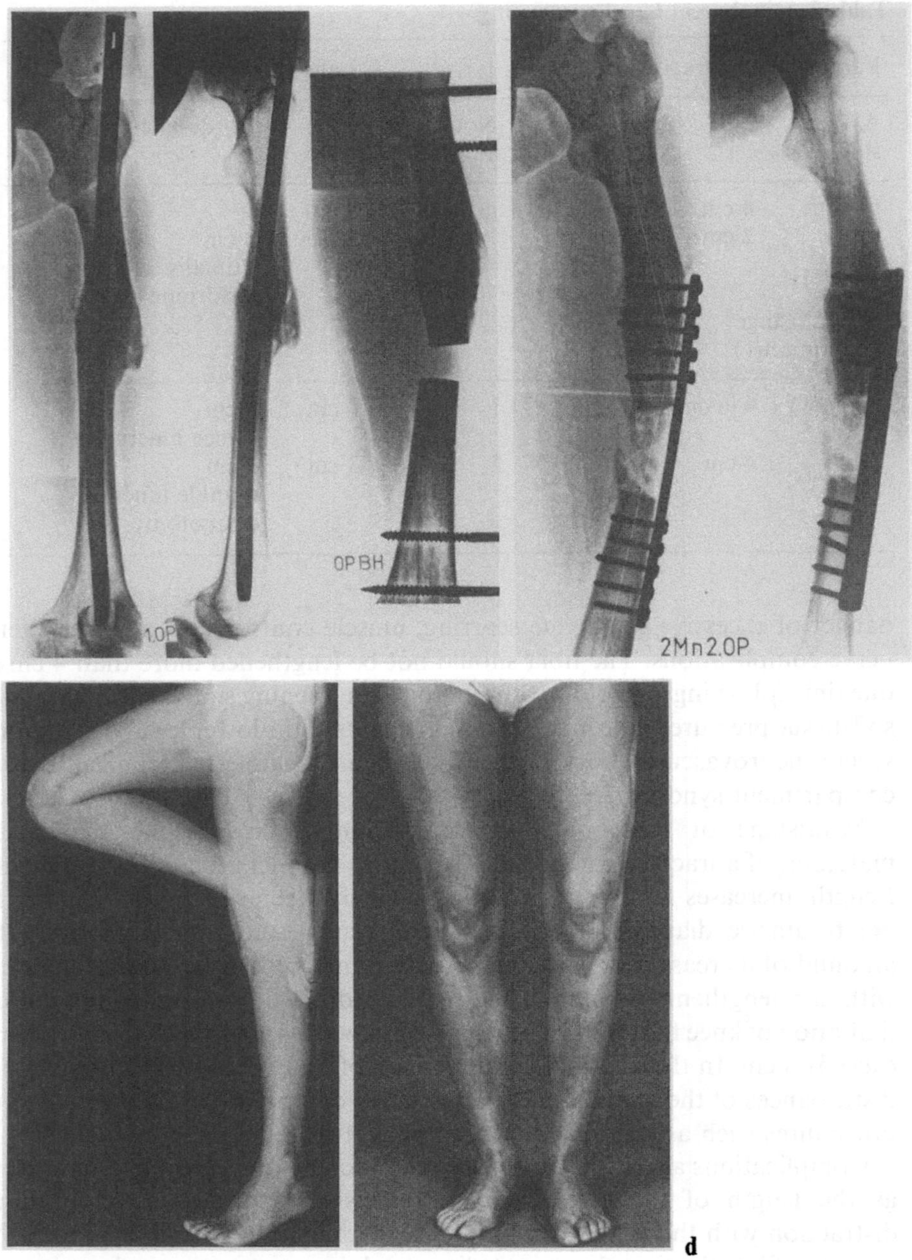

Fig. 6. a Femoral fracture that healed with shortening (type II) in woman 24 years of age, managed by transverse osteotomy and continuous distraction. **b** and **d** Two months after plating and cancellous grafting: proximal plate dislodgment and varus bowing of the femur. The fixation was revised and combined with cancellous grafting. **c** Function of the left leg at conclusion of treatment

infection or at least a soft-tissue irritation around the Schanz screws as continuous distraction is carried out. Even with regular screw tract care and the judicious use of skin relaxing incisions, the constant muscular unrest and rising pressure in the soft tissues around the Schanz screws lead to some degree of local infection that aggravates the risk of bone infection during subsequent plating of the fragments.

Leg Shortening

Diaphyseal leg shortenings are considerably less problematic than leg lengthenings, although their cosmetic result is not always as good. The main advantage of the shortening operation is that it can be done on the healthy limb. When faced with a disturbance of wound healing, bone infection, or impaired fracture healing, we prefer to shorten the uninvolved leg rather than attempt a risky lengthening procedure on the injured leg. The femur can be safely shortened by up to 4 cm. Shortening of 4–6 cm may be considered borderline due to the resultant loss of tension in soft tissues. Shortening of more than 10 cm is no longer advised in the femur, because the muscle and soft-tissue excess would create a compressing effect that would prevent primary wound closure and jeopardize active extension of the knee.

In the tibia, diaphyseal shortening of 2–3 cm is considered to safe, although tibial osteotomies are associated with a higher incidence of postoperative complications than femoral shortenings. The limited mobility of the soft tissues of the lower leg makes wound closure difficult. The increase in soft-tissue pressure poses a threat to the deep peroneal nerve in its course through the tense, compressed soft tissues. Furthermore, the disturbance of gait that results from a tibia that is too short relative to the femur makes it inadvisable to shorten the tibia by more than 4 cm.

Special considerations apply to osteomyelitis on the femur associated with bone loss. Cases are known in which a series of operations utilizing all possible modes of stabilization and their combinations (femoral plate, intramedullary nail, external half frame or joint-spanning frame, plaster) failed to bring the osteomyelitis under control (Fig. 7). Any instability will serve to perpetuate the infection. The bone becomes sequestered or sclerotic and, at least in the infected area, its blood supply becomes deficient. If no more autogenous cancellous bone is available at that point because of numerous prior grafts, it is possible to control the infection and promote fracture union by resecting the necrotic bone and plating the fragments under axial compression according to accepted technique. The overriding concern in these rare cases is to save the leg through surgical shortening and internal fixation. Cosmetic aspects relating to unsightly shortness of the limb are less important in these "hopeless" cases. Postoperatively, the patient will have to rely on orthopedic aids. In most cases the joint function of the affected limb is already seriously compromised after the numerous prior operations.

It should be stressed that this type of shortening operation of the femur is appropriate only in rare cases of intractable osteomyelitis. It is by no means

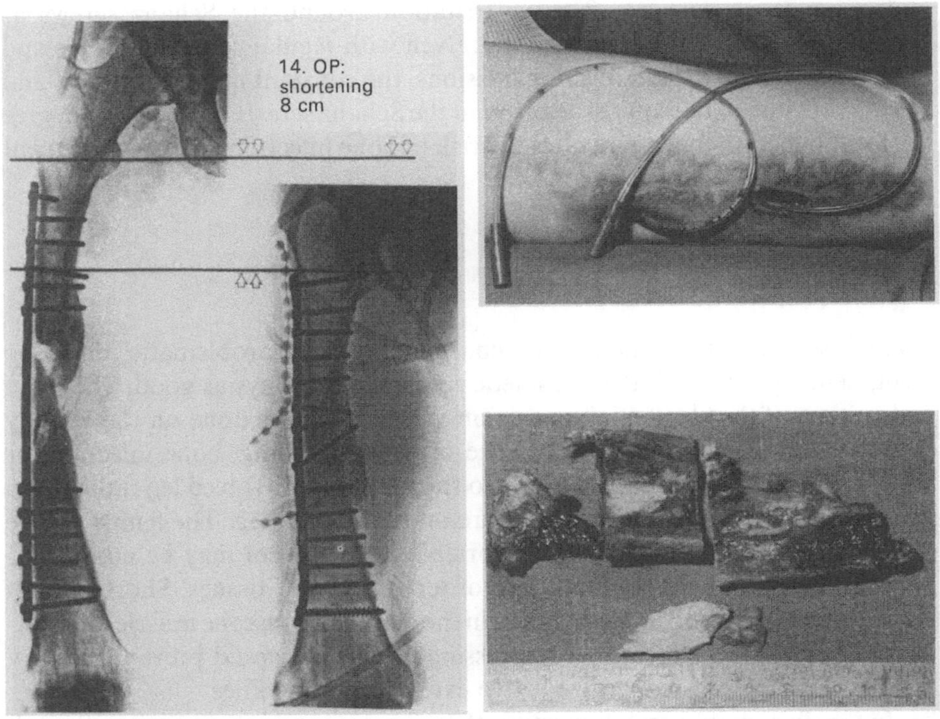

a b c

Fig. 7 a – c. Despite 13 operations in a 2-year period, the bone infection failed to clear and the fracture failed to unite in this 35-year-old man. **a** A 14th operation was done in which all necrotic bone was resected (**c**) and the bone was replated with 8 cm of shortening. Afterward the infection subsided, and progressive osseous bridging of the osteotomy was achieved. **b** Appearance of the soft tissues before the shortening operation

Table 4. Comparison of Surgical Lengthening and Shortening

	CORRECTION OF DEFORMITY	
	▲	
	(Affected leg)	Slow consolidation
Soft tissues	↑	Adjunctive surgery
Increased tension	Lengthening	● Cancellous grafting
→ restricted movement		● Replating
	or	● Tendon lengthening
		→ Younger patients
Decreased tension	Shortening	Quick consolidation
→ restricted movement	↓	Operation safer and easier
	(Healthy leg)	No adjunctive surgery
		→ Also suited for older patients
	▼	
	"Bilateral deformity"	

the treatment of choice for osteomyelitis of the femur. It should be considered only when all other treatment measures have been tried and have proved unsuccessful.

A sparing resection may also be considered for a highly unstable avascular nonunion if it will create the conditions necessary for a stable internal fixation.

Today several effective procedures are available for the operative correction of significant posttraumatic leg length discrepancies. Each type of operation, diaphyseal leg lengthening and shortening, has its special indications, advantages and disadvantages (Table 4). By knowing the different procedures that are available, the surgeon will be able to plan a treatment suited to the needs of the individual patient. Taking into account the age of the patient, local conditions and the desired result, the surgeon must decide whether to choose the more difficult, more risky, and more time-consuming lengthening operation or the technically easier, safer and less time-consuming shortening operation. He must understand that the latter procedure will produce a bilateral deformity, and that this may have noticeable effects on body proportions.

References

1. Abbott LC (1927) The operativ lengthening of the tibia and fibula. J Bone Joint Surg 9:128
2. Anderson WV (1952) Leg lengthening. J Bone Joint Surg 34:150
3. Bailey RW, Dubow HI (1963) Studies of longitudinal bone growth resulting in an extensible nail. Surg Forum 14:455
4. Bier A (1922) Aussprache 46. Tg. Dt. Ges. f. Chirurgie. Arch Klin Chir 121:119
5. Cisar J, Rehm J, Schumacher W, Walter E (1979) Zur Varusverbiegung des Femur bei der Verlängerungsosteotomie. Aktuel Traumatol 9:105
6. Götz J, Schellmann WD (1975) Kontinuierliche Verlängerung des Femur bei intramedullärer Stabilisierung. Arch Orthop Unfallchir 82:305
7. Hähnel H (1977) Die Distraktionsepiphyseolyse – erste Erfahrungen bei der operativen Beinverlängerung nach Ilisarow. Beitr Orthop Traumatol 24:594
8. Lange M (1962) Orthopädische-chirurgische Operationslehre, 2. Aufl. Bergmann, München
9. Leong JCI, Ma RYP, Clark JA, Cornish LS, Yau ACMC (1979) Viscoelastic behavior of tissue in lengthening by distraction. Clin Orthop 139:102
10. Lezius A (1947) Der stabile osteoplastische Ersatz großer Knochendefekte der unteren Gliedmaßen. Chirurg 17/18:162
11. Lukeš J (1965) Möglichkeiten der Unterschenkelverlängerung. Beitr Orthop Traumatol 12:142
12. Rettig HM (1977) Indikationen zur operativen oder konservativen Behandlung von Beinlängendifferenzen. Schriften Unfallmed Tagung Landesverb Gewerbl Berufsgen 29:33
13. Soukup P, Hofmann W (1977) Mitteilung über die Anwendung einer Gleitplatte bei der Verlängerungsosteotomie. Beitr Orthop Traumatol 24:232
14. Wagner H (1971) Operative Beinverlängerung. Chirurg 42:260
15. Wagner H (1977) Prinzipien der Korrekturosteotomie am Bein. Orthopäde 6:145
16. Wagner H (1982) Ermüdungsfrakturen nach der Verlängerungsosteotomie des Oberschenkels. Orthopäde 11:86

17. Witt AN, Jäger M (1977) Tierexperimentelle Ergebnisse mit einem voll implantierbaren Distraktionsgerät zur operativen Beinverlängerung. Arch Orthop Unfallchir 88:273
18. Witt AN, Jäger M (1978) Die operative Oberschenkelverlängerung mit einem voll implantierbaren Distraktionsgerät. Arch Orthop Trauma Surg 92:291

Complications after Corrective Osteotomies: Persistent Deformity, Nonunion, Infection

S. Decker and H. Strosche

Despite many improvements in techniques of operative and nonoperative fracture management, posttraumatic deformities are not uncommon and can cause serious problems in the lower extremity due to the large static and dynamic loads that exist in that region. The necessity of correcting posttraumatic deformities of the lower extremity is well established, for even small deviations of axial alignment can change the lever arms of the muscles and alter the physiologic positions of the joints, creating an incongruity that leads to osteoarthritis.

The risks and potential complications of corrective osteotomies are similar to those encountered in general surgery of the musculoskeletal system. The main difference with respect to operations for the treatment of acute injuries, for example, is that many patients selected for corrective osteotomy may be only mildly symptomatic or even asymptomatic, and they must be convinced of the need for corrective surgery whose intent is prophylactic rather than curative. Given this situation, it is essential that the patient be counseled as to the possible complications of a corrective osteotomy, for the level of expectations and cooperativeness of the patient will have a significant bearing on the end result, especially in elective procedures.

Thus, the prospect for success in a corrective osteotomy sould be carefully weighed against the risks and should be thoroughly discussed with the patient, giving attention to the local and general features of the specific case. To avoid serious complications such as persistent or secondary deformity, nonunion, and postoperative infection, the surgeon should be highly experienced and have a clear understanding of the functional anatomy and biomechanics of the musculoskeletal system.

As mentioned above, posttraumatic deformities are relatively common after fractures, and a large percentage of them are serious enough to warrant treatment.

A total of 389 corrective osteotomies of the lower extremity were performed at the Bergmannsheil Surgical Clinic in Bochum over a 10-year period. 285 of these operations were performed in patients with deformity or osteoarthritis secondary to trauma.

Several instances of serious local complications occurred in this series, some of which caused permanent damage of necessitated secondary surgery. There were six persistent or secondary deformities, five postoperative infections, two vascular injuries, one irreversible peroneal nerve palsy, and two nonunions, one of which was associated with avascular necrosis of the femoral head. We disregard early, local complications such as hematomas, seromas, wound

Corrective Osteotomies of the Lower Extremity
Edited by G. Hierholzer, K. H. Müller

dehiscence, necrotic wound margins, swelling, etc. that were managed primarily and left no sequelae.

Of the six iatrogenic deformities that were noted, four were corrected by a second operation. One patient declined to have a second operation, and in the remaining case of a failed lengthening osteotomy it was felt that a previous infection contraindicated further surgery. The five postoperative infections resolved after repeated surgical interventions. Three of these patients were left with significant residual disability of the affected limb in addition to extensive scarring. Both vascular injuries were discovered at operation and were immediately repaired with sutures. The one case of irreversible peroneal nerve palsy was caused by pressure from a plaster dressing applied after surgery. In one of the two nonunions the occcurred, a second operation is pending. The other was a subcapital nonunion with avascular necrosis of the femoral head, which was managed by total hip arthroplasty.

Below we shall present several examples illustrating the complications that may arise after corrective osteotomies of the lower extremity. Some were taken from the Bergmannsheil series and others from medical evaluation files and the files of the Friederik Foundation in Hannover.

One of the most frequent corrective osteotomies of the upper femur is the intertrochanteric osteotomy for nonunion or posttraumatic deformity of the femoral neck [2]. The reasons for failure after this procedure may relate to errors of indication or errors of operative technique. While a total hip arthroplasty would be preferred over a proximal femoral osteotomy in an elderly patient, the osteotomy would be preferred in the middle-aged patient who shows no evidence of avascular necrosis.

The example presented here (Fig. 1) shows a nonunion of the femoral neck that developed after the faulty operative treatment of a medial femoral neck fracture. While an intertrochanteric repositioning osteotomy was definitely indicated and was performed, several technical errors occured that were at

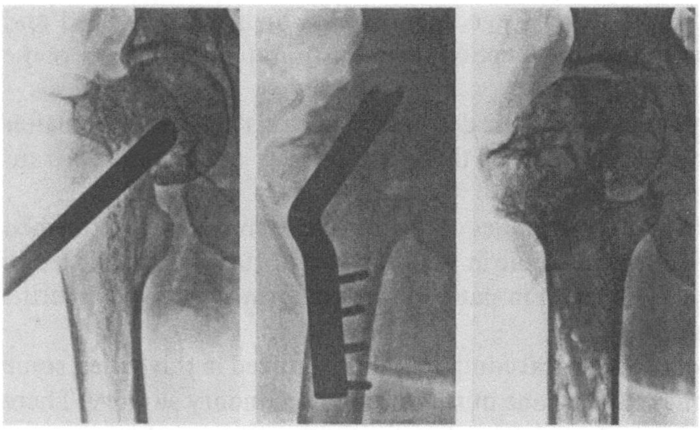

a b c

Fig. 1. a Nonunion of the femoral neck following inadequte operative treatment of a medial femoral neck fracture. **b** Faulty intertrochanteric repositioning osteotomy. **c** Unsatisfactory result two years after osteotomy

least partly responsible for the unsatisfactory roentgenographic result and poor functional outcome: 1) The tip of the blade engaged the upper hemisphere of the femoral head instead of the lower hemisphere; 2) the distance between the proximal osteotomy and site of blade entry was too small, allowing the blade to penetrate the osteotomy surface; 3) the femoral shaft was displaced medially instead of laterally, resulting in an undesired lateral shift of the mechanical axis that placed abnormal loads on the distal joints; 4) an external rotation deformity of 40° was present postoperatively; 5) the 1.5 cm of leg shortening caused by medial and distal angulation of the femoral head was not corrected as it should have been, but was actually increased to 2.5 cm by the surgery.

In retrospect, it is clear that the foregoing technical errors could have been avoided by precise planning and by careful referral to preoperative drawings indicating the steps of the procedure in their proper sequence. Planning of this type, which must take into account the normal axial relations of the limb, is the key to avoiding complications referrable to errors of technique.

Another of the many errors that are possible in intertrochanteric osteotomies is illustrated by the case of a medial femoral neck fracture. First, the indication for a primary corrective osteotomy in this case was questionable. Second, the blade of the implant was too long and was placed too far proximally and anteriorly. After the plate was replaced in a second operation, a segmental avascular necrosis developed, and the blade again perforated the femoral head. In a third operation an attempt was made to ameliorate the situation by repositioning the blade and supplementing the fixation with a cancellous screw. Even then the situation failed to improve significantly, and the result was a nonunion of the femoral neck with complete avascular necrosis that necessitated total hip arthroplasty.

It is known that even a technically flawless internal fixation or osteotomy for a medial femoral neck fracture has a relatively high association with late complications in the form of nonunions and avascular necrosis. The incidence of these complications is variously reported in the literature as being between 20% and 50% [5]. Nevertheless, it is apparent that an already doubtful prognosis can be made even worse by technical errors of the type described.

Leg length discrepancies give rise to compensatory mechanisms which place unphysiologic loads on the joints of the lower limb and spine. Some type of correction is mandatory in such cases and may be done conservatively by applying elevation to the shoe or operatively through surgical lengthening of the affected leg or sortening of the unaffected leg [4].

In the present case (Fig. 2) the intramedullary nailing of a fracture of the proximal femoral shaft was followed by a telescope-like impaction of the fragments, causing the limb to become shortened by 4 cm. The femur can be lengthened up to 4 cm at one time without risk of neurovascular injury, and this was done here by means of a step-cut osteotomy followed by distraction with the Müller apparatus. The distal step of the osteotomy broke off during the operation, the desired amount of lengthening could not be obtained, and varus angulation of the femur developed. In addition, a pyogenic infection became manifest in the early postoperative period.

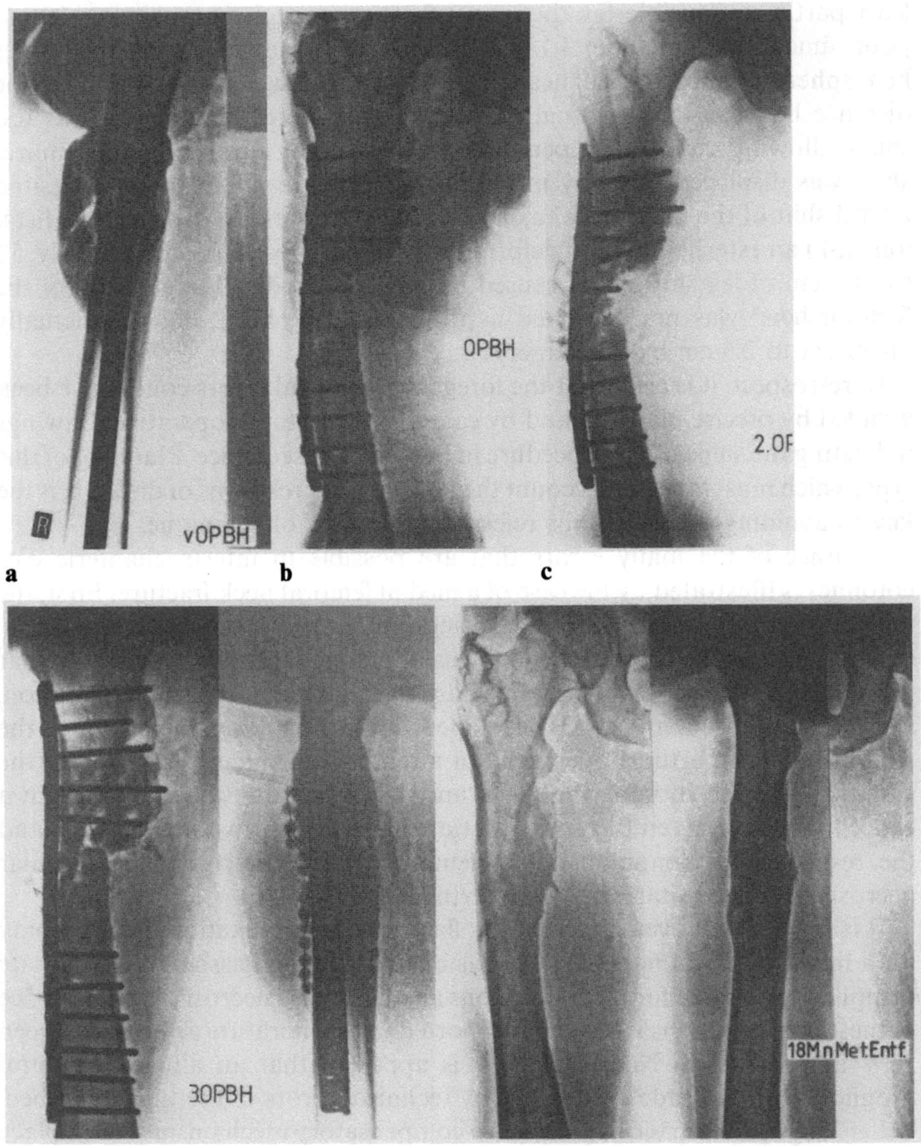

a b c

d e

Fig. 2. a Limb shortened 4 cm after intramedullary nailing of the femur. **b** Unilateral lengthening osteotomy. **c** Early pyogenic infection with varus deformity; re-exposure, implantation of gentamycin-impregnated PMMA beads. **d** Third operation: sequestrectomy, cancellous bone grafting, and revisionary fixation with correction of varus deformity, sacrificing the length previously gained. **e** 18 Months after removal of metal: Healing of the osteotomy and infection with 4 cm of residual shortening

At first reoperation the plate was left in place, and the screws were simply retightened. Two months later a revisionary fixation was carried out, at which time the varus deformity was corrected, but some limb length had to be sacrificed. The infection was brought under control, and consolidation of the osteotomy endued. However, the original 4 cm of shortening was still present, and so, quite apart from the complicated course, the lengthening osteotomy must be regarded as a failure.

A lengthening osteotomy of the lower extremity, whether done in one stage or by continuous distraction with the Wagner apparatus, is generally more technically complex than a shortening osteotomy of the contralateral limb and thus carries a higher risk of complications. In considering treatment, the surgeon should carefully weigh the possibility of shortening the healthy leg and should discuss this option with the patient.

One 24-year-old woman whose femoral shaft fracture was treated by primary intramedullary fixation was left with 4.5 cm of limb shortening combined with an external rotation deformity of 45°. The patient insisted, mostly for cosmetic reasons, on a lengthening osteotomy of the shortened left femur. This was effected by continuous distraction with the Wagner apparatus following osteotomy and correction of the rotational deformity. At the end of the distraction phase the fragments were plated in a position of marked varus, which increased with passage of time and led to loosening of the proximal screws. The fragments were realigned and fixed with a longer plate, and additional cancellous bone grafts were applied. However, varus bowing recurred, and a fall left the patient with severe pain and evidence of plate loosening, necessitating yet another operation. Eighteen months after osteotomy the fragments still have not consolidated. Part of the initial 4.5-cm length increase was lost during the subsequent operations, and there is marked residual varus deformity. This case dramatically illustrates the serious problems that can arise during bony consolidation after lengthening.

Leg length discrepancies after femoral fractures are frequently accompanied by angular or rotational deformities. A 42-year-old woman who sustained a supracondylar femoral fracture exhibited 3 cm of leg sortening, marked varus deformity, and slight backward displacement in association with delayed fracture union (Fig. 3). The osteotomy performed one year after injury apparently was designed to correct only the varus deformity. It neglected the limb shortening, which can be particularly detrimental about the knee, although a length correction would have been relatively easy to accomplish via an oblique displacement osteotomy. During passive postoperative extension of the knee joint, the patella engaged against anterior projecting bone, which was removed in a subsequent operation. The patient was still left with a 20° deficit of active extension and 3 cm of limb shortening, and so the result cannot be considered satisfactory.

Angular deformities of the tibia are just as damaging to neighboring joints as femoral deformities – varus more so than valgus [1]. Varus deformities of the proximal and distal tibia of 5° or more, and varus deformities of the shaft of 10° or more, are considered to be an indication for prophylactic corrective osteotomy [3].

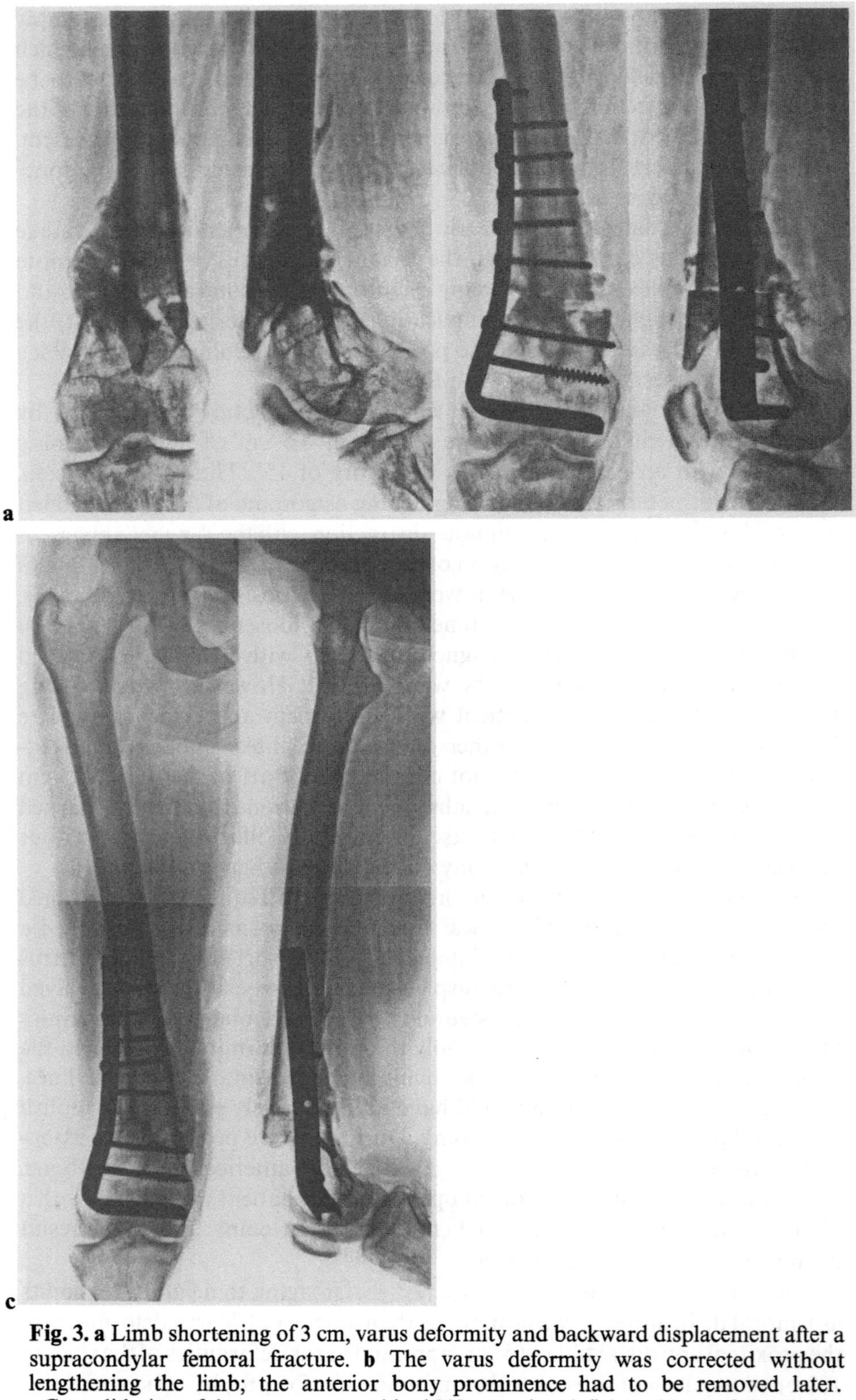

a b c

Fig. 3. a Limb shortening of 3 cm, varus deformity and backward displacement after a supracondylar femoral fracture. **b** The varus deformity was corrected without lengthening the limb; the anterior bony prominence had to be removed later. **c** Consolidation of the osteotomy; residual 20° extension deficit and 3 cm of shortening

A corrective osteotomy in a 50-year-old man was performed for a "minimal" indication, i.e., a distal tibial varus deformity of 5°. Osteotomy and plate fixation resulted in a valgus angulation of approximately 5°, which the surgeon obviously had not intended, even though this amound to valgus is insufficient to warrant correction.

Even with precise planning and execution, an "overcorrection" of this kind can easily occur if too much primary tension is applied to the plate used to stabilize the osteotomy. One such error (Fig. 4) occurred in a 51-year-old woman who had a corrective osteotomy for a 15° valgus deformity of the tibia. Apparently the overcorection was not detected on intraoperative roentgenograms, but it was discovered on an AP film taken two months after surgery. This was accompanied by a marked recurvatum deformity, which also was missed intraoperatively because the operator failed to obtain a lateral roentgenogram.

The complications described thus far were mainly the result of inadequate planning and faulty technique. Most were avoidable. While it is true that the

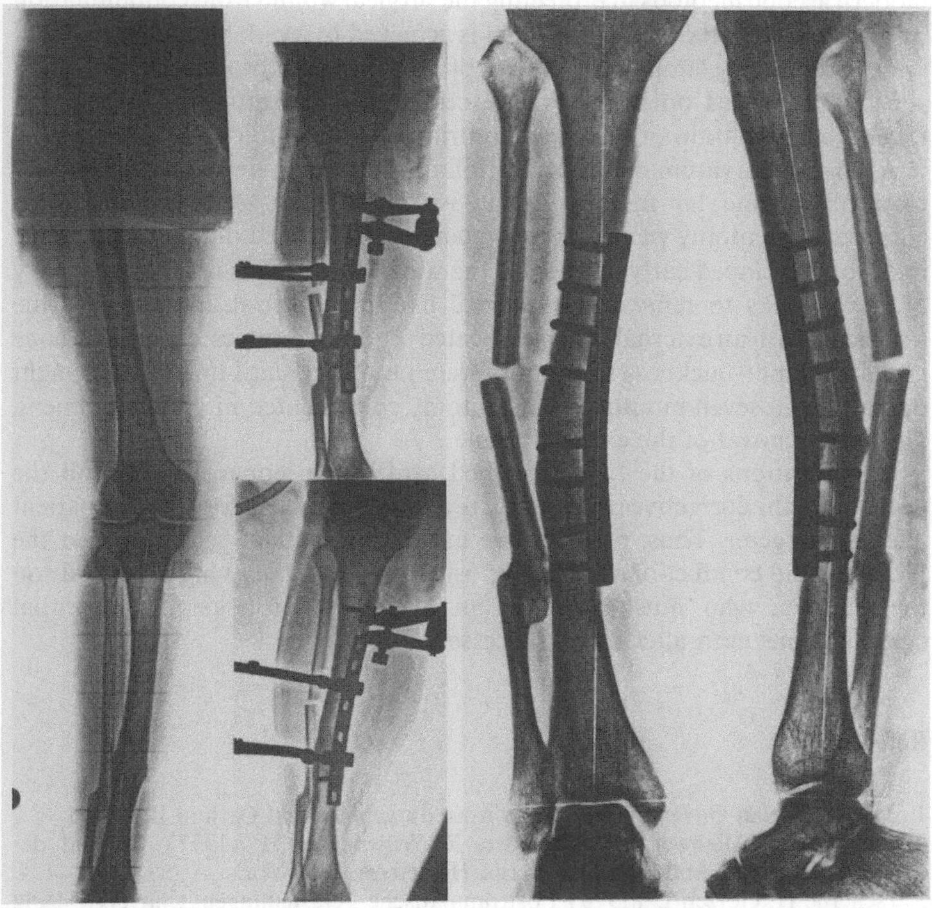

a b

Fig. 4. a Tibial valgus deformity of 15°, corrected by osteotomy and compression plating. **b** "Overcorrection" caused by excessive plate tension; recurvatum is also present

outcome of an operative procedure cannot be predicted with absolute certainty, the danger of complications of the type described above can be virtually eliminated through proper planning and conduct of the corrective osteotomy. This includes all diagnostic measures that are relevant to patient selection, such as special radiographic techniques, as well as detailed preoperative drawings indicating the operative steps and end result of the osteotomy, and an experienced surgeon who understands the functional anatomy and biomechanics of the musculoskeletal system.

The very fact that corrective osteotomies for posttraumatic deformity must be carried out on a previously traumatized and possibly dystrophic limb already poses a greater surgical risk than the operative treatment of most acute injuries, for example, and the patient should be made aware of this. The prospect for a successful osteotomy depends on local osseous and soft-tissue conditions as well as on such general factors as the age of the patient, coexisting disorders, and occupational habits.

Perhaps the most serious complication of skeletal surgery, postoperative infection, cannot be excluded with absolute certainty, despite the efficacy of modern aseptic methods in protecting the surgical wound from contamination by airborne bacteria. The asepsis that is achieved by available techniques and systems, including laminar airflow, is optimum but not absolute. Other factors such as prolonged operating time, excessive traumatization of tissues, and excessive denudation of bone can contribute to the etiology of infection.

A varus-recurvatum deformity with limb shortening developed secondary to a tibial condylar fracture in a 23-year-old man. A two-dimensional corrective osteotomy was accurately planned and carried out, but a pyogenic infection developed early in the postoperative course. This made it necessary at three weeks to remove the internal fixation material and stabilize the fragments with an external frame. Repeated sequestrectomies, cancellous bone grafts and split-thickness skin grafts were necessary until finally, after eight operations in seven months, the osteotomy consolidated in good alignment, allowing removal of the external frame.

Complications of the type described, which can jeopardize or spoil the outcome of the corrective procedure, are a serious problem for both the patient and the surgeon. Thus, peroperative evaluation, patient selection, and the planning and conduct of a corrective osteotomy place very high demands on the surgeon, who must maintain an awareness of risks and potential complications even after many successes.

References

1. Bouillet R, van Gaver P (1961) Arthrose du genou. Acat Orthop Belg 27:5
2. Müller ME, Allgöwer M, Schneider, R, Willenegger H (1977) Manual der Osteosynthese, 2 Aufl. Springer, Berlin Heidelberg New York
3. Tscherne H, Gotzen L (1978) Posttraumatische Fehlstellungen. Chir Ggw 4a:52
4. Wagner H (1972) Technik und Indikation der operativen Verkürzung und Verlängerung von Ober- und Unterschenkel. Orthopäde 1:59
5. Weber BG, Cech O (1973) Pseudarthrosen. Huber, Bern Stuttgart Wien

Corrective Osteotomies of the Lower Extremity in the Presence of Infection

C. Burri and O. Wörsdörfer

The goal in the treatment of trauma patients with fractures is the complete restoration of anatomy and function. In fractures, this is most readily achieved by adequate internal fixation. But the most frequent and dreaded complication of internal fixation is infection. Posttraumatic osteitis, in turn, remains a great therapeutic challenge and makes the control of infection the first priority of treatment, even at the expense of limb shortening or deformity. It is our view that even in patients with posttraumatic osteitis, serious attention should be given to the possibility of a complete functional and anatomic restoration as stated above.

The surgical treatment of bone infection consists of stabilization, debridement, local therapy, and repair of the defect. The purpose of these measures is to control the infectious process, make the bone stable under loading, and reconstruct bony anatomy if at all possible.

The *stabilization* of an infected bone by external splinting was a practice known to the ancient Egyptians. Celsus, in the first century A.D., was the first author to describe the radical debridement of necrotic or affected tissue, while the technique of local irrigation was introduced by Sir Henri de Mondeville (1260–1320). Numerous methods have been described for repairing an existing or iatrogenic defect: Senn was probably the first, in 1889, to recommend the use of bone transplants in the form of decalcified chips. With the introduction of autologous cancellous bone by Matti in 1932, this treatment method assumed basically the form that is familiar today.

We may persume that the first three steps in the surgical treatment of osteitis are generally known and recognized, noting that suction irrigation can today be replaced by the use of PMMA beads [3] or other antibacterial agents such as Taurolin [1,4]. We shall focus our attention on the problem of bone grafting in the management of osteitis. Two factors are of fundamental importance: the recipient bed and the bone graft [2,5]. With regard to the bed, it is obvious that a range of conditions may exist between the least favorable case of instability, deficient blood flow and active infection and the most favorable case of stability, good blood flow and very low-grade infection. The graft may consist of heterologous, homologous or autologous material in the form of cortex or cancellous bone. We share the view of many authors that only a graft of highest biological quality composed of autologous cancellous bone or autologous corticocancellous bone (e.g., for femoral defects) is appropriate for osseous infection, and that there is a reasonable prospect of incorporation only if the recipient bone is stable, adequately perfused, and free of aggressive infection

Corrective Osteotomies of the Lower Extremity
Edited by G. Hierholzer, K. H. Müller

[2,5]. Hence a bone graft should be attempted in the presence of osteitis only if favorable conditions have been established in the recipient bed.

The question of stability is moot in the consolidated fracture, but it is extremely important in unstable situations such as an infected nonunion with bone loss. In long tubular bones that have good muscular and soft-tissue coverage, stability is best achieved by plate osteosynthesis. In the tibia or any other area with a precarious soft-tissue envelope, external skeletal fixation is preferred. It need hardly be said that the establishment of normal length and axial alignment of the lower extremity is critical in cases of this type.

The second important step is debridement, at which time all devitalized bone is resected to a healthy, bleeding surface.

Finally, the infectious process should be controlled before bone grafts are applied. This may be accomplished by means of open suction irrigation [6] or by the implantation of PMMA beads. The latest innovation in this area is the use of denatured collagen impregnated with an antibacterial agent such as Taurolin. This new method has two main advantages over the widely used PMMA beads:

1. Taurolin is bactericidal and does not induce resistance; this contrasts with reports of increasing bacterial resistance to gentamycin.
2. The collagen mass with the Taurolin completely fills the infected cavity, and the Taurolin is slowly released as the collagen dissolves. This obviates the need for removal of the antibiotic material, which is usually necessary with PMMA and often necessitates anesthesia. In the past 2 years we have treated more than 150 patients with this agent, and the results have been comparable to those obtained with PMMA beads [4].

In most cases the three preliminary treatment measures described above will be sufficient to transform an aggressive bone infection with instability and poor blood flow into a bed of good quality that can incorporate and remodel an autologous cancellous graft. If these measures also effect a satisfactory anatomic restoration, the result after bony consolidation will be a useful limb in which recovery is virtually complete.

However, if the osteitis is cured but residual deformities persist which impair the function of the limb either directly or indirectly through unphysiologic loading of the distal joints, serious consideration should be given to a corrective osteotomy.

In these cases it is generally preferable to avoid the original focus of the infection and perform the osteotomy in uninvolved bone (Fig. 1).

In cases where instability coexists with active bone infection, it is preferable to correct the deformity at the site of the infection, provided this can be done concurrently with stabilization. In young patients with leg length discrepancies we accomplish this by using the Wagner apparatus both for limb lengthening and for external skeletal fixation. Of course this increases the size of the osseous defect that must be filled later, which in turn places greater demands on the recipient bed and especially on the necessary length of the bone graft.

When limb deformity exists in the presence of chronic infection, and stable bridging of the affected bone has failed to occur during the course of treatment,

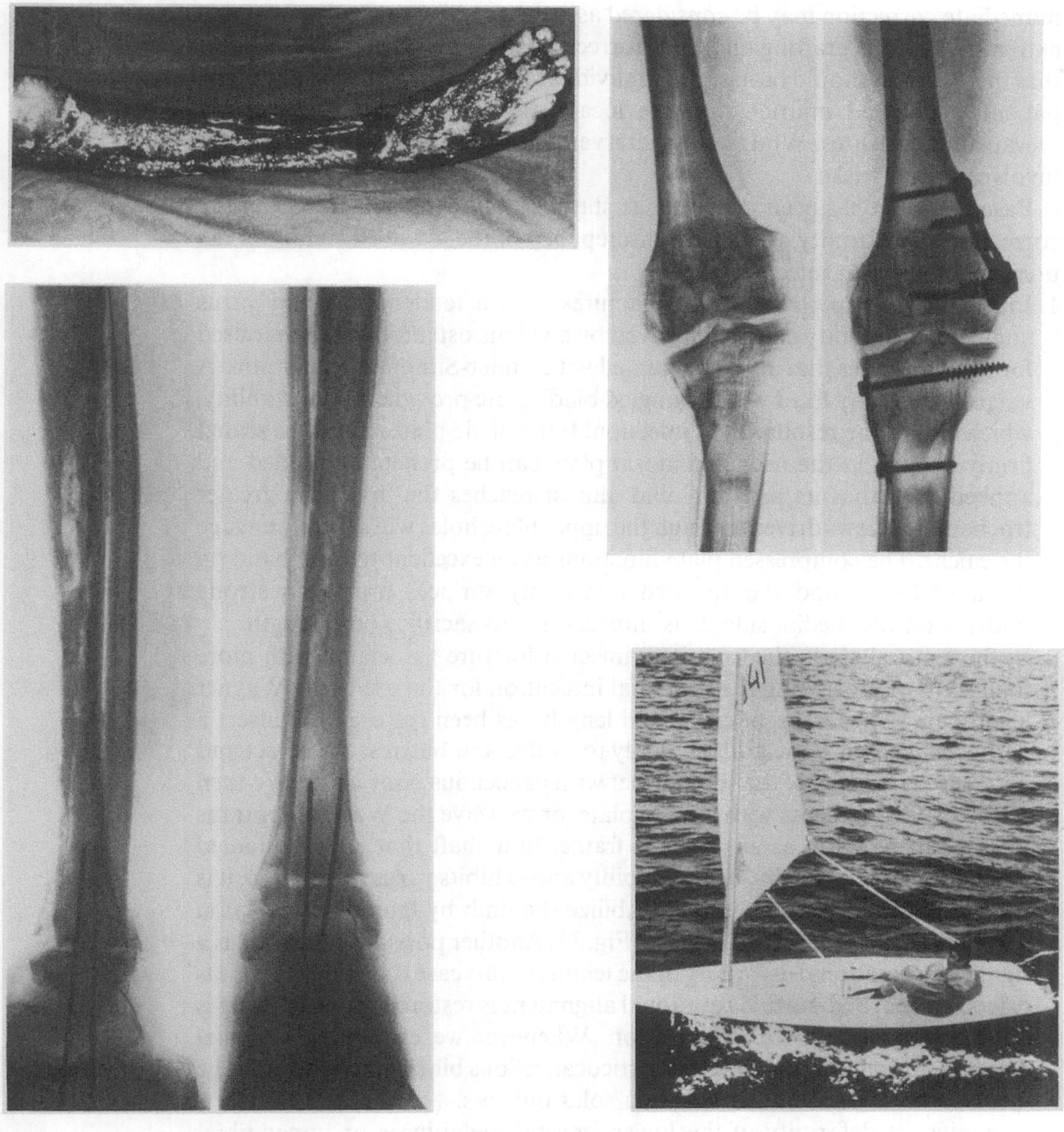

a b c d

Fig. 1 a–d. Osteotomy after clearing of infectious process about the knee. **a** Appearance of the limb at referral (patient had been run over by a bus). Tibial necrosis with pyogenic gram-negative infection of the lower leg. **b** Roentgenograms taken as referral, showing transfixion of the ankle and subtalar joints (open dislocation); the proximal and distal epiphyseal plates are involved by infection. **c** After infection subsided, deformity at the knee was corrected by valgus osteotomy of the femur and varus osteotomy of the tibia. The osteotomies were opened, and autologous grafts were inserted to equalize leg lengths. **d** The young patient is again active athletically

immediate correction may be considered as an alternative to creating a stable extremity by bone grafting and then correcting the limb secondarily. We feel that this decision should be based on individual factors including the age of the patient, associated injuries, and the localization and extent of necessary therapeutic measures. While active intervention can save time, it necessarily involves greater risks.

Based on what has been said, we may state the following indications for the correction of deformity and length discrepancy of the lower extremity in the presence of osseous infection:

1. Internally fixed pertrochanteric fractures with a tendency toward varus angulation. Stability can be improved by a valgus osteotomy like that used for fresh fractures that are to be treated with Ender-Simon-Weidner pins. A valgus osteotomy fixed with an angled blade plate provides better stability, which aids in the resolution of infection. If the blade plate cannot be seated firmly enough in the neck, a femoral plate can be prebent as needed and applied such that its proximal end almost reaches the tip of the greater trochanter. Screws driven through the upper plate holes will securely engage the calcar. The compressed plate functions as an excellent tension band on the lateral side, and the apposed osteotomy surfaces provide a strong buttress on the medial side. It is unnecessary to sacrifice limb length.
2. In the femoral shaft, the ununited, infected fracture associated with more than 2 cm of shortening is a potential indication for the use of the Wagner lengthening apparatus. after normal length has been restored, we insert a corticocancellous bone graft medially to bridge and buttress the defect and pack the remainder of the shaft defect with cancellous bone chips. We then stabilize the fragments with a wave plate, or we leave the Wagner appratus in place to function as an external frame. In a shaft that is consolidated medially but lacks weight-bearing ability and exhibits varus angulation, it is sometimes possible to align and stabilize the limb by lateral compression without the need for an osteotomy (Fig. 2). Another possible indication is a significant rotational deformity of the femur. In this case the bridging zone is osteotomized, and normal rotational alignment is restored. Bone grafting is done concurrently with stabilization. Whenever we encounter a medial defect in this region, we harvest a corticocancellous block and screw it to the medial side of the femur to create a solid buttress.
3. A significant deformity of the lower femoral metaphysis or upper tibial metaphysis in the presence of infection may be corrected early if the bone is well vascularized. The limb is stabilized with an external compression frame.
4. In empyema of the knee following a severely comminuted intra-articular fracture that has destroyed the joint, the lines of resection for arthrodesis can be made so as to correct for angular deformity. Again, the limb is stabilized externally with a compression frame.
5. With deformity of the tibia, a consolidated fibula can sometimes interfere with realignment. In this case we do not hesitate to osteotomize the fibula when the main fragment is stabilized (Fig. 3). We first cover the infected area with a sterile compress and plastic film. We can then osteotomize the fibula away from that area without much risk of spreading the infection.

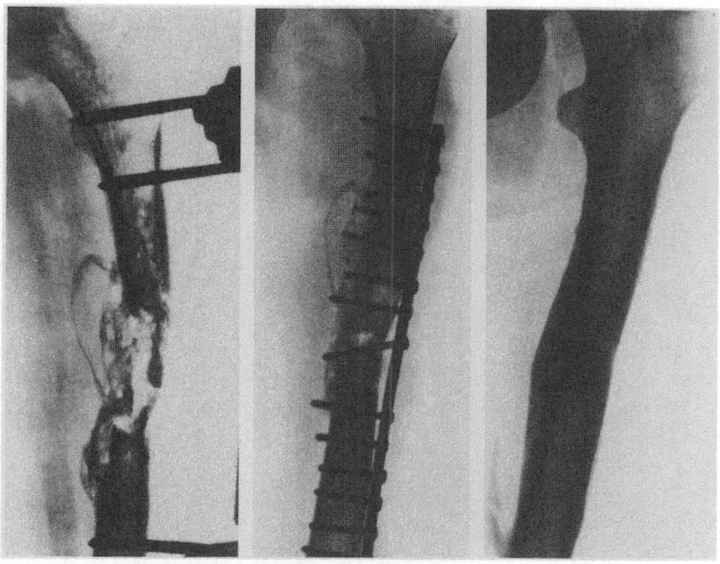

Fig. 2 a–c. Axial correction of a femur that consolidated medially in the presence of osteitis with bone loss. **a** Status with Wagner apparatus in place. **b** Valgus correction with a tension band plate and medial corticocancellous bone graft. **c** Consolidated bone 18 months after surgery

Another indication for correction of the tibia is shortening. The principles are the same as in the femur (Figs. 3 and 4).

In recent years we have performed limb corrections in 39 patients who had coexisting osseous infection. The patients consisted of 33 men and 6 women ranging in age from 17 to 56 years. Follow-ups were conducted in 35 patients at intervals of 1 to 7 years after surgery (Table 1).

A total of 32 patients had deformities of the lower extremity, 10 involving the femur and 22 th tibia; 7 patients had deformities of the upper extremity. With allowance for combined deformities, we noted 32 instances of angular deformity, 11 instances of rotational deformity, and 8 instances of shortening. The infection was markedly pyogenic in 10 cases and low-grade in 22 cases; a draining sinus was present in 7 patients (Table 2).

Table 3 shows the therapeutic procedures that were employed in this series. As the Table indicates, 9 osteotomies were performed on the femur, 21 on the

Table 1. Patient Population

Limb corrections in the presence of infection	
Number of patients	39
Men	33
Women	6
Age	17–56 years
Follow-up	1– 7 years
Number	35

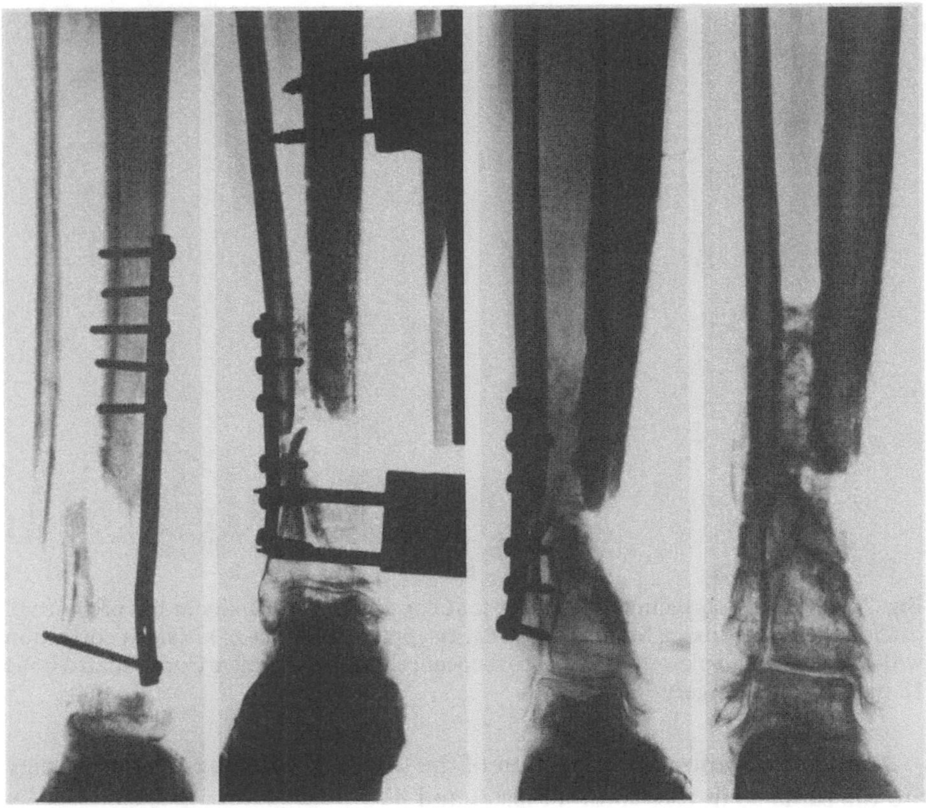

a b c d

Fig. 3 a–d. Length equalization and axial correction in tibial osteitis with bone destruction after plate osteosynthesis with callous bridging of the fibula. **a** Initial status with 3 cm of limb shortening and 25° valgus deformity of the ankle joint. **b** Fibular osteotomy (callus), 3 cm lengthening, and correction of valgus deformity; interosseous cancellous bone graft. **c** At 3 months after the first operation the cancellous bone is largely incorporated, and progressive weight bearing is initiated. **d** Result at 1 year after corrective surgery

Table 2. Initial Status (n = 39)

Site	Femur	10	32
	Tibia	22	
	Humerus	3	7
	Forearm	4	
Deformity	Angulation	32	
	Rotation	11	
	Shortening	8	
Infection	Pyogenic	10	
	Low-grade	22	
	No sinuses	7	

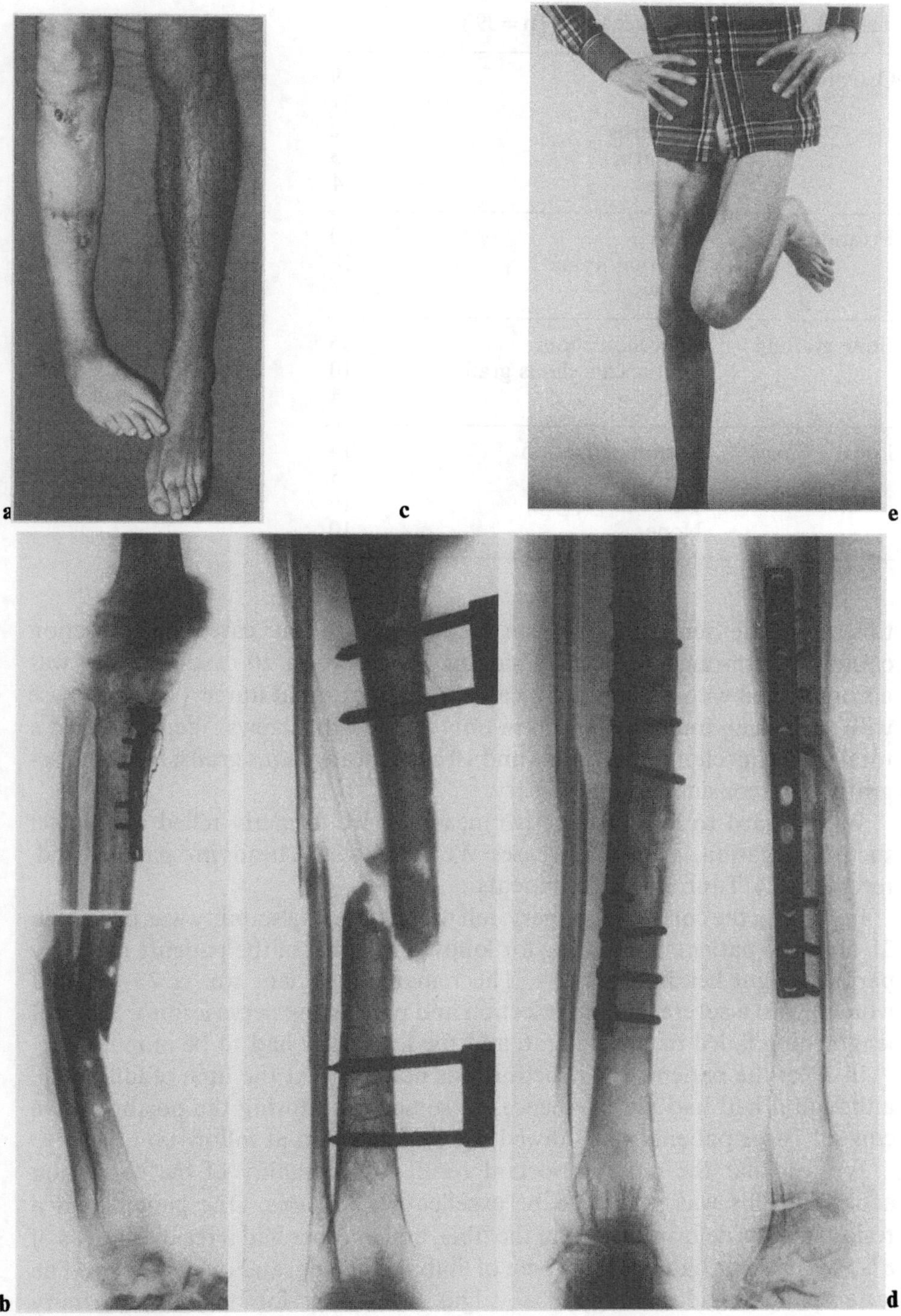

Fig. 4 a – e. Axial and length correction of the tibia in the presence of infection after plate osteosynthesis and peroneal nerve palsy. **a** Clinical appearance with proximal and midshaft sinuses and peroneal paralysis. **b** Preoperative roentgenogram showing the bridging callus on the tibia and fibula. **c** The callus was sectioned, and the fragments were distracted with the Wagner apparatus to restore normal length and alignment. **d** Radiologic result at 7 months after corrective surgery. **e** Functional result at 12 months. The peroneal palsy has regressed completely

Table 3. Therapeutic Procedures (n=39)

Osteotomy	Femur	9
	Tibia	21
	Humerus	2
	Forearm	3
	None	4
Fixation	Plate	20
	External frame	18
	Screws	1
Bone grafting	Cancellous bone	35
	Corticocancellous graft	10
	None	4
Local adjunct	Suction irrigation	14
	PMMA beads	5
	Taurolin [1,4]	10
	None	10

tibia, 2 on the humerus, and 3 on the forearm. In four cases the correction could be performed without sectioning the bone. In 20 cases fixation was accomplished with a plate, in 18 cases with an external frame (which we use with increasing frequency), and in only 1 case with screws. We performed a total of 35 cancellous bone grafts and 10 corticocancellous grafts. In four cases grafts were considered unnecessary.

With regard to local adjunctive measures, we formerly relied mainly on suction irrigation, using it in 14 cases. We used PMMA beads in 5 patients and, recently, 4% Taurolin in 10 patients.

Following the corrective surgery, full weight-bearing stability was present in 31 of the 35 patients presenting for follow-up. Three of the patients had only partial weight-bearing stability. The remaining patient was a 23-year-old woman with a severe femoral infection and preexisting nerve lesions. Surgical lengthening failed in this patient, and the leg finally had to be amputated.

In 32 of the patients the infection was not active at the time of follow-up, although 6 had had recrudescences at some point during the postoperative course. Three patients still showed signs of infection at follow-up.

We feel that the most important result is the quality of the correction achieved. This was judged to be excellent in 30 cases. One patient had a residual varus deformity of 5° in the tibia, and another had a residual varus of 8°. Two patients had less than 2 cm of limb shortening, and one had 3 cm. The latter patient had undergone a valgus osteotomy for angular deformity secondary to an infected pertrochanteric fracture. After surgery a persistent sepsis developed which necessitated an extended Girdlestone resection of the hip. Two years later a total hip arthroplasty was performed at the urging of the patient, resulting in 3 cm of leg sortening (Table 4).

Evaluation of our results indicates that in appropriately selected cases and especially in young patients, a carefully planned osteotomy may be performed

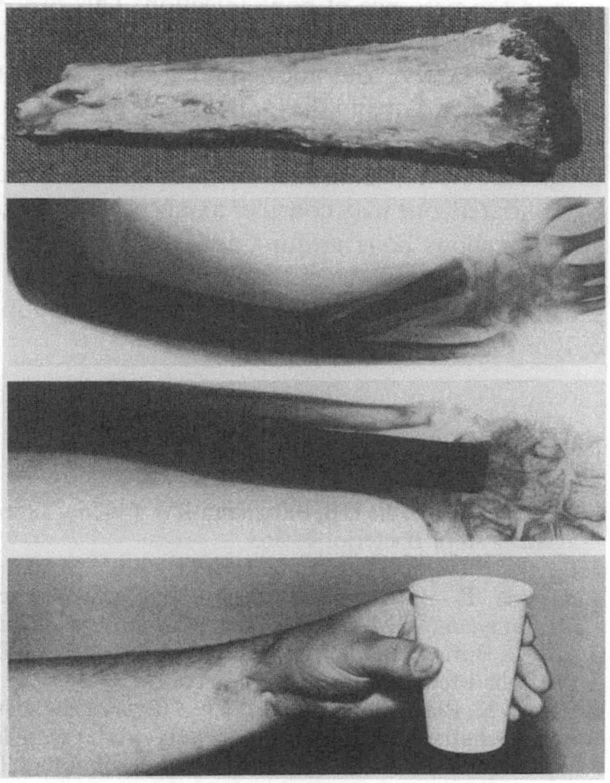

Fig. 5 a–d. Axial and length correction of the radius for shortening and angular deformity. **a** Resection of the distal third of the radius in the region of the former epiphyseal plate. **b** Radilogic status. **c** Three months after alignment, plating, and placement of a corticocancellous graft. The graft is completely integrated. **d** The functional result is shown. The hand is fully useful for ordinary functions

Table 4. Results of Treatment (n=35)

Weight-bearing ability	Full	31
	Partial	3
Amputation		1
Infection	None at follow-up	32
	Prior recrudescence	6
	Present at follow-up	3[a]
Position	Excellent	30
	Varus 5°	1
	Varus 8°	1
	Shortening <2 cm	2
	Shortening 3 cm	1[b]

a One amputation
b Total hip replacement after Girdlestone

even in the presence of bone infection. This procedure is not without risks, however, and is a reasonable option only under the conditions stated above. We do not believe that infected bone should be osteotomized once consolidation has occurred and the limb is stable enough to bear weight. In these cases it is best to wait for the infection to subside and then perform the corrective osteotomy at a site distant from the former infection. If the bone has not consolidated, one may consider axial correction with concurrent stabilization and cancellous bone grafting as well as limb lengthening with the Wagner apparatus. We are aware that corrections of this type may be riskier in the presence of osteitis, and so they are appropriate only in exceptional cases and only if the bone is well vascularized.

References

1. Browne MK, Leslie GB, Pfirrmann RW (1976) Taurolin, a new chemotherapeutic agent. J Appl Bacteriol 41:363
2. Burri C (1979) Posttraumatische Osteitis, 2. Aufl. Huber, Bern Stuttgart Wien
3. Klemm K (1976) Die Behandlung chronischer Knocheninfektionen mit Gentamycin-PMMA-Ketten und -Kugeln. Unfallchirugie Sonderheft
4. Lob G, Burri C (1983) Lokale Chemotherapie der Osteitis mit Taurolin-Gel 4%. Fortschr Med 101:88
5. Parsch K, Plaue R (Hrsg) (1982) Hämatogene Osteomyelitis und posttraumatische Osteitis. Medizinisch Literarische Verlagsgesellschaft, Uelzen
6. Willenegger H, Roth W (1962) Die antibakterielle Spüldrainage als Behandlungsprinzip bei chirurgischen Infektionen. Dtsch Med Wochenschr 87:1

Results after Surgical Correction of Posttraumatic Leg Length Discrepancies

W. Baur

The permanent correction of leg length discrepancies is essential for the prevention of painful osseous and soft-tissue sequelae. This correction may be effected conservatively with an orthopedic shoe or suitable orthosis, or operatively by means of a shortening or lengthening osteotomy [1,3,4]. An extremity that is elongated as a result of trauma should be surgically shortened if at all possible. In cases of posttraumatic shortening, the treatment of choice depends of four main factors:

1. *The degree of shortening*: For leg length discrepancies less than 3 cm, conservative orthopedic correction is recommended.
2. *The location of the shortening*: Shortening of the tibia is adequately managed with a shoe or orthosis. If the femur is involved, conservative methods are less satisfactory because they place the knees at different levels and affect the length of the stride.
3. *The condition of the soft tissues*: Surgical lengthening is nor recommended in the presence of extensive cutaneous and soft-tissue scarring.
4. *The age and sex of the patient*: In juvenile patients and women concerned with cosmesis, one can be more liberal in the election of lengthening osteotomies than in adult men. A length-equalizing orthosis is much easier to use in men then in women because it is more easily concealed by clothing.

In addition to the points above, one should follow the principle of limiting reconstructive surgery to the affected limb if at all possible. In special cases it may be advantageous to combine treatment modalities, such as partially correcting a shortened limb by surgical means and then correcting the remaining length discrepancy with an elevated shoe. It is rarely necessary to perform a shortening osteotomy on one limb and a lengthening osteotomy on the other.

Results of Lengthening Osteotomies

At Wichernhaus Orthopedic Hospital we correct leg length discrepancies by the technique of Wagner [2,3,4], i.e., a diaphyseal osteotomy followed by continuous distraction and then internal fixation, possibly combined with bone grafting (Table 1). In some length discrepancies secondary to shaft fractures the osteotomy can be performed through the former fracture site. Angular and rotational deformities of the shaft can be corrected immediately or during the lengthening process (Fig. 1).

Corrective Osteotomies of the Lower Extremity
Edited by G. Hierholzer, K. H. Müller

Table 1. Lengthening Osteotomies of the Lower Extremities

		Femur	Tibia
Total number of all lengthening osteotomies		255 (100%)	169 (100%)
Lengthening osteotomies after trauma		49 (19.2%)	8 (4.3%)
Average age of patients		19.8 years	19.0 years
Patients with prior epiphyseal fractures		29	2
Supplementary axial correction		18	0
Amount of lengthening	maximum	11.3 cm	5.5 cm
	minimum	3.0 cm	3.5 cm
	average	6.55 cm	4.1 cm
End result:			
Equal leg lengths		42 patients	7 patients
Residual shortening		5 patients less than 2.5 cm	1 patient less than 1 cm
Further lengthening		2 patients	0
Problems:			
Delayed union		5 patients, 3 with history of infection	0
Plate fatigue fracture		3 patients	1 patient
Replacement of plate		11 patients	2 patients
Soft-tissue revision		0	1 patient (lengthening of Achilles tendon)

From 1966 to 1981 we performed 49 lengthening osteotomies of the femur for posttraumatic leg length discrepancies. This represents 19.2% of the total of 225 femoral lengthening osteotomies performed. The average age of the patients at examination was 19.8 years. More than half the patients with posttraumatic leg shortening had sustained epiphyseal plate injuries, very often resulting in concomitant angular deformity. Eighteen patients required axial correction in addition to leg lengthening. The average amound of lengthening needed after trauma was 6.5 cm , with a maximum of 11.3 cm. At the conclusion of treatment 42 patients had equal leg lengths. Five patients had residual shortening of less than 2.5 cm. In two patients residual shortening is sufficient to require additional lengthening measures.

Delayed consolidation was noted in five patients, but in three of these an old infection became reactivated during the course of lengthening. All infections were controlled by surgical treatment. In three patients the special lengthening plate sustained a fatigue fracture during consolidation of the defect. In each case the fixation was revised and cancellous bone grafts were applied. In 11 patients the broad femoral plate was replaced with a narrower, more elastic plate to accelerate bone remodeling in the area of lengthening.

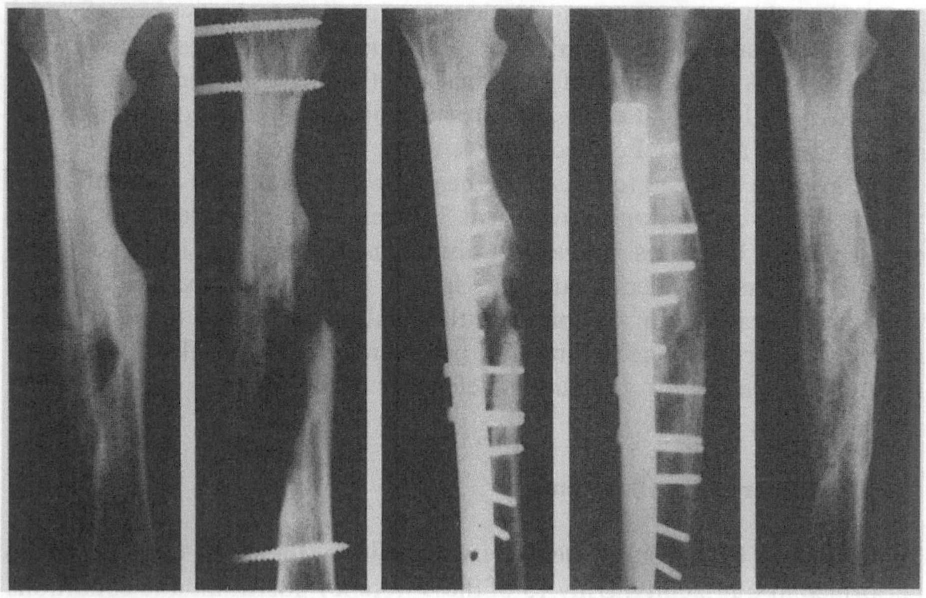

a b c d e

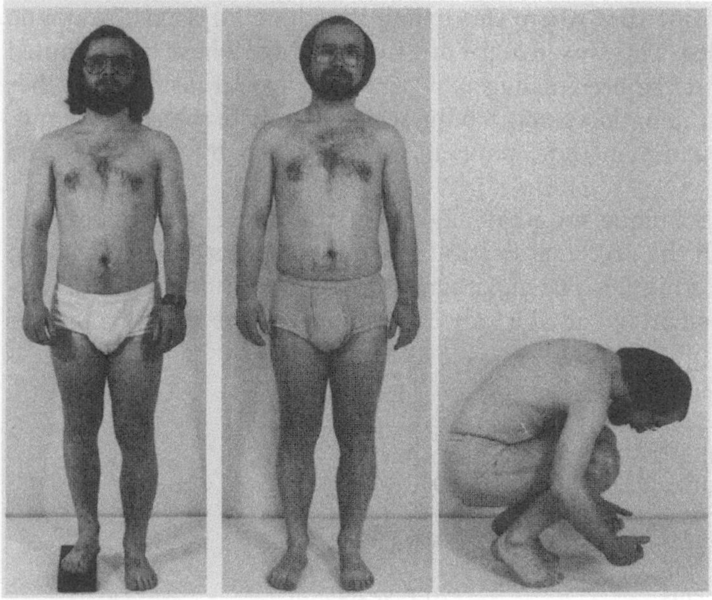

f g

Fig. 1 a – g. Lengthening osteotomy in a 22-year-old man for a malunited femoral shaft fracture with 4.5 cm of shortening and 15° of external rotation. **a** Preoperative roentgenogram on 2/25/75. **b** Appearance at completion of distraction on 5/20/75. **c** After plate osteosynthesis on 7/17/75. **d** After initial consolidation of defect on 11/23/75. **e** Status on 4/17/80 after complete ossification of the lengthening defect. **f** Preoperative appearance on 3/2/75. **g** Postoperative appearance on 11/24/77 with equality of leg lengths and unrestricted joint motion

Considerably fewer posttraumatic lengthening osteotomies were performed in the tibia than in the femur. The 8 patients who had these osteotomies represent 4.3% of the total of 169 tibial lengthening osteotomies that were performed. Only two patients had limb shortening secondary to an epiphyseal plate fracture, and axial corrections were not required.

The average amound to tibial lengthening was 4.1 cm, with a maximum of 5.5 cm. At the conclusion of treatment 7 patients had equal leg lengths, and only 1 patient had a residual length discrepancy, which was less than 1 cm.

As in the femur patients, one plate fatigue fracture ocurred and required revisionary fixation. In two patients the fixation plate had to be replaced during the course of bone healing. One patient required surgical lengthening of the Achilles tendon for an equinus deformity of the foot.

Results of Shortening Osteotomies

From 1967 to 1982, 100 shortening osteotomies of the lower extremity were performed at out facility. Only 13 of these were for posttraumatic conditions (Table 2). The average age of the patients was 31.6 years.

There was only one case where shortening was done for a posttraumatic elongation of the leg. This was in a girl of 14 years of age whose comminuted fracture of the femur had been managed by wire traction and casting. All other patients had posttraumatic leg shortening, which mainly involved the femur. The length discrepancy in these patients was corrected by shortening the uninvolved limb.

With regard to technique, the great majority of shortening osteotomies were performed through the proximal femoral metaphysis and stabilized with an angled blade plate (Fig. 2). The maximum amount of shortening was 6.5 cm. Performing the osteotomy in the cancellous bone of the proximal femur

Table 2. Shortening Osteotomies of the Lower Extremities

Total number of all shortening osteotomies		100 (100%)
Shortening osteotomies after trauma		13 (13%)
Average age of patients		31.6 years
Patients with prior epiphyseal fractures		5
Amount of shortening	maximum	6.5 cm
	minimum	1.5 cm
	average	3.9 cm
Site of osteotomy:		
Proximal femoral metaphysis		9 patients
Femoral shaft		2 patients
Proximal tibia		1 patient
Tibial shaft		1 patient

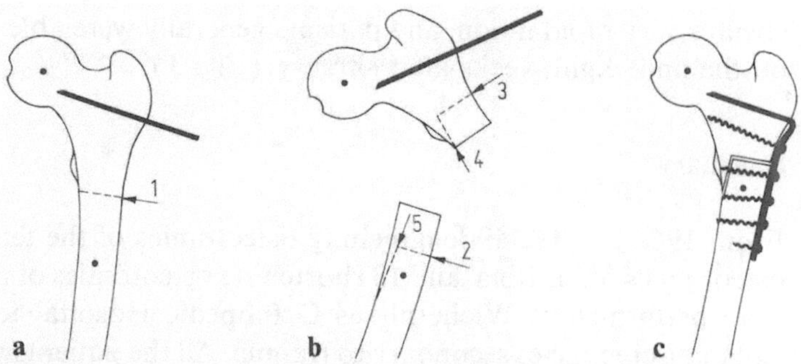

Fig. 2 a–c. Schematic representation of the shortening osteotomy of the proximal femoral metaphysis [4]

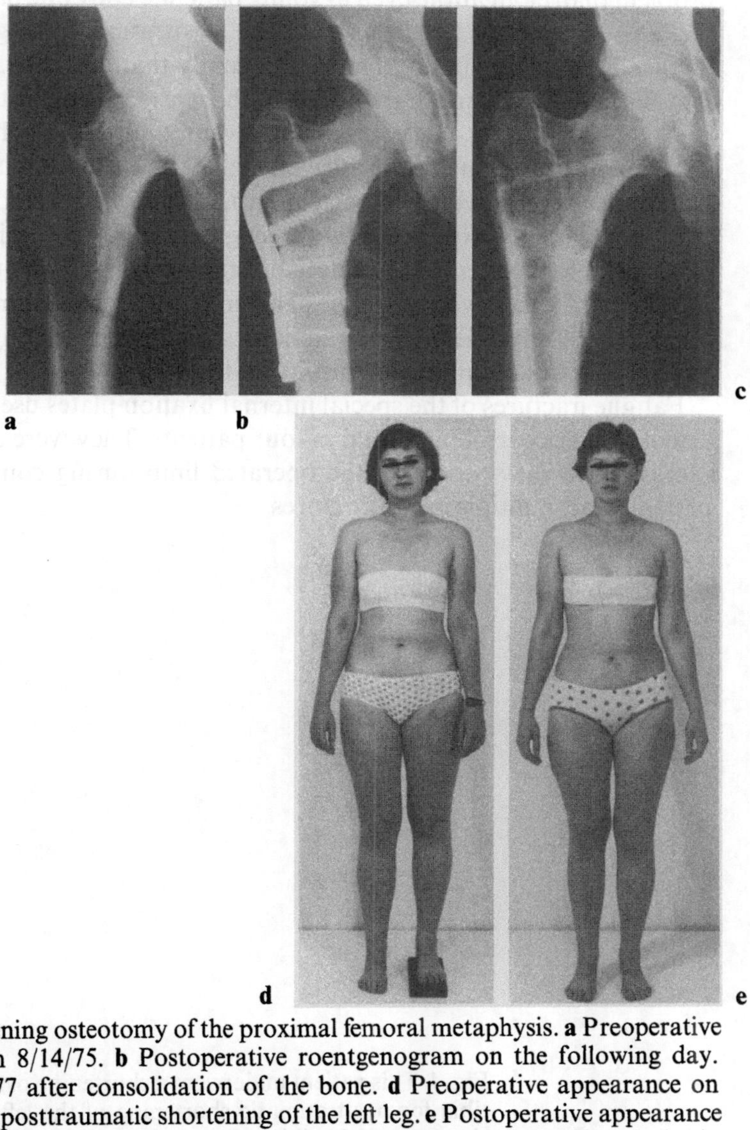

Fig. 3 a–e. Shortening osteotomy of the proximal femoral metaphysis. **a** Preoperative roentgenogram on 8/14/75. **b** Postoperative roentgenogram on the following day. **c** Status on 1/13/77 after consolidation of the bone. **d** Preoperative appearance on 8/14/75 with 3-cm posttraumatic shortening of the left leg. **e** Postoperative appearance on 8/31/76 following a shortening osteotomy of the right proximal femoral metaphysis. Leg lengths are equal

ensures very rapid union, and patients generally were able to bear full weight on the limb eight weeks after surgery (Fig. 3).

Summary

From 1966 to 1982 49 lengthening osteotomies of the femur, 8 lengthening osteotomies of the tibia, and 13 shortening osteotomies of the lower extremity were performed at Wichernhaus Orthopedic Hospital for deformities and length discrepancies secondary to trauma. All the patients were followed after surgery.

It was found that posttraumatic limb shortening was a far more common problem than elongation, even in young patients. Only one patient was treated for a posttraumatic length excess. The posttraumatic length discrepancies involved the femur six times more frequently than the tibia. It is noteworthy that 36 patients, or more than half of those examined, sustained epiphyseal plate injuries during the traumatizing event, and that all these patients had subsequent shortening of the affected leg. Half of all patients with epiphyseal plate injuries required axial correction in addition to length correction.

In contrast to experience with lengthening osteotomies of the lower extremities for congenital leg length discrepancy, we encountered virtually no problems of excessive soft-tissue tension in our posttraumatic lengthening operations. Only one patient required surgical lengthening of the Achilles tendon due to an equinus deformity of the foot.

Fatigue fractures of the special internal fixation plates used for lengthening osteotomies occurred in a total of four patients. They were mainly caused by excessive weight-bearing on the operated limb during consolidation. Some patients had multiple plate froctures.

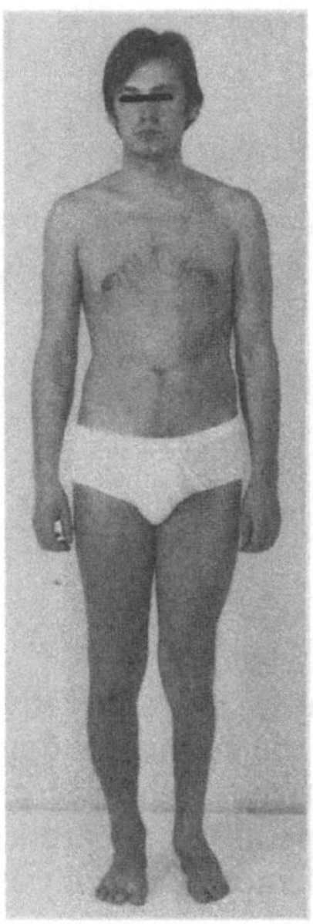

Fig. 4. This patient underwent a shortening osteotomy of the right tibia for posttraumatic shortening of the left tibia. The relative shortness of the tibiae alter the body proportions and shorten the stride

In 13 patients the original fixation plate was replaced with a thinner and more elastic implant to encourage remodeling of the new bone.

The advantage of the lengthening osteotomy in the correction of posttraumatic leg length discrepancy is that it enables the surgery to be done on the injured leg, thereby preserving the body proportions, a normal gait, and an adequate step length. These cannot be obtained when lengths are equalized by shortening the unaffected limb (Fig. 4). For this reason, and with regard for the criteria listed earlier, we made an effort to limit surgery to the injured limb whenever possible in patients with posttraumatic leg shortening. This effort is reflected in the relatively small number of shortening osteotomies (12) performed on the uninjured limb.

The great majority of shortening osteotomies were performed through the upper femoral metaphysis. This permits axial corrections and reduces the time to consolidation (Fig. 3). Two shortening osteotomies were performed through the femoral shaft, one through the upper tibia, and one through the tibial shaft. We did not perform any closed diaphyseal osteotomies with intramedullary fixation.

References

1. Müller ME, Allgöwer M, Willenegger H (1977) Manual der Osteosynthese-AO-Technik. Springer, Berlin Heidelberg New York
2. Wagner H (1971) Operative Beinverlängerung. Chirurg 42:260
3. Wagner H (1971) Technik und Indikation der operativen Verkürzung und Verlängerung von Ober- und Unterschenkel. Orthopäde 1:59–74
4. Wagner H (1976) Prinzipien der Korrekturosteotomie am Bein. Orthopäde 6:145

Summary: Corrective Osteotomies of the Diaphyses after Trauma

J. Müller-Färber

Most deformities of the *femoral shaft* are secondary to fractures that were treated conservatively or by intramedullary nailing. They are less common after plate osteosynthesis.

The main techniques of corrective osteotomy are the transverse osteotomy, the closed wedge osteotomy, and the oblique and step-cut displacement osteotomy.

The oblique closed wedge osteotomy has several important advantages over the transverse wedge osteotomy. First, it provides a relatively simple means of correcting limb length discrepancy. Second, good compression of the large osteotomy surfaces can be obtained by the use of lag screws and a neutralization plate.

Malunited fractures of the *tibial shaft* are considered to be preosteoarthritic beyong a certain degree of deformity.

Rotational deformities of the tibia are manifested radiologically by excessive obliquity of the talar baseline. An external rotation deformity produces a valgus inclination of the talar baseline, while an internal rotation deformity causes a varus inclination.

With malunited fractures of the tibial shaft, local circumstances often make it necessary to perform the osteotomy in the metaphysis. But the farther the osteotomy is from the point of intersection of the shaft axes above and below the deformity, the more difficult it is to center the mechanical axis of the limb without also altering the physiologic position of the articular baselines.

Because a proximal metaphyseal osteotomy for a varus deformity of the diaphysis will shift the mechanical axis into the lateral compartment, it is appropriate to perform the operation near the knee joint. A valgus deformity in the same location is corrected by an osteotomy near the ankle joint.

The preferred type of osteotomy is the *closed wedge* or wedge resection osteotomy. The oblique form is generally preferred for the reasons stated above.

The method of choice for the stabilization of corrective osteotomies is plate osteosynthesis. If soft-tissue conditions are poor or there has been previous bone infection, external skeletal fixation is preferred.

In cases where there is generalized bowing of a long bone that would require osteotomies at multiple levels to obtain satisfactory alignment through wedge resection, the *displacement osteotomy* of Wagner is a valuable alternative. It can also be used to correct angular deformities of the shaft.

The classic application of the displacement osteotomy is in the supracondy-

Corrective Osteotomies of the Lower Extremity
Edited by G. Hierholzer, K. H. Müller

lar region of the femur, expecially when a large amount of angular correction is needed.

A closed wedge osteotomy may create bony surfaces that differ markedly in size. In the displacement osteotomy the bone is divided transversely, the fragments are aligned, and the cortical edge of one fragment is impacted into the medullary cavity of the other. This interlocking of the cortices provides good primary stability and creates a secure foundation for internal fixation.

A posttraumatic *leg length discrepancy* requires permanent correction, for it causes cosmetic as well as functional effects with painful sequelae in the skeleton and soft tissues.

Discrepancies of less than 3 cm are best managed conservatively with orthopedic footwear. If surgical treatment is indicated, a lengthening osteotomy of the affected limb is preferred over a contralateral shortening osteotomy, as the former operation will preserve body proportions.

More than 50% of cases of posttraumatic leg shortening with tissue loss are the result of epiphyseal plate injuries.

Leg shortening that exceeds 6 cm in the femur or 4 cm in the tibia should not be corrected in one stage due to the possibility of nerve injury and excessive soft-tissue tension. These cases should be managed by diaphyseal osteotomy and continuous distraction followed by internal fixation according to the Wagner technique.

When lengthening surgery is indicated, one must be aware of potential complications such as delayed union and loosening or fatigue fracture of the special internal fixation plates.

When surgical shortening of the unaffected leg is indicated, the procedure is usually performed throught the proximal femoral metaphysis and stabilized with an angled blade plate.

When deformity exists in the presence of osseous *infection* with instability, the deformity should be corrected at the site of the infection, and the bone concurrently stabilized to promote resolution of the infection. If the fragments have already united and the limb can bear weight, the infected bone should not be osteotomized. It is better to wait until the infection subsides and then perform the corrective osteotomy through bone that has not been involved by infection.

The risks and potential *complications* of the corrective osteotomy are basically the same as those associated with the treatment of fresh musculoskeletal injuries.

A major difference is that patients who are selected for corrective osteotomy are relatively asymptomatic and must be convinced of the need for corrective surgery. As a result, they are likely to be less accepting of complications than acutely injured patients. It is essential that these elective patients be thoroughly counseled as to the risks that are involved, the results that may reasonably be expected, and the importance of a cooperative attitude.

Besides the "avoidable" complications referrable to poor planning of the operation or faulty technique, the complications most frequently encountered are delayed union, nonunion, and the most serious complication of all, infection.

IV. The Distal Femur and Proximal Tibia

Indications, Localization and Planning of Posttraumatic Osteotomies about the Knee

K. H. Müller and J. Müller-Färber

Introduction

When the lower limb is in normal alignment, the articular surfaces of the femur and tibia act in concert with ligamentous and muscular stabilizers to minimize shear forces on the knee joint and transmit compressive forces evenly and symmetrically across the largest possible area of joint surface (Fig. 1 a) [7,8,9,12]. The complex anatomy, statics and dynamics of the lower extremity explain why the knee joint reacts so sensitively to deviations of axial alignment [10,12,14], and why deformities associated with malunited fractures alter the pattern of loads on the knee and predispose to degenerative disease (Fig. 1 b–e). The traumatic causes of these deformities include anatomically and

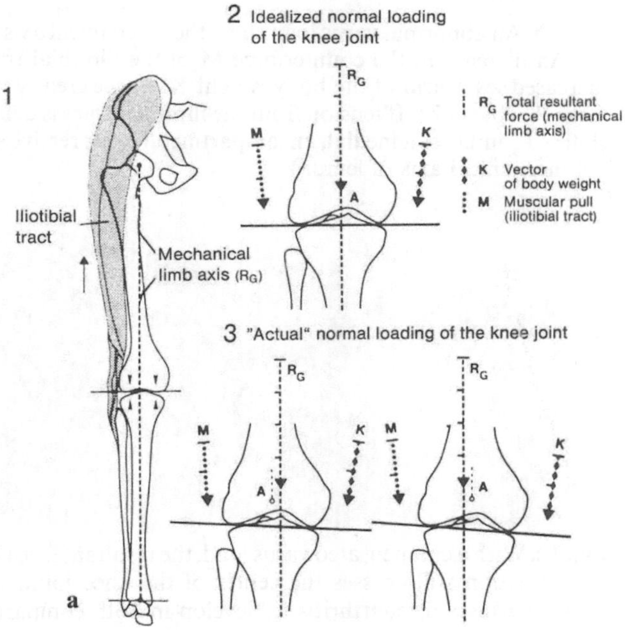

Fig. 1 a–e. Diagrams and roentgenograms depicting the forces acting on the knee joint in the frontal plane under normal, varus and valgus loading
a With a normal alignment the mechanical axis of the leg passes through the center of the knee joint. The total resulting force R_g along the mechanical axis is the vector sum of the body weight K and the counterpull M of the iliotibial tract (panels 1 and 2). Although the force vary functionally, a net varus load tends to act on the knee joint under physiologic conditions (panel 3) (*A* mechanical axis of femur)

Corrective Osteotomies of the Lower Extremity
Edited by G. Hierholzer, K. H. Müller

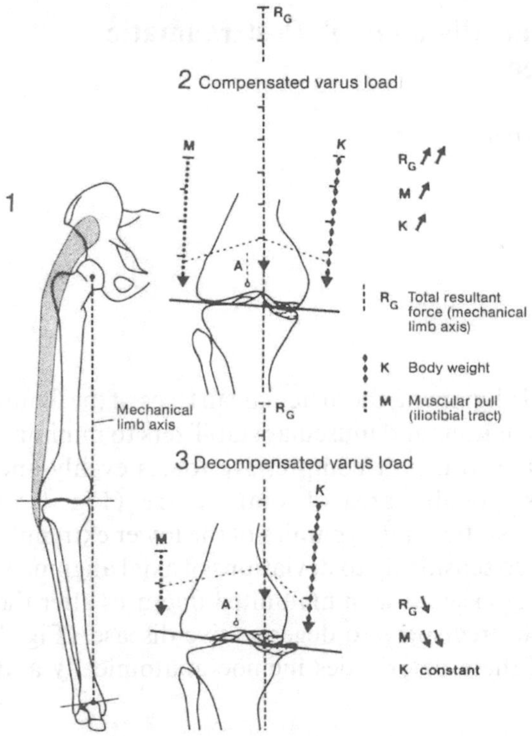

Fig. 1 b. An abnormal varus load shifts the mechanical axis of the limb medially (panel 1). An increase in the counterforce M of the iliotibial tract can compensate for the increased lever arm of the body weight K, but it greatly increases the total resultant force R_g (panel 2). If tension from the iliotibial tract is deficient, the increasing medial shift of R_g imposes a medial, uncompartmetal compressive stress on the joint (panel 3) (*A* mechanical axis of femur)

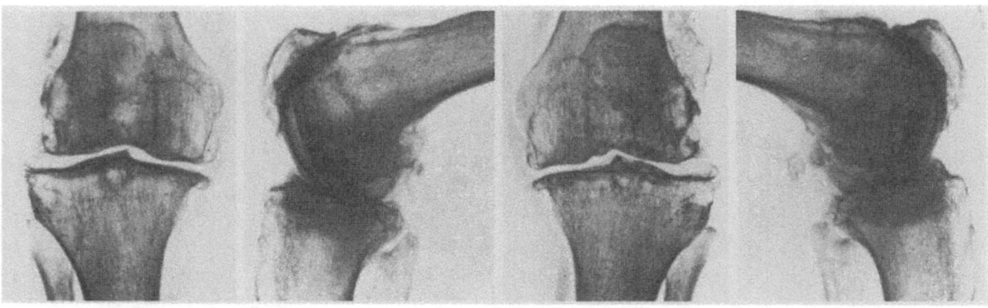

Fig. 1 c. With a compensated varus load, the resultant force R_g is increased. Although its line of action still crosses the center of the knee joint, the increased intraarticular pressure causes osteoarthritis to develop in both compartments of the knee

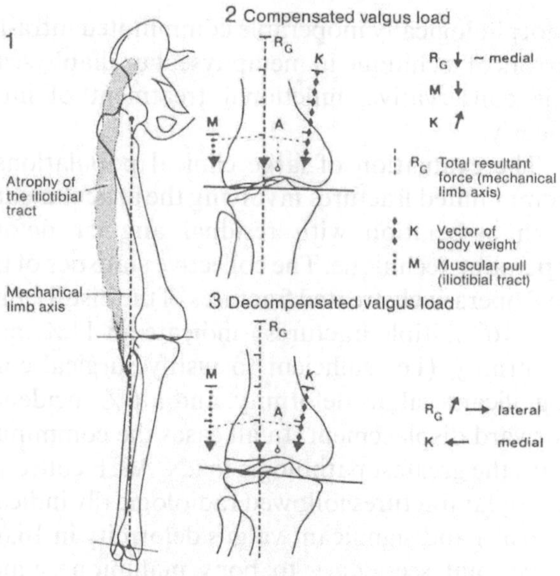

Fig. 1 d. A valgus load shifts the mechanical axis laterally (panel 1). With a compensated valgus stress, the tension M of the iliotibial tract decreases. This opposes the medially displaced vector of the body weight K and keeps the resultant force R_g nearer the center of the knee (panel 2). As the valgus deformity increases, R_g moves laterally while the body-weight vector K approaches the center of the knee. The result is a lateral, unicompartmental stress with stretching of the medial collateral ligament (panel 3) (*A* mechanical axis of femur)

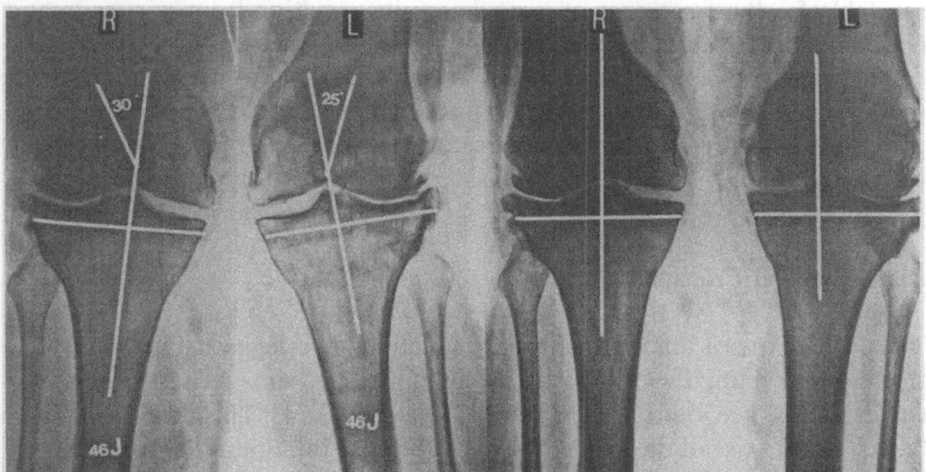

Fig. 1 e. The films at left show decompensated valgus loading of both knee joints with osteoarthritis of the lateral compartment. The filme at right, taken 3 years after corrective osteotomy, show an arrest and partial regression of osteoarthritic changes

morphologically inoperable comminuted intra-articular fractures of the knee; errors of technique in metaphyseal or diaphyseal internal fixations; as well as the conservative, functional treatment of intra-articular fractures in the elderly.

The evaluation of large clinical populations proves that segmental and comminuted fractures involving the articular surfaces of the knee have a fairly high association with residual angular deformity despite a satisfactory operating technique; The collective statistics of the ASIF [22] on the results of 199 operatively treated fractures of the distal femur (including 91 comminuted and 16 multiple fractures) indicate an 11% incidence of "significant" varus deformity (i.e., sufficient to justify surgical correction), a 7% incidence of significant valgus deformity, and a 6% incidence of significant backward or forward displacement. In all cases the comminuted fractures were associated with the greatest pathologic loads. ASIF collective statistics [16] on 225 tibial condylar fractures followed radiologically indicate significant varus deformity in 6.6% and significant valgus deformity in 16.6%. Besides deformities of the knee joint secondary to bony malunions, functional posttraumatic angulations caused by ligamentous and capsular lesions or by a combination of osseous and soft-tissue lesions can lead to cartilage damage and an osteoarthritic pattern of stress transmission [1,2,10,12]. Axial deformities in the sagittal plane, such as periarticular fractures that have healed with backward or forward displacement, can be compensated by muscular action up to a certain point, but this, too, is a preosteoarthritic condition in which the articular surfaces are no longer fully utilized, and symptoms develop as a result of muscle strain [2]. Occasionally, corrective osteotomy may be the only means available for the treatment of joint deformity resulting from posttraumatic contracture or ankylosis and for limitations of knee motion (especially extension) that are not correctable by arthrolysis. Finally, many patients with multiple injuries require a prioritized management that may have to neglect a primary anatomic and functional restoration of the articular surfaces by internal fixation.

Biomechanical Principles

The normal knee is loaded axially in symmetrical two-legged stance, provided the line connecting the centers of the hip and ankle joints passes through the center of the knee joint (Figs. 1 a and 2) [7–10,13,14]. This line is called the "mechanical axis" of the lower extremity (Fig. 1) [14]. For us, it is the guide to selecting patients for corrective osteotomies about the knee and for planning the operative procedure (Figs. 2 and 9). To understand how this line is used, it is necessary to understand the biomechanics of knee loading under conditions of normal and abnormal limb alignment.

Numerous studies confirm [1,7,8,9,14] that the complex motor sequences that occur during gait constantly alter the loads on the knee. The mechanical axis no longer passes through the center of the joint.

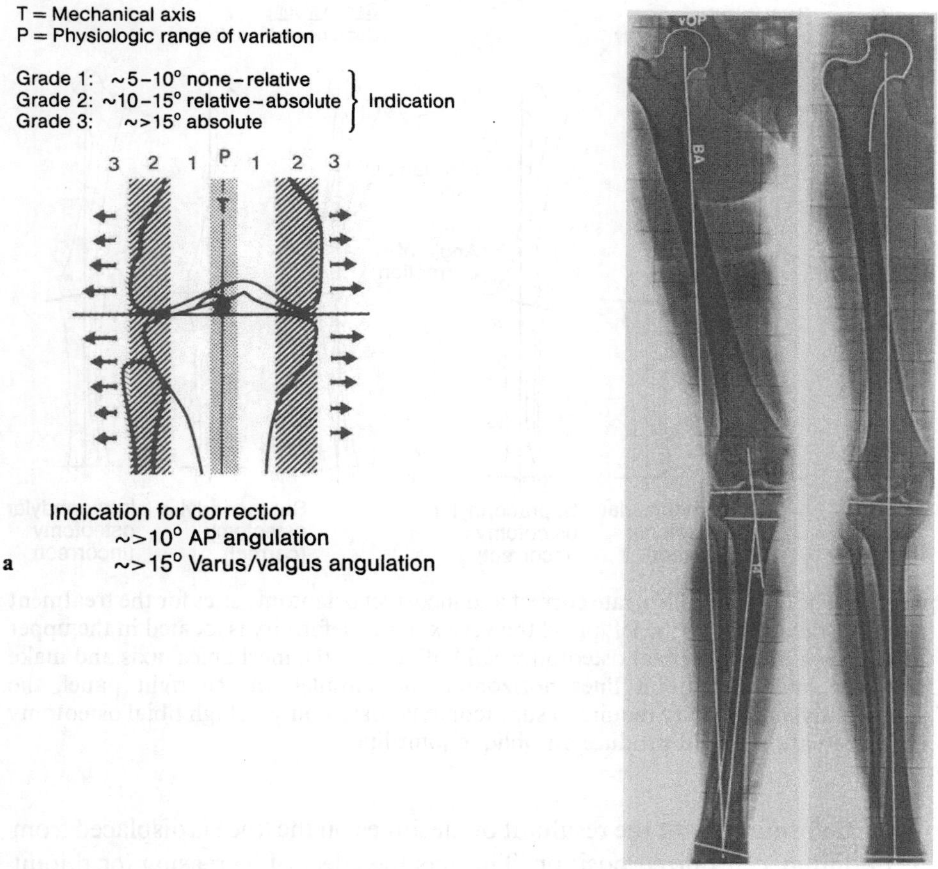

Fig. 2 a – c. Indications for corrective osteotomy after trauma, and determination of the exact site of the correction
a Grades of severity of genu valgum or genu varum based on the position of the mechanical axis. If the axis crosses the extended joint line outside the joint, a Grade 3 deformity exists. It is an absolute indication for corrective osteotomy

As a result, the functional loading of a joint is described in terms of the vectorial sum ("resultant") of the forces acting on that joint. The magnitude of the resultant R_g of all forces acting on the knee joint in the frontal plane is a functional variable [8,9]. It represents the balance that is established between all the forces exerted on the knee. Normally R_g is shifted toward the medial side of the knee joint (Fig. 1 a, panel 3), with the result that the knee is subjected to a slight varus stress under physiologic conditions. The joint can easily cope with this stress owing to the trajectorial design of its articular surfaces and the natural load-bearing ability of its cartilage cells [18]. During walking, the knee joint of the supporting leg eccentrically bears the entire body weight minus the weight of the supporting leg. At this moment the vector of the body weight, K, imposes an extreme varus load on the knee. This load is opposed by the force M of the ilitibial tract, which serves as a lateral checkrein [8,9]. Thus, for a given magnitude of body weight, the balance of forces at the knee depends on the opposing force produced by the tension of the iliotibial tract (Fig. 1).

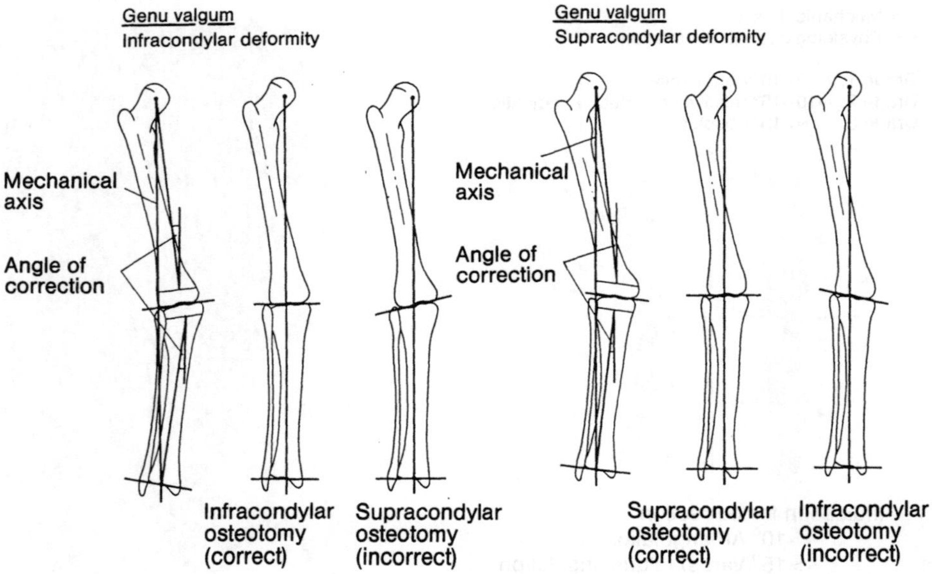

Fig. 2 b. The diagrams illustrate correct and incorrect osteotomy sites for the treatment of valgus deformity. In the left panel the vertex of the deformity is located in the upper tibia; only a proximal tibial osteotomy can both center the mechanical axis and make the knee and ankle joint lines horizontal and parallel. In the right panel, the supracondylar deformity requires a supracondylar osteotomy. A high tibial osteotomy in this situation would produce an oblique joint line

When deformity exists, the resultant of the forces on the knee is displaced from its optimum, centralized position. This has the effect of increasing local joint stresses and reducing the load-bearing area of the articular surfaces (Figs. 1 b and d). With *varus angulation* of the limb, the lever arm of the body weight is increased (Fig. 1 b, panel 2). This increase in K can be compensated by an augmentation of the muscular force of the iliotibial tract. However, vector addition shows that even though the line of action of R_g still passes through the center of the knee in this situation, the absolute magnitude of R_g is substantially increased. The resulting increase of compressive stress within the joint causes cartilaginous lesions that promote osteoarthritis. This theory is supported by the clinical observation of Debrunner that genu varum is frequently accompanied by degenerative changes affecting both the medial and lateral compartments of the knee (Fig. 1 c) [1,14]. If the iliotibial tract is deficient, it will allow R_g to become displaced medially, producing asymmetrical intra-articular stresses (Fig. 1 b, panel 3). This increases local compressive stresses both absolutely and through the dwindling area of load-bearing surface, and a vicious cycle is established.

With *valgus angulation* of the limb, the knee joint approaches the line of action of the body weight (Fig. 1 d). Relaxation of the iliotibial tract enables the joint to adapt to the altered load to some degree (Fig. 1 d, panel 2), the initial result being a decrease in the total load on the joint. But if the valgus deformity increases, the lack of a strong checkrein on the medial side of the knee will cause stresses to become concentrated laterally, leading to local

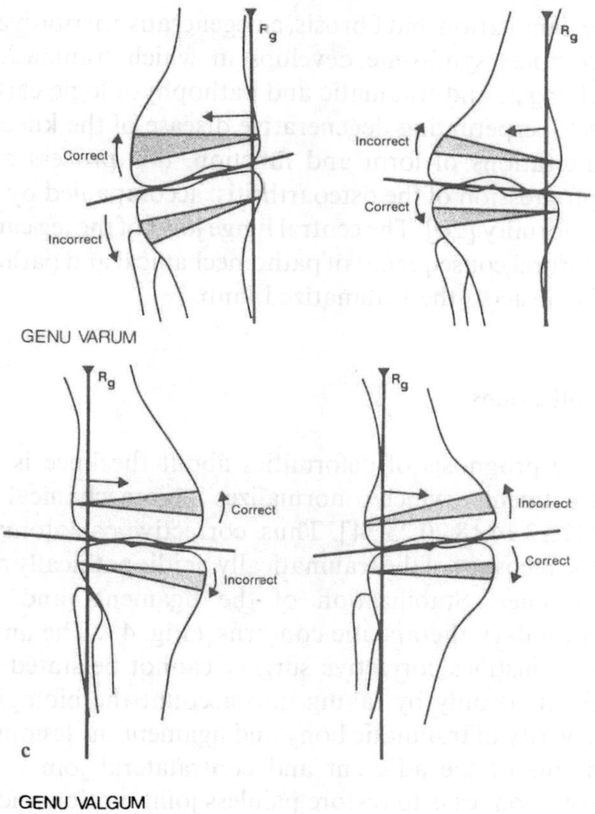

Fig. 2 c. Every corrective osteotomy about the knee that removes a wedge whose base is on the convex side shifts the resultant force R_g toward the center of the joint. As R_g is centered, it is also necessary to rotate the part of the joint adjacent to the osteotomy such that R_g and the joint surface are mutually perpendicular

osteoarthritic change (Fig. 1 d, panel 3, and 1 e) [7,8]. Finally the obliquity and subluxation of the articular surfaces give rise to shear forces for which the joint is not structurally equipped [13,14]. The part of the joint on the concave side [sic] of the deformity even comes under tensile stress during weight bearing, resulting in further loss of stability through stretching of the ligaments and through exacerbation of preexisting ligamentous lesions [2,21]. Disuse atrophy of the muscles is yet another source of instability in the malaligned and pathlogically loaded joint. Thus, the changes that result from trauma of the lower extremity are transmitted and compounded in a highly intricate manner.

In portraying the biomechanics of posttraumatic axial deviations of the knee joint, we must necessarily begin with an analysis of static conditions. Also, we must take into account the change in the metabolism and structure of the synovial system – i.e., the articular cartilage, synovial fluid and joint capsule regarded as a functional unit – that results from unphysiologic loading of the cartilaginous surfaces [3]. As synovial metabolism is disrupted and chondrocytes are destroyed, a synovitis develops. With continued inflammation and fibrosis, a degenerative, irritative condition is established. A complex syndrome develops in which traumatic deformities, ligamentous changes, and traumatic and pathophysiologic cartilage destruction lead to a self-perpetuating degenerative disease of the knee. Aside from the traumatic alterations of form and function, this process alone is sufficient to cause progression of the osteoarthritis, accompanied by a worsening of the original deformity [20]. The central hinge joint of the leg can do nothing to prevent this natural consequence of pathomechanical and pathomorphologic laws that are intrinsic to the traumatized limb.

Indications

The prognosis of deformities about the knee is dramatically improved by treatment which normalizes biomechanical parameters (Fig. 3) [12,13,14,18,20,23,24]. Thus, corrective osteotomy is the prime requisite for the recovery of the traumatically or idiopathically malaligned and osteoarthritic knee. Stabilization of the ligaments and muscle strengthening are secondary therapeutic concerns (Fig. 4). The amount of angular deformity that justifies corrective surgery cannot be stated in absolute terms. We can define it only by taking into account the biological age of the patient, the severity of traumatic bony and ligamentous lesions, residual stability, and the status of the adjacent and contralateral joints. The goal of all corrective osteotomies is to restore painless joint motion and normal axial alignment in order to halt the progression of joint wear and tear or delay its onset. Authors are virtually unaminimous in declaring that more than 10° of angular deformity in the frontal plane will precipitate a posttraumatic osteoarthritis and ought to be corrected (Fig. 2) [1,2,5,6,10,14,15,19,20,22–24]. Besides angular deformity, the election of osteotomy also requires the presence of reasonably stable ligaments and at least 50–60° of knee motion. If necessary, this range of motion should be placed in a biomechanically favorable position when the osteotomy is performed.

The time elapsed since the injury will determine the nature of the corrective procedure for posttraumatic deformities about the knee. If it is still possible to identify the old fracture line and mobilize its fragments, causal treatment by *corrective internal fixation* is preferred (Fig. 5). This is most easily done after monocondylar fractures or comminuted fractures whose fragments can be mobilized en bloc. Nonunions in such cases are rare but when present will permit a late realignment and internal fixation of the fragments.

If the fracture has become fully consolidated in a position of deformity, a *corrective osteotomy* is necessary (Tables 1 and 2) [1,5,6,8,10,14,19,20,21, 23,24]. We try to perform the osteotomy as soon as possible after muscular strength has returned, the ligaments are stabilized, and optimum function has been restored (Table 1). The intent of early corrective osteotomy is to prevent secondary disease and encourage reparative processes (Figs. 6–8). This applies equally to isolated traumatic lesions of the articular surfaces that might benefit from a normalization of loads. In many cases the

a

b

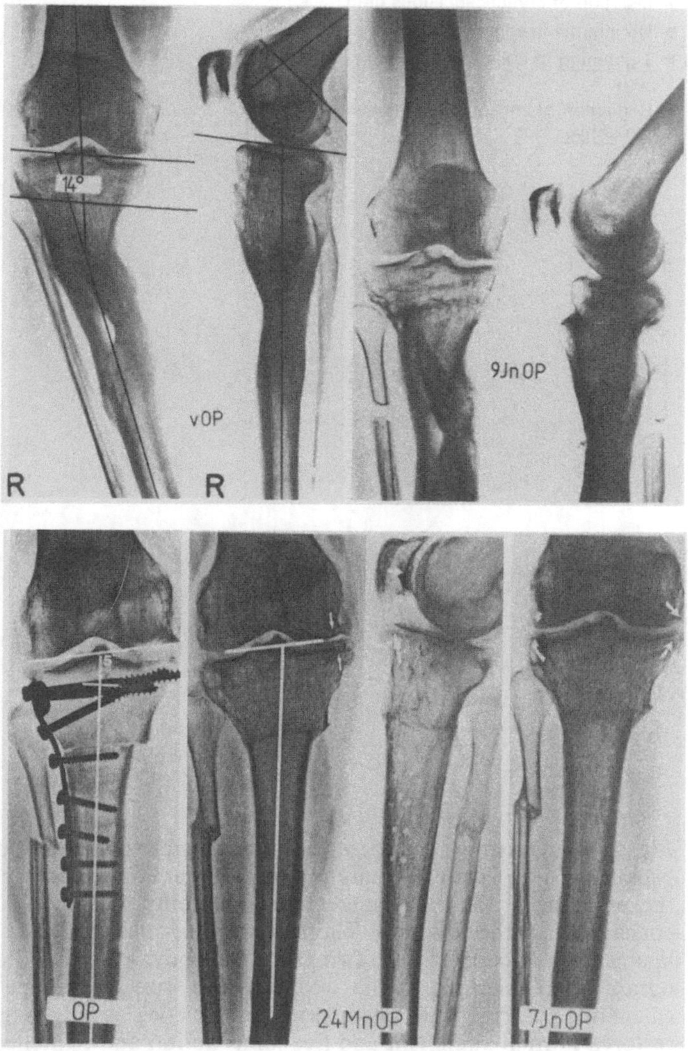

Fig. 3 a,b. Roentgenograms showing the late results of two high tibial osteotomies –one biomechanically correct, the other faulty. **a** Man 42 years of age 3 years after a proximal tibial fracture with posttraumatic varus. After corrective osteotomy, the centered mechanical axis crosses the joint line at right angles. Progression of osteoarthritis was halted, and knee motion at 9 years was unrestricted. **b** Inappropriate proximal tibial osteotomy for valgus deformity in woman 76 years of age. The mechanical axis crosses the joint line obliquely, leading to a shifting of the tibial plateau on the femoral condyles. At 7 years postoperatively the resulting shear forces have caused marked progression of osteoarthritis despite a centered mechanical axis

improvement of metaphyseal blood flow alone will be beneficial. A *late* corrective osteotomy is used to treat severe posttraumtic (or idiopathic) osteoarthritis of the knee (Table 2). Accordingly, the goal of this surgery is not to prevent joint wear and tear, but to arrest or retard its progress. Because the progression of osteoarthritis is intermittent rather than continuous, one should not undertake surgical correction during the asymptomatic phase,

- ▶ Insertion of corticocancellous graft
- ▶ No internal fixation
- ▶ Tightening of collateral ligament on concave side
- ▶ Reduction of tension on collateral ligament on convex side

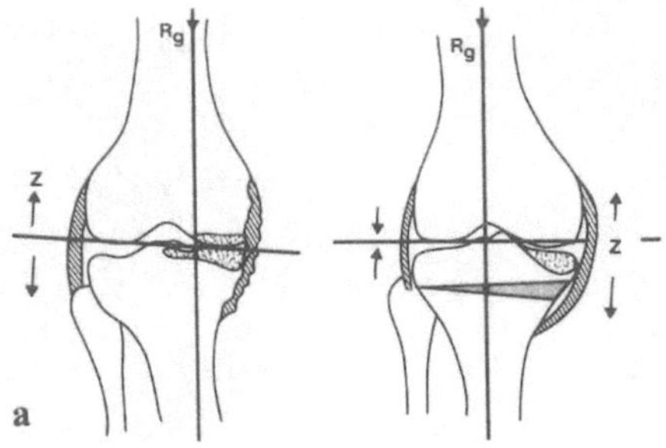

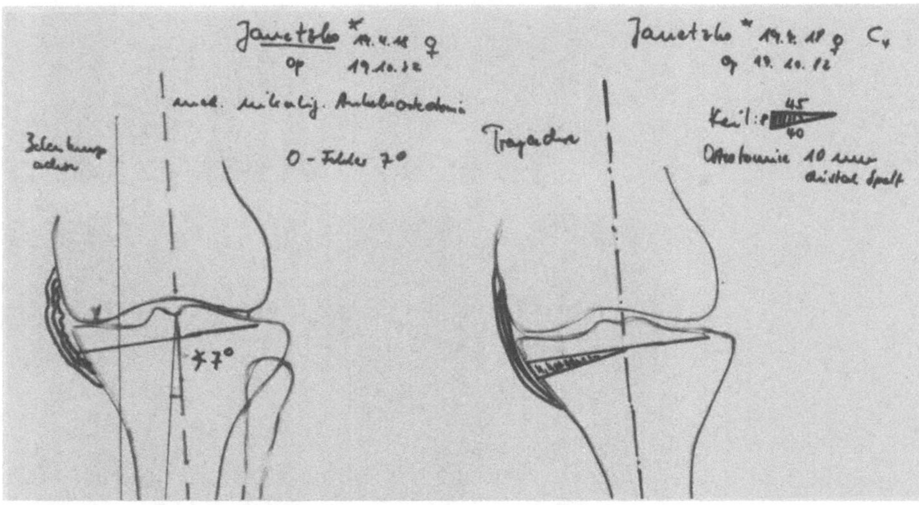
b

Fig. 4 a – e. Drawings and roentgenograms used to plan an intraligamentous elevating osteotomy. I. J., female, 62 years, injured while at home. **a** Schematic diagrams showing the principle of the intraligamentous osteotomy with insertion of a wedge on the concave side of the deformity. The procedure elevates the tibial plateau and tightens lax ligaments. **b** Preoperative drawings for the above patient. **c** Postoperative roentgenogram after insertion of the wedge, whose size and shape had been accurately calculated. **d** Pre- and postoperative whole-leg reontgenograms. The operation restored normal alignment and free joint motion and tightened the medial collateral ligament. **e** Sequence of photos showing the prepared corticocancellous bone wedge, the opened intraligamentous osteotomy made 1 cm distal to the medial tibial plateau, insertion of the prepared wedge, and final impaction of the graft

Table 1. Early Corrective Osteotomy for Posttraumatic Angular Deformities of the Knee

After bone healing and after physical therapy	● Muscular force ● Ligament stabilization ● Therapeutic range of motion
Before secondary changes	● Prevention (amelioration) of osteoarthritis ● Reduction of load ● Replacement tissue ● Adjacent joints

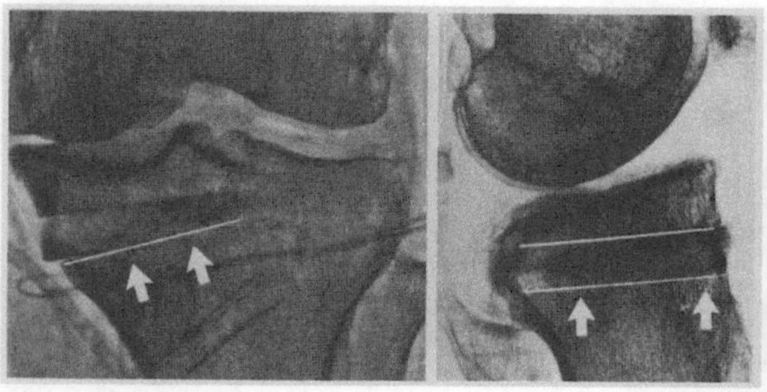

c

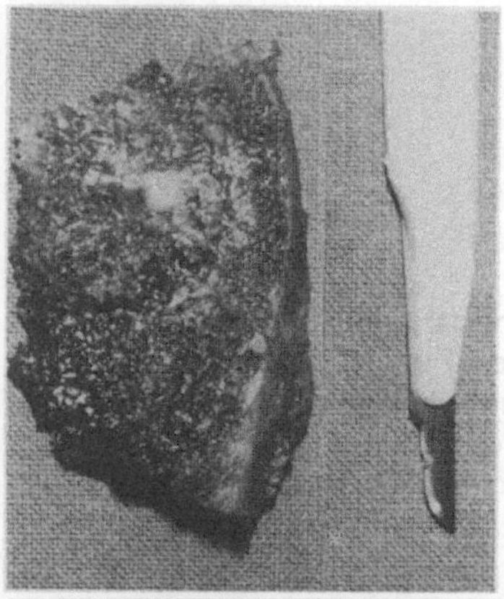

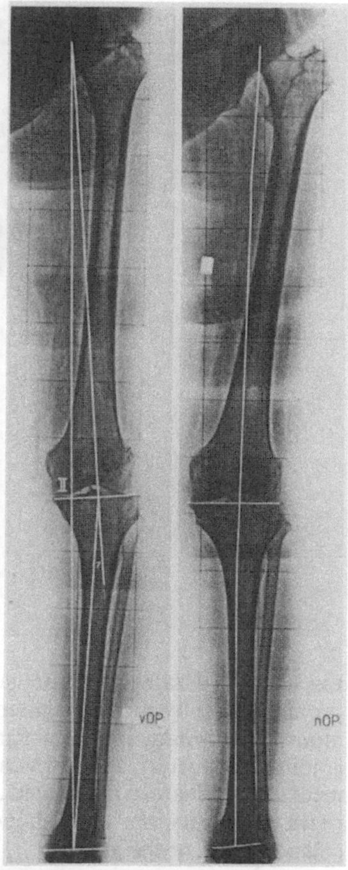

d

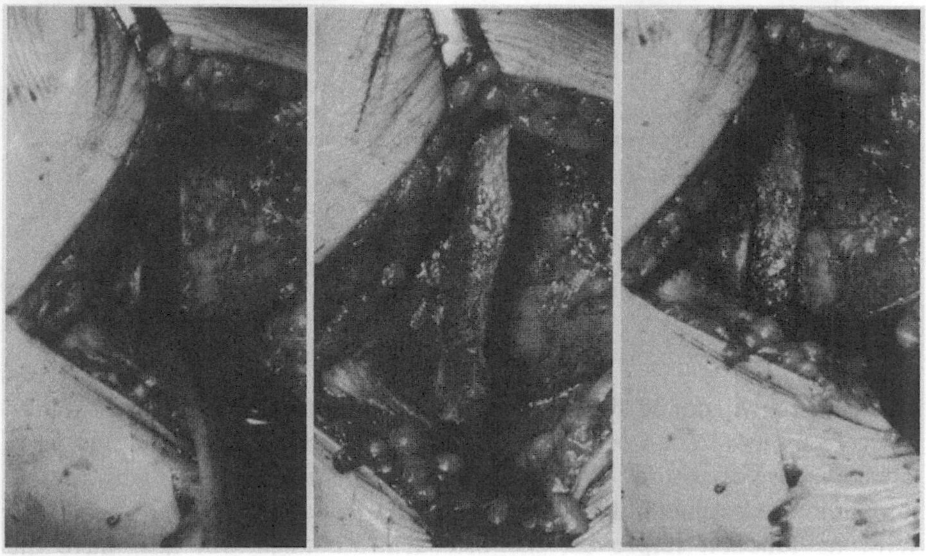

e

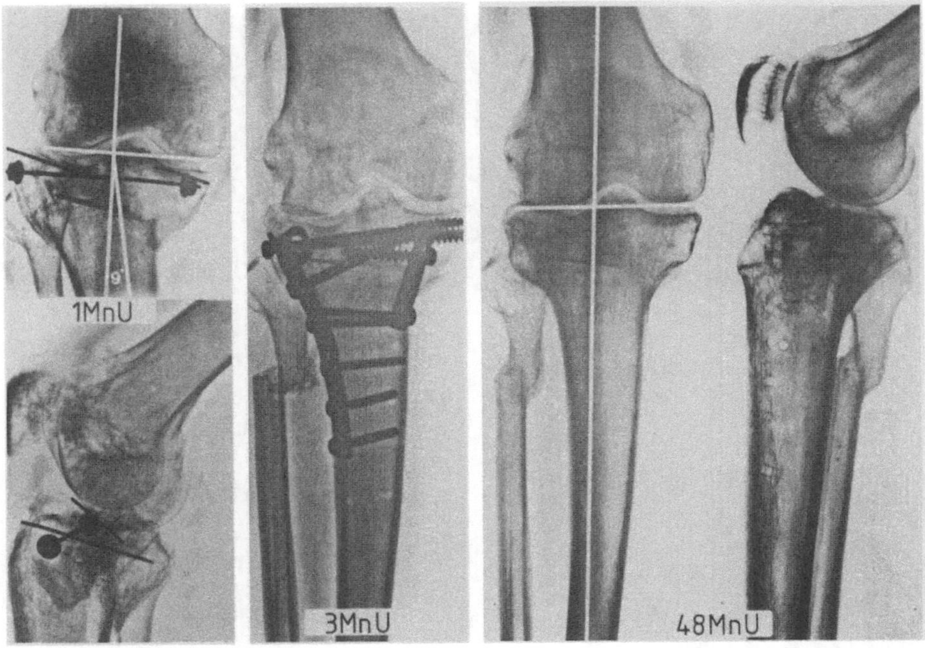

a b c

Fig. 5 a–c. Example of the causal treatment of a posttraumatic deformity of the proximal tibia by corrective internal fixation. F. B., male, 37 years, athletic injury. **a** One month after minimal internal fixation of an intraarticular tibial condylar fracture there is joint incongruity and varus angulation. **b** Stable, corrective internal fixation. The medial tibial plateau is elevated and supported by insertion of cancellous bone. **c** Four years postinjury the limb shows excellent alignment with moderate posttraumatic osteoarthritis of the knee

Table 2. Late Corrective Osteotomy for Posttraumatic Angular Deformities of the Knee

After years of deformity and after development of osteoarthritis of the knee	
Osteotomy is performed when increase is noted in:	● Subjective complaints ● Angulation ● Disability ● Instability

when surgery will not be of subjective benefit, unless the deformity or disability is severe enough to compel intervention [23]. The most favorable time for a late corrective osteotomy is when obvious deterioration is noted with regard to pain, radiographic findings, angulation and instability (Figs. 3,5 and 8). With its function improved, the osteoarthritic knee will also have an opportunity for structural recovery. This is manifested in a fibrocartilage regeneration of the articular surfaces, a regression of circumscribed sclerosis due to stress concentration, and a more uniform structure of the periarticular cancellous bone (Fig. 8) [23].

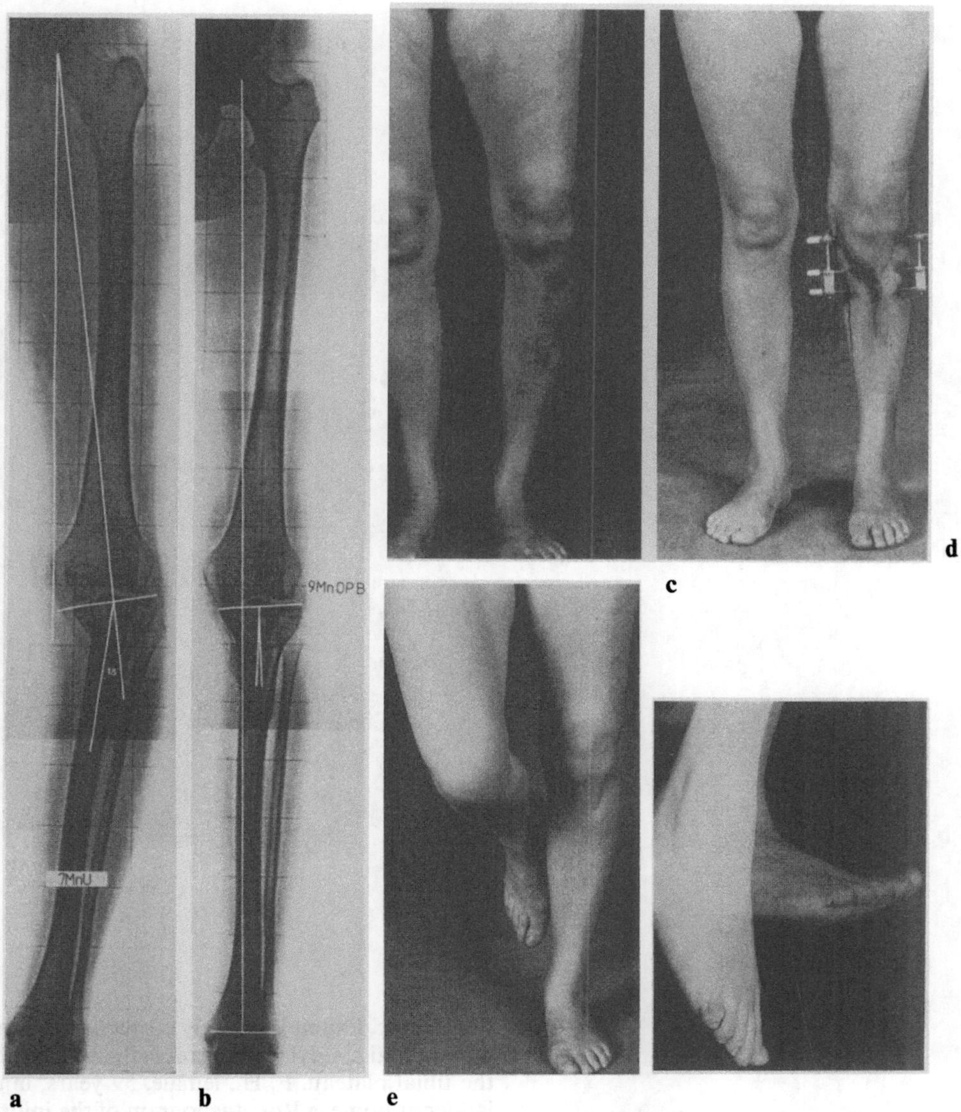

Fig. 6 a – e. Example of an early corrective osteotomy. D. H., female, 44 years, injured in a bicycle accident. **a** A 15° varus deformity is present 7 months after conservative treatment of proximal tibial fracture not involving the joint. **b** Whole-leg roentgenogram 9 months after union of the corrective osteotomy in good alignment. **c** Clinical appearance on admission. **d** Postoperative clinical appearance after proximal tibial osteotomy stabilized with a threaded-rod external fixator. **e** The functional result at 9 months is shown. Knee and ankle motion are unrestricted, and the leg is stable during stance; subjective complaints are mild

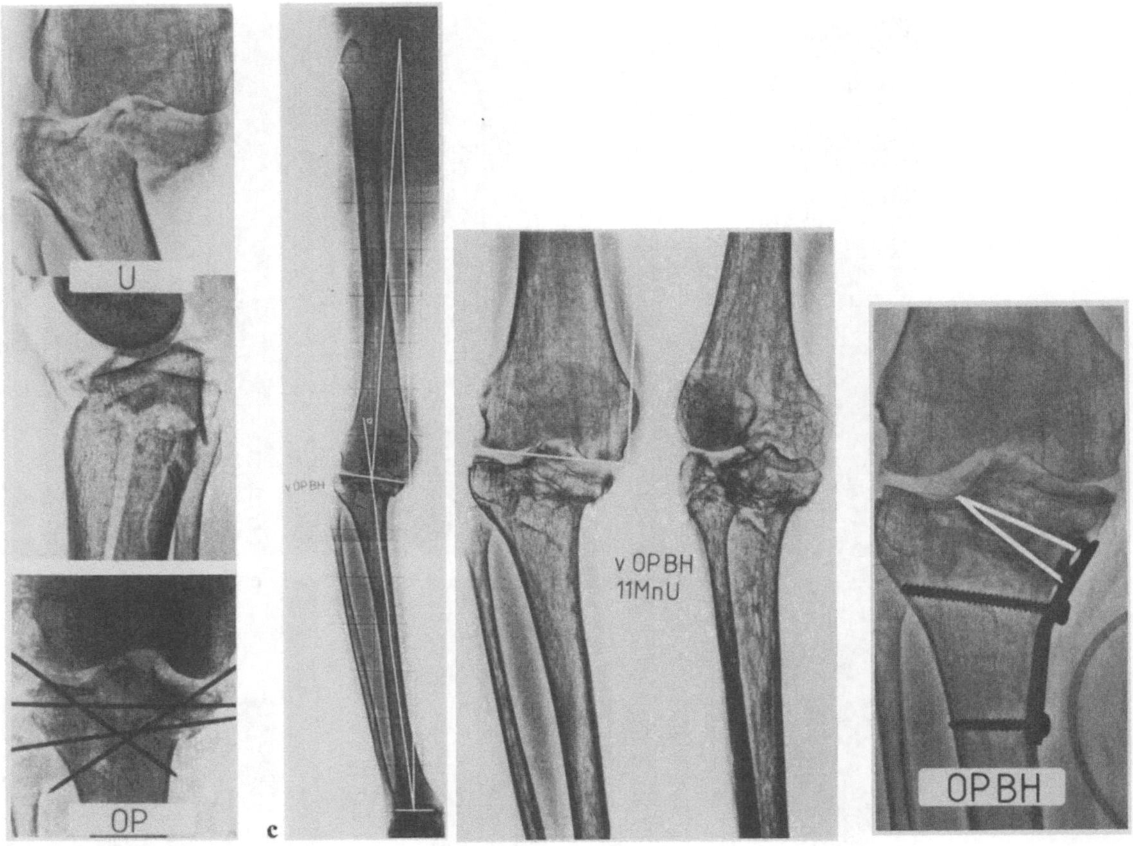

a b c d

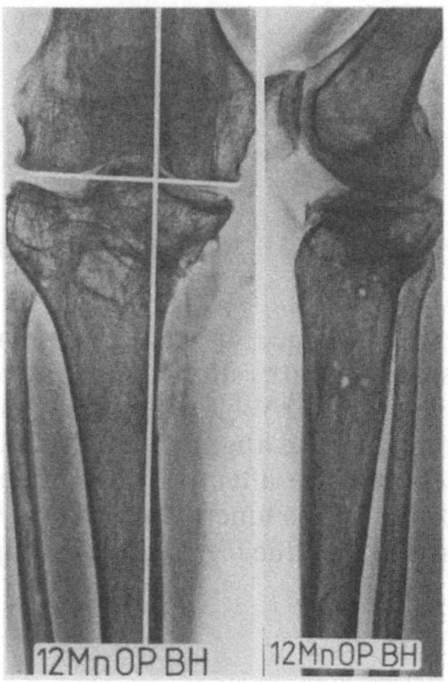

e

Fig. 7 a – c. Example of early corrective osteotomy after comminuted tibial condylar fracture and osteoplastic reconstruction of the tibial plateau. F. H., female, 59 years, injured in fall from a ladder at home. **a** Roentgenogram of the injury showing marked dislocation. **b** Minimal internal fixation was carried out elsewhere. **c** Whole-leg roentgenograms and close-ups of the knee show significant posttraumatic deformity of the tibial condyle and plateau with 18° varus deformity at 11 months postinjury. **d** Status after open wedge osteotomy with insertion of wedge, cancellous grafting, and internal fixation with a buttress plate. **e** Satisfactory reconstruction of the upper tibia with residual traumatic deformity of the medial plateau at 12 months after surgery. The patient has a 0 – 0 – 120 range of knee motion, a stable leg, and moderate subjective complaints

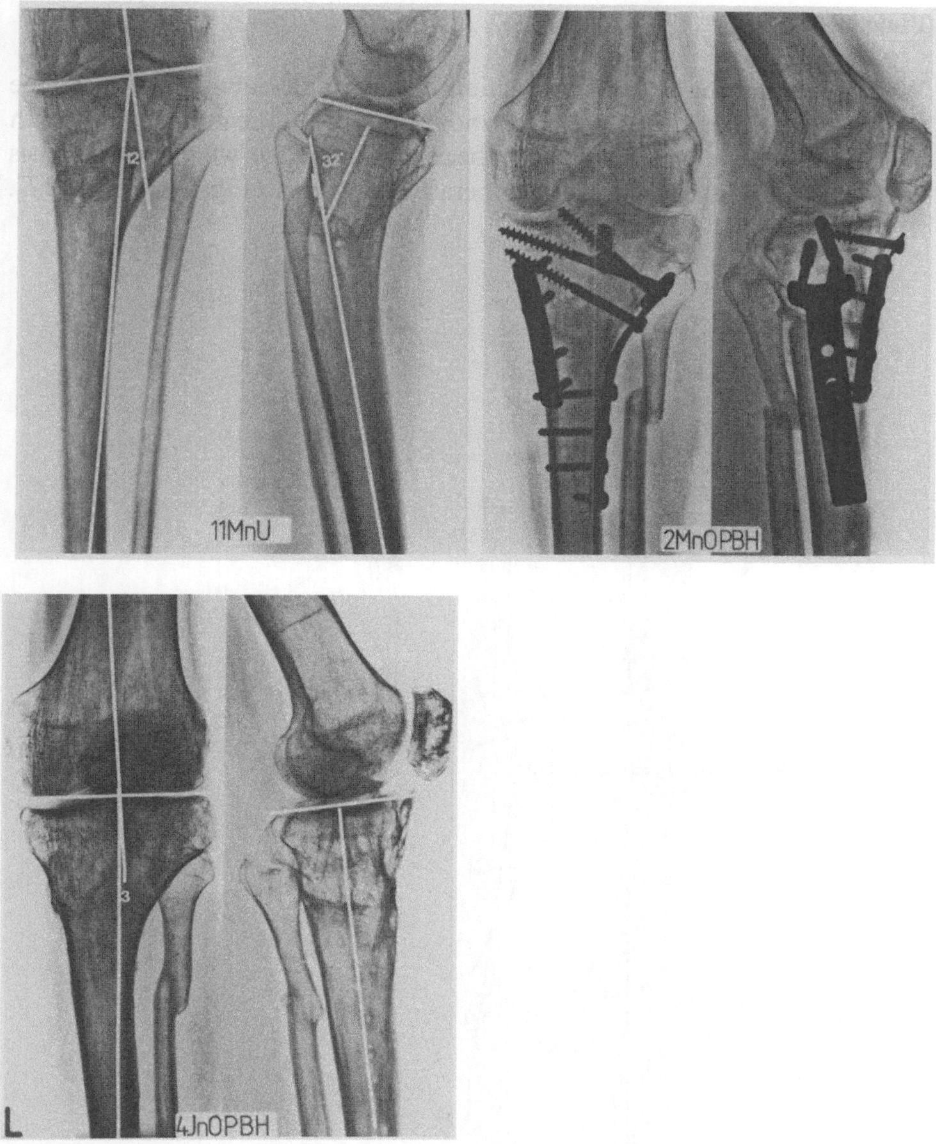

a b c

Fig. 8 a – c. Example of early corrective osteotomy of the proximal tibia in two planes. D. W., male, 19 years, injured in motorcycle accident. **a** Roentgenograms on admission 11 months postinjury show significant deformity of the upper tibia in both planes. **b** Two months after proximal tibial osteotomy. **c** Fourteen years after surgery there is normal alignment in both planes, mild osteoarthritis, and excellent knee motion; the patient has no subjective complaints

Planning

When planning the surgical correction of deformities about the knee, one should obtain roentgenograms in standard projections as well as full-length axial films of both legs under weight bearing. These films will provide a basis for the preparation of accurate preoperative drawings (Fig. 9) [4,12,13,17].

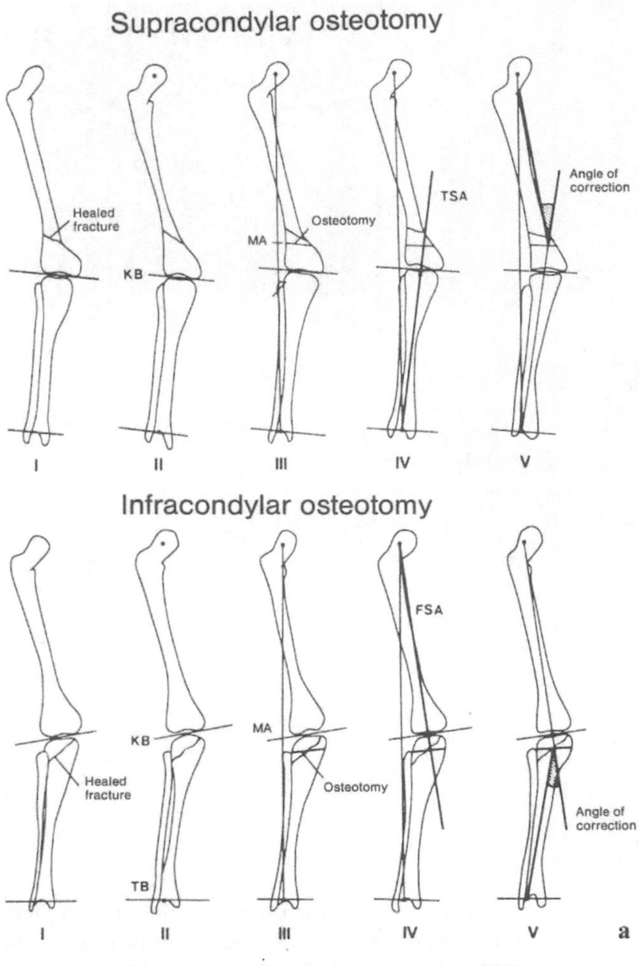

Fig. 9 a – d. Planning the surgical correction of deformities about the knee in the frontal plane.
a Diagrams illustrating the planning of supracondylar and infracondylar osteotomies for posttraumatic genu valgum: Whole-leg roentgenograms are used to determine the site of the osteotomy and the numerical correction angle in relation to the level of osteotomy. After the mechanical axis and proposed line of supracondylar osteotomy are drawn (upper panel), the correction angle is found by extending the line connecting the centers of the ankle and knee joints, finding its point of intersection with the line of osteotomy, and drawing a line from that point to the center of the femoral head. In the infracondylar osteotomy (lower panel), the numerical correction angle is determined at the osteotomy site by finding the intersection of the mechanical axis of the intact bone with the osteotomy surface, and drawing a line from that point to the center of the ankle joint

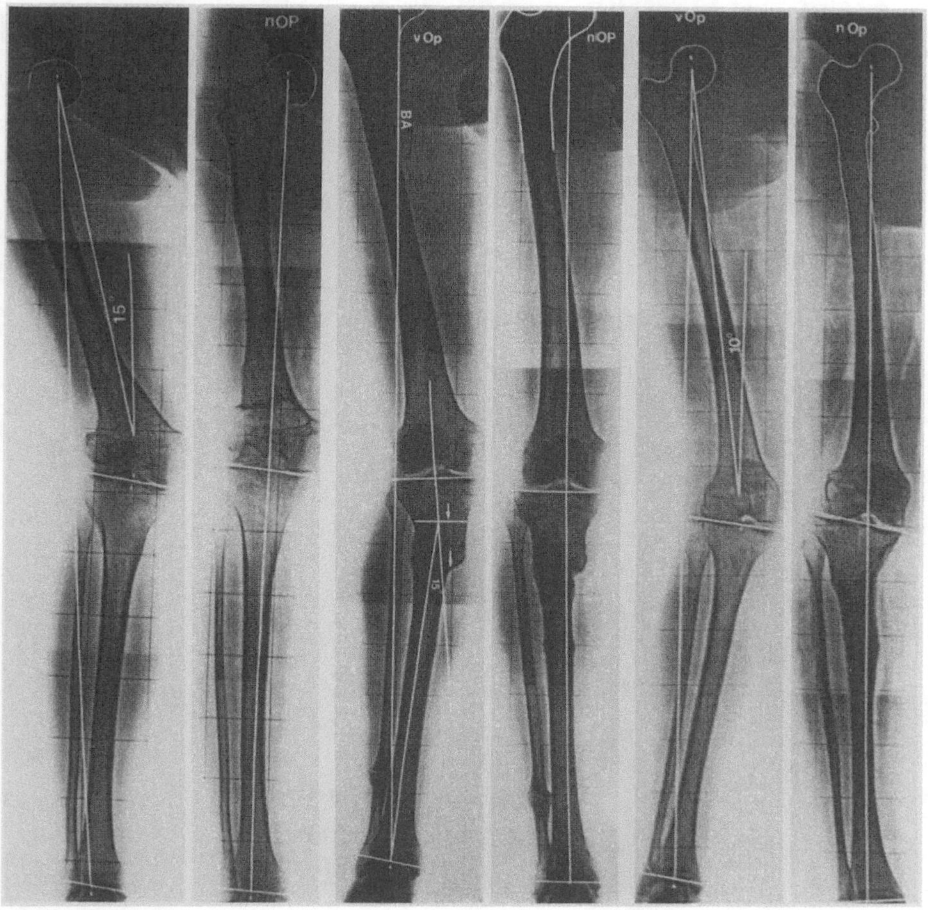

b **c** **d**

Fig. 9 b–d. b Example of a supracondylar closed wedge osteotomy to correct a 15° posttraumatic deformity. **c** Example of an infracondylar closed wedge osteotomy to correct a posttraumatic 15° valgus deformity of the upper tibia; normal alignment is restored. **d** Example of an inappropriate proximal tibial osteotomy: The 10° supracondylar valgus deformity (secondary to a lateral condylar fracture) was corrected in the upper tibia, necessarily resulting in abnormal obliquity of the knee and ankle joints despite a centered mechanical axis. This caused aggravation of subjective complaints

The whole-leg roentgenograms are used to determine the proper angle of correction and the site of the osteotomy (Figs. 2 and 9 a) [4,17]. When obtaining these films, it is essential that the knee joints be frontalized with respect to the film plane to avoid apparent errors of projection [13,17,19]. This danger is present with flexion deformity of the knee. Leg lengths must be equalized before the films are taken. Significant rotational deformities should be accurately measured. Lately, computed tomography has gained increasing importance in the evaluation of rotational limb deformity. The full-length roentgenograms of the legs will provide information on the numerical value of the correction angle in relation to the level of the osteotomy (Figs. 2 and 9). First the mechanical axis of the intact bone (femur or tibia) is drawn on the

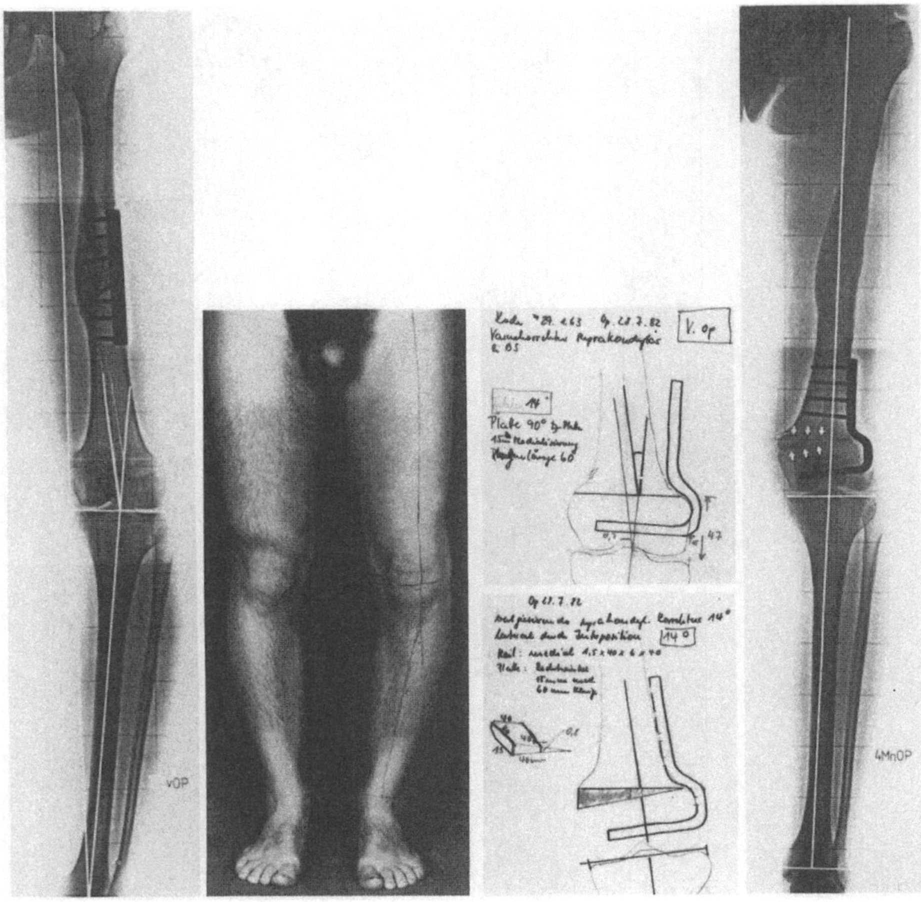

a b

Fig. 10 a – f. Roentgenograms and drawings used in the planning of supracondylar corrective osteotomies for posttraumatic deformity.
a Clinical and roentgenographic appearance of a 14° varus deformity 12 months after a motorcycle accident in which the patient sustained a femoral shaft fracture and an ipsilateral medial condylar fracture, which was treated conservatively. **b** Preoperative drawings of the valgus supracondylar osteotomy with medial insertion of a corticocancellous wedge and lateral placement of a right-angle plate. Bony consolidation, good axial alignment and unrestricted knee motion are present 4 months after surgery

film, and its point of intersection with the proposed line of osteotomy (osteotomy surface) is located. Then a line is drawn from that point to the center of the hip joint (for a supracondylar deformity) or to the center of the ankle joint (for an infracondylar deformity). The angle formed by that line with the mechanical axis of the intact bone will equal the necessary angle of correction (Fig. 9 a) [4,13,17]. The actual operative procedure is planned with the help of scale drawings that indicate the sequence of operative steps, the location and size of the bone wedge that is to be resected or interposed, the technique for fixation of the fragments, and the result of the correction (Figs.

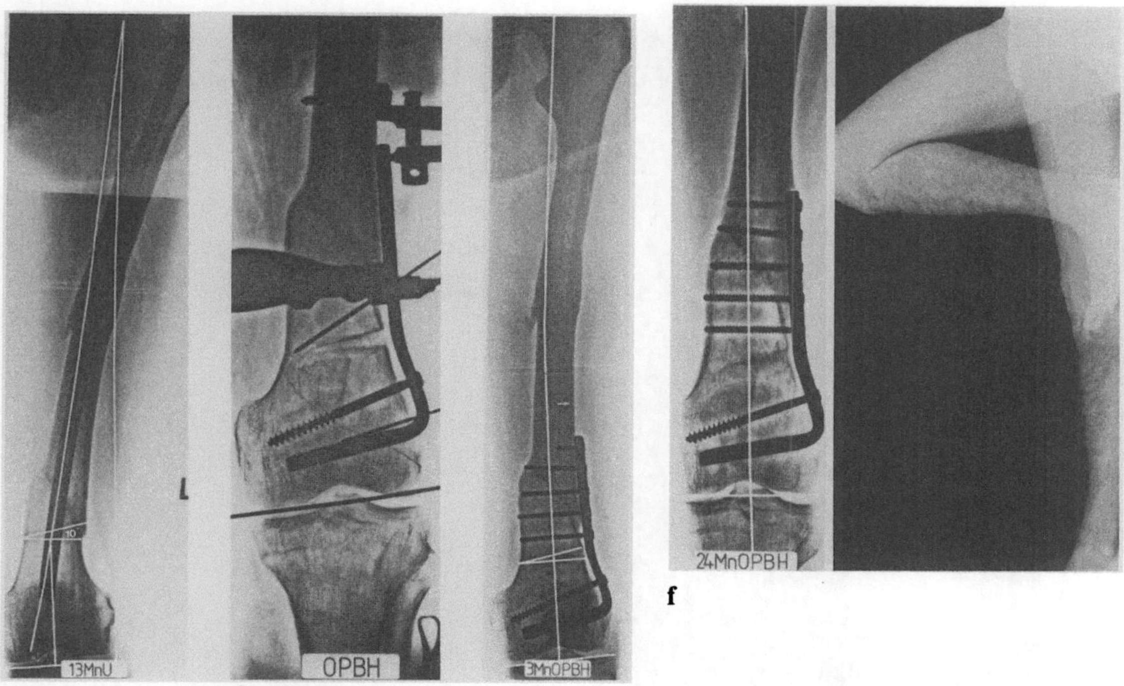

c d e f

Fig. 10 c – e. c Supracondylar valgus deformity of 10° after the intramedullary nailing of a double femoral fracture (performed elsewhere). **d** Intraoperative roentgenogram to check alignment after lateral insertion of a corticocancellous wedge; the internal fixation was stabilized under compression with a condylar plate. **e** Good axial alignment at 3 months after surgery. **f** Roentgenographic and clinical result with proper limb alignment at 2 years after surgery

4, 10 – 12). Complex deformities require a staged planning in which one joint member is aligned first before proceeding to the other. This simulation of the operative steps will help even the experienced surgeon to prepare difficult steps, shorten operating time, and obtain a better end result (Fig. 12). Any difficulties that are identified preoperatively should be presented to the patient in terms he can understand.

With posttraumatic angular deformity, the fractured joint member or traumatically bowed shaft near the joint will indicate the vertex of the deformity (Fig. 9 b). The location of this vertex determines whether a supracondylar or infracondylar osteotomy will be required. It is important to note that the site of the osteotomy and the site of the former periarticular fracture rarely coincide. In principle, osteotomies above and below the knee may by equally effective in centering the mechanical axis of the limb (Figs. 2 b,c and 9). However, every axial correction must ensure that the baselines of the knee and ankle joints remain parallel. If a supracondylar osteotomy or high tibial osteotomy results in obliquity of the joint line of the knee relative to the ankle joint with relative displacement of the articular surfaces of the femoral condyle and tibial plateau, the resulting shear forces will exacerbate the asymmetric loads on the knee, and stretching of the collateral ligaments

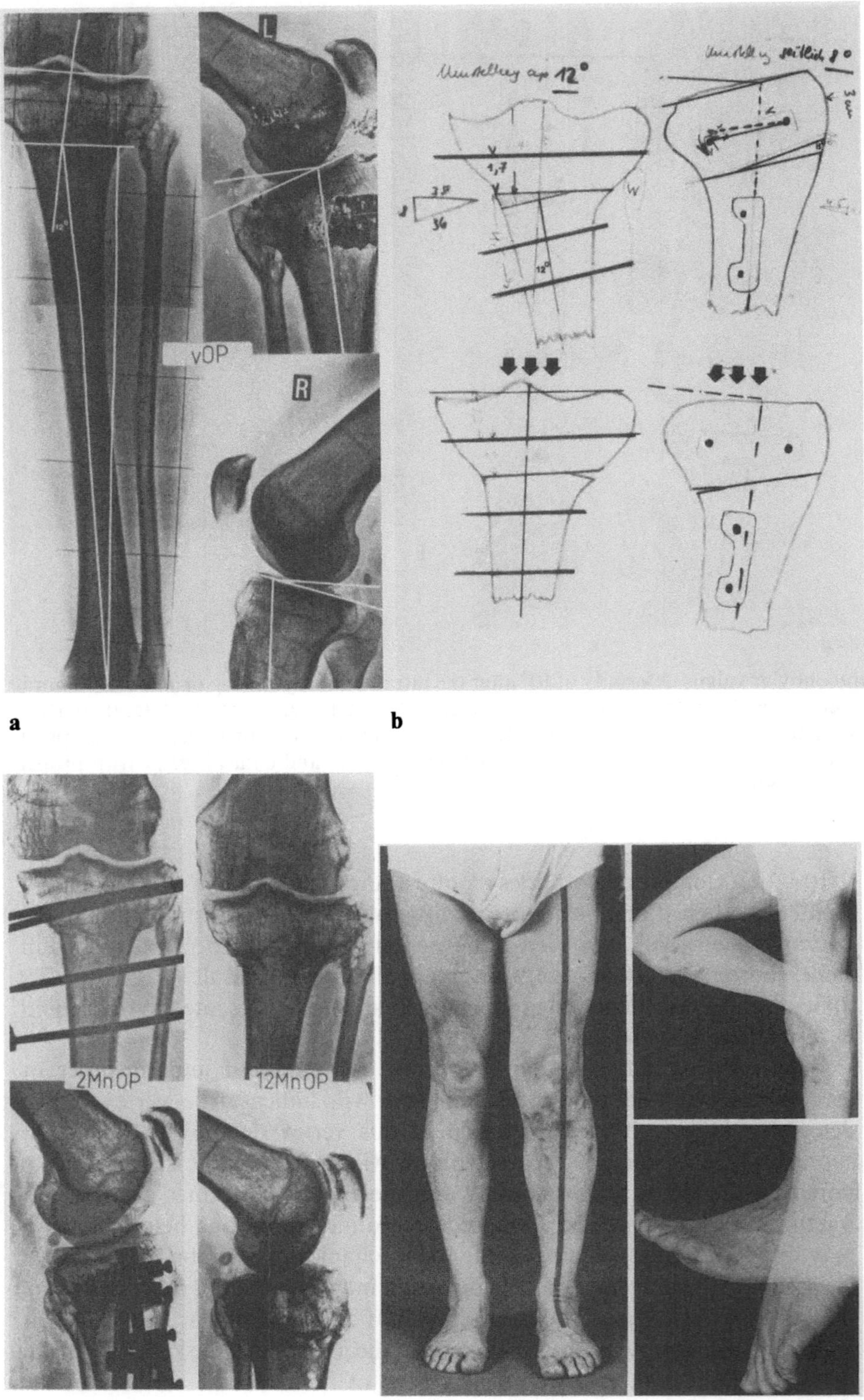

a b

c d e

will destabilize the joint. Despite centering of the mechanical axis, the operation must be considered a failure because it aggravates pathologic symptoms and osteoarthritic disease (Figs. 2 b and 9 d). To state this in biomechanical terms: The line of action of the resultant R_g will pass lateral or medial to the center of the knee, depending on whether a valgus or varus deformity exists. The resection of a wedge based on the convex side of the deformity shifts R_g toward the center of the joint. The articular surfaces in turn will alter their position according to whether a supra- or infracondylar correction is performed. The correction must not only center the resultant R_g, but must also rotate the articular baseline such that it is perpendicular to R_g (Fig. 2 c) [8,9]. This will expose the articular surfaces to pure compressive forces, and the compressive stresses will be distributed over surfaces of equal size. Given the variety of biomechanical changes that can occur, the surgeon who deals with angular deformities about the knee requires a mastery of all relevant operative procedures [1,2,5,6,10,15,19–21,23,24). Yet even with traumatic deformity proximal to the axis of the knee, many surgeons continue to prefer the technically easier *high tibial osteotomy* (infracondylar osteotomy) over the supracondylar osteotomy (Fig. 9 d) [12,13]. When a high tibial osteotomy is indicated, we presently stabilize it with the special threaded external fixator of the ASIF (Figs. 5,11 and 12). Certainly, *supracondylar* femoral osteotomies are among the most technically demanding operations about the knee (Figs. 9 a,b and 10) [23]. Meticulous operating technique and a sound program of physical therapy are necessary to prevent disability due to adhesions of mobile soft-tissue layers. The medial approach often selected for supracondylar correction of a valgus deformity by medial wedge resection is unfavorable due to the proximity of major blood vessels, the likelihood of significant wound and scar pain on the sensitive medial surface of the thigh, and impairment of wound healing by adipose tissue. These problems can be avoided, even with a valgus deformity, by using a lateral approach and applying a lateral right-angle or condylar plate. At this time a wedge may be resected medially, or a supracondylar open wedge osteotomy may be performed laterally and corticocancellous wedge graft inserted (Figs. 10 c–f). In any event this is the more rational option in posttraumatic states due to the necessity of a lateral approach.

Axial corrections about the knee must also take into account the condition of capsular and ligamentous structures. A closed wedge osteotomy often fails

Fig. 11 a–e. Roentgenograms and drawings used to plan a proximal tibial osteotomy for deformity in two planes. K. H., male, 49 years, sustained a closed intraarticular tibial condylar fracture in a fall from scaffolding. **a** Preperative roentgenograms showing 12° valgus deformity and 8° posterior slope of tibial plateau at 7 months postinjury. **b** Preoperative drawings of the correction in two planes, indicating the placement of the Steinmann pins and the size of the lateral and anterior wedges to be removed. **c** Roentgenograms at 2 months postoperatively showing the external fixator in place. **d, e** The roentgenographic, clinical and functional result at 1 year after surgery: no subjective complaints, unrestricted joint motion, moderate osteoarthritis from traumatic deformity of the medial tibial plateau

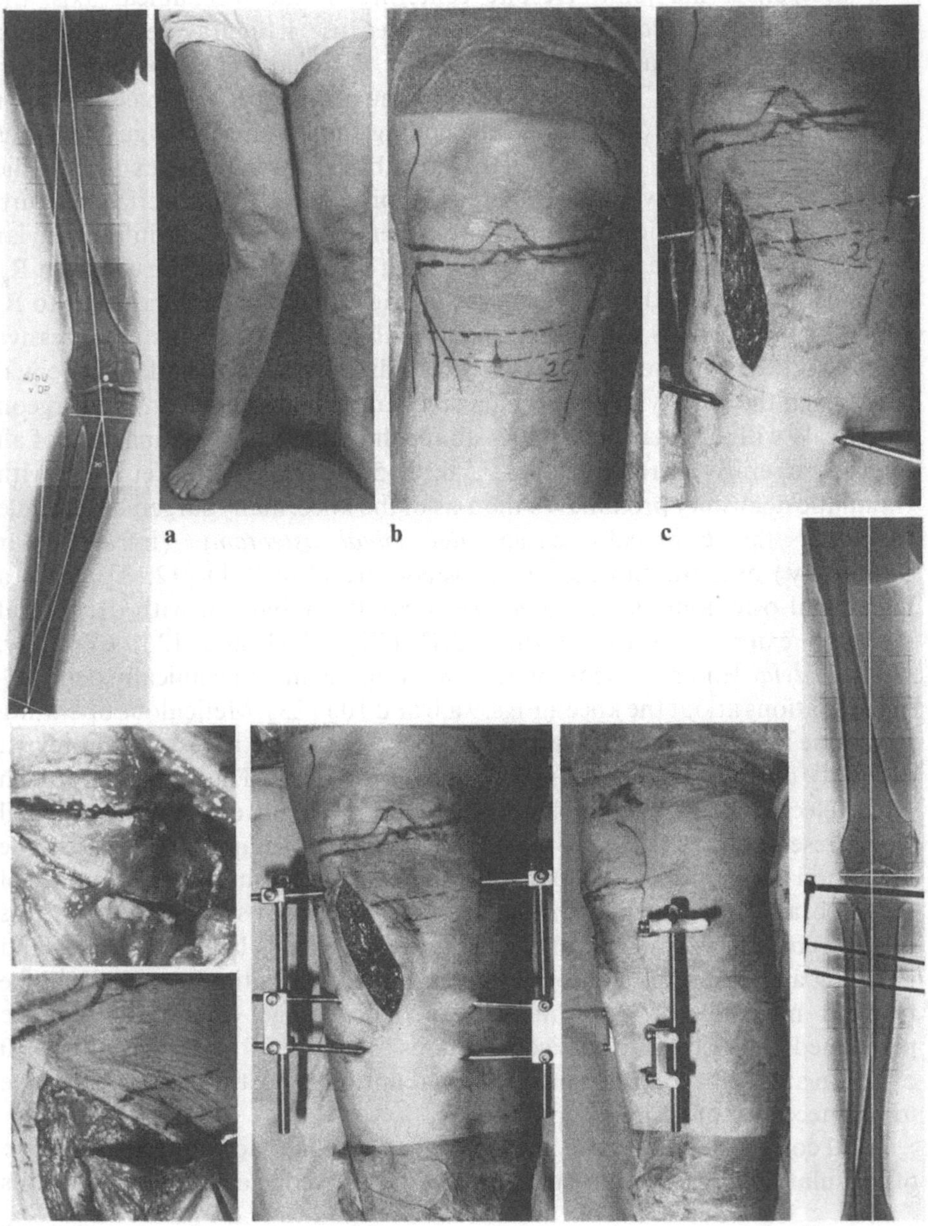

d e f

Fig. 12 a–f. a Whole-leg roentgenogram and clinical appearance of 20° valgus deformity. **b** The joint space and position of the proximal Steinmann pin, which is parallel to the joint space, are marked on the skin under image intensifier control. **c** The Steinmann pin proximal to the osteotomy is inserted parallel to the articular surface of the tibial plateau; the distal pin is inserted at an angle corresponding to the valgus deformity measured preoperatively. **d** Through a lateral incision, the wedge size determined preoperatively is marked on the periosteum with a chisel, and the wedge is restricted. **e** The distal fragment is aligned, the clamps of the external fixator are attached to the pins, a supplementary pin is inserted, and medial compression is applied. **f** Postoperative roentgenogram showing restoration of axial alignment with good placement of the external fixator

to relieve instability because the ligaments remain lax on the concave side of the deformity (Fig. 1 a, b). In patients under 50 years of age, we solve this problem by performing an intraligamentous open wedge osteotomy on the concave side and inserting a corticocancellous wedge graft, which both elevates the tibial plateau and restores tension to the collateral ligaments (Fig. 4) [3]. With irreversible laxity of the ligamentous attachment, neither an open wedge nor closed wedge osteotomy can restore stability to the malaligned knee, because the dynamic muscular stabilizers are absent and cannot be reactivated by conditioning [12]. Posttraumatic deformities of the femoral and tibial shaft can likewise be corrected near the knee [12,23]. The advantage of this is the more favorable healing potential of the metaphyseal bone. The metaphyseal correction of a shaft deformity is necessary in the presence of local soft-tissue damage or a prior midshaft infection that would preclude a direct diaphyseal correction. The disadvantage is that valgus and varus corrections involve more than simply noting angular deviation from the mechanical axis. A metaphyseal correction that takes into account only the shaft deformity will cause a lateral or medial displacement of the limb axis distant from the osteotomy and will produce functional malalignment of the knee joint. For this reason a femoral shaft deformity that is to be corrected by a distal osteotomy needs a slightly greater angle of correction than the shaft deformity itself would require. Conversely, a tibial shaft deformity corrected by proximal tibial osteotomy requires a somewhat smaller correction angle than would otherwise be the case [4,11,12]. Because of these difficulties, we try to correct the deformity at the site of the old shaft fracture in younger patients if local conditions are satisfactory.

It should be emphasized that idiopathic angular limb deformities can be corrected with a high degree of accuracy, and that the treatment of traumatic angular deformity about the knee with intact articular surfaces has a very high success rate when biomechanical and technical principles are observed (Figs. 3, 10 and 13). By contrast, deformity that is secondary to comminuted fractures of the femoral condyle and upper tibia is already so serve that, regardless of associated cartilage damage, osseous defects, and capsular and ligamentous lesions, the goal of treatment is simply to restore an alignment that approximates the normal weight-bearing axis (Figs. 7, 8 and 11). The status of the limb may be so poor that residual deformities of less than 10° will be tolerated rather than subject the patient to another osteotomy (Fig. 14). In the presence of multiple intra- and extra-articular lesions at various levels, a corrective osteotomy of the knee joint after trauma may not always be entirely satisfactory in terms of function and subjective outcome. However, this should not prevent the surgeon from exhausting all reasonable corrective and osteoplastic options, especially in young patients (Fig. 14).

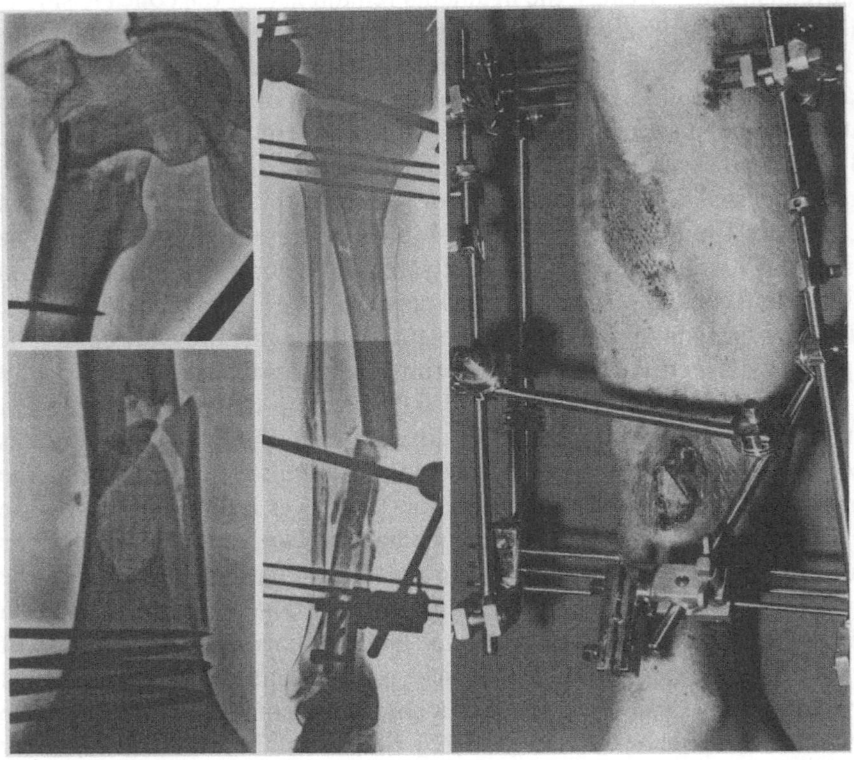

a

Fig. 13 a – c. Example of the need for compromise in treating posttraumatic angular deformities in a leg with multiple injuries. J. L., male, 55 years, injured in traffic accident while driving a truck. **a** The patient presented with a subtrochanteric and distal femoral fracture and segmental tibial shaft fracture that had been fixed externally abroad. There was posttraumatic osteomyelitis of the distal tibia

Fig. 13 b. The femoral shaft fractures were managed by open reduction and internal fixation. The tibial osteomyelitis was treated by stable external fixation, debridement, autologous cancellous bone grafting, and the application of split-thickness skin grafts
Fig. 13 c. Roentgenographic, clinical and functional status 18 months postoperatively. There is an S-shaped bowing of the limb axis, but the joint axes are excellent, and the leg bears weight normally. The patient was left with 2 cm of residual shortening, a slight limitation of terminal motion in the hip, and a greater restriction of motion in the knee and ankle

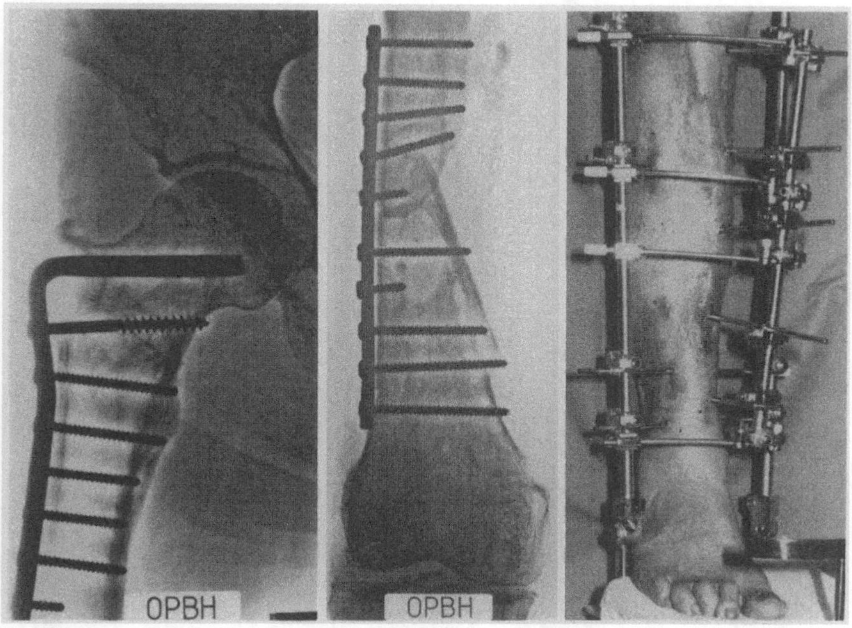

b

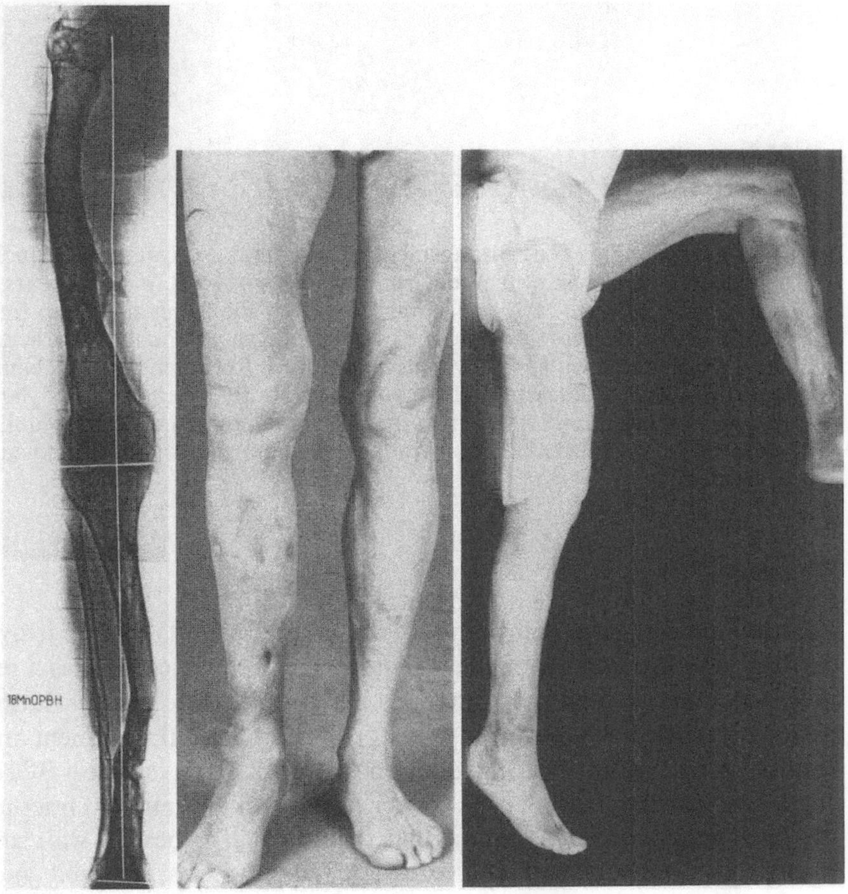

c

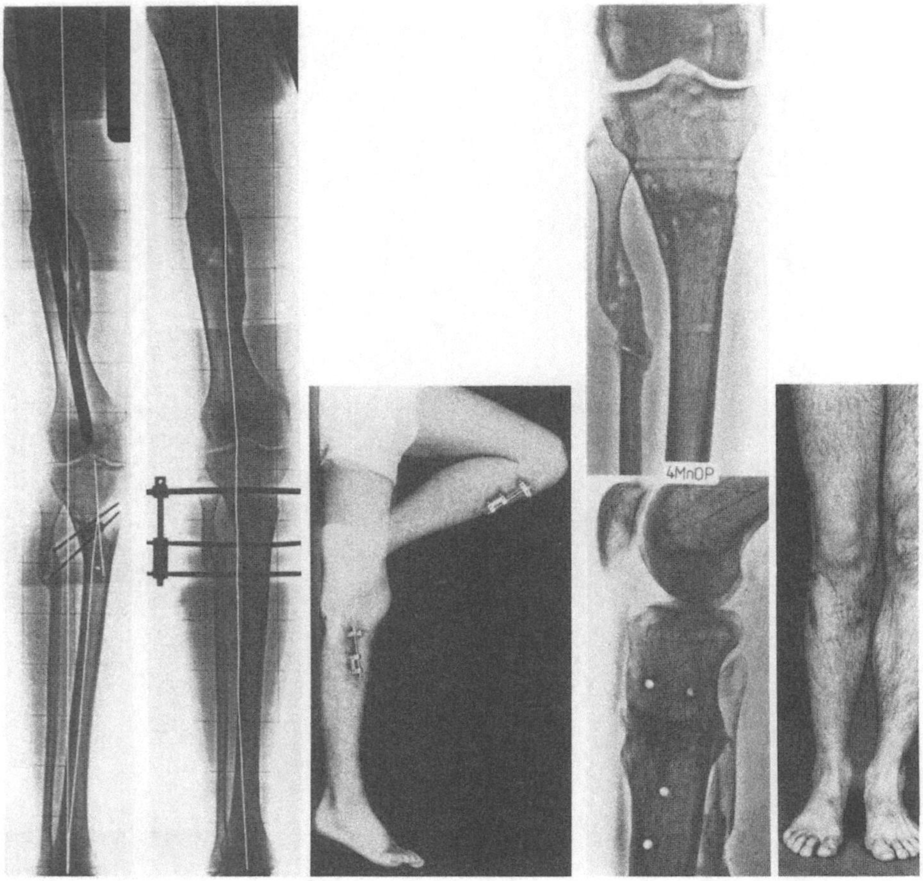

a b c

Fig. 14 a–e. Example of the management of ipsilateral posttraumatic sequelae with shortening of the femur and valgus deformity of the tibia. M. F., male, 18 years, injured in a motorcycle accident. **a** A segmental fracture of the femur had been treated by intramedullary nailing, resulting in 5 cm of shortening; a proximal tibial fracture fixed with drill wires healed with 14° of valgus deformity. **b** Roentgenographic, clinical and functional result after correction of the valgus deformity by an infracondylar medial wedge-resection osteotomy stabilized with an external frame (the intramedullary nail was removed). **c** At 4 months postoperatively the limb shows good alignment with 6 cm of shortening

Summary

Posttraumatic angular deformities of the lower extremity lead to irreversible cartilage damage and traumatic osteoarthritis of the knee joint as a result of excessive, concentrated pressure loads on the joint. The goal of the surgical treatment of these conditions is to restore a normal axial alignment and thus restore normal weight-bearing loads on the cartilaginous surfaces. If a causal, corrective internal fixation is no longer possible in an ununited fracture near the knee with accompanying angular deformity, it is best to wait until the fracture has consolidated and adequate function has returned and then

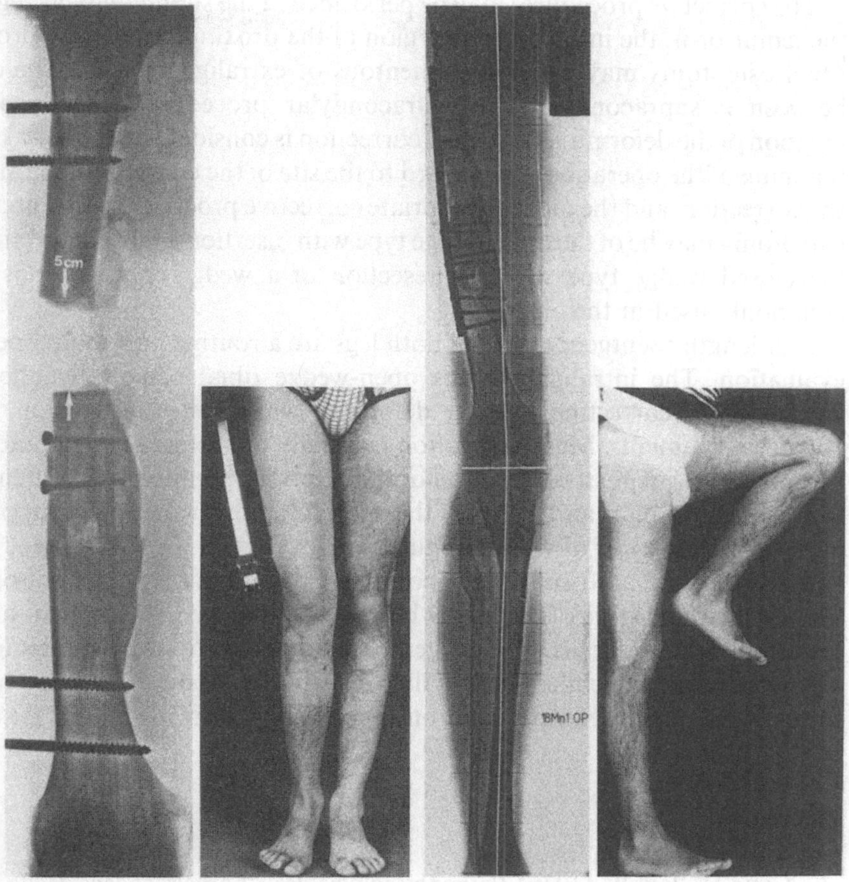

d e

Fig. 14 d, e. d Roentgenographic and clinical result of a femoral lengthening osteotomy using the Wagner distraction apparatus. **e** Result at 18 months after initial treatment. Angular deformity has been corrected with 1 cm of shortening. The lengthening defect is largely consolidated, and motion is unimpaired

perform an "early" corrective osteotomy. With regard to the late correction of posttraumatic deformity, which is somewhat rare in comparison with idiopathic deformity, pain is the main criterion in the election of corrective osteotomy. On the whole, the following factors should be considered when selecting cases for posttraumatic osteotomies about the knee:
– subjective complaints
– the nature and location of the angular deformity
– the stability of the ligaments
– the range of joint motion
– the condition of traumatically damaged joint surfaces and periarticular osseous structures
– the location and severity of osteoarthritis
– biological age
– the status of adjacent and contralateral joints.

The corrective procedures may be performed in the supracondylar region of the femur or in the infracondylar region of the proximal tibia. The proximal tibial osteotomy may be intraligamentous or extraligamentous. The choice between a supracondylar and infracondylar procedure depends on the location of the deformity. If surgical correction is considered necessary, careful planning of the operation with regard to the site of the correction, the angle of the correction, and the most appropriate corrective procedure is essential. The osteotomy may be of the open wedge type with insertion of a wedge graft, or of the closed wedge type with the resection of a wedge. The latter is more commonly used in the elderly.

Full-length roentgenograms of both legs are a routine part of preoperative evaluation. The intraligamentous open-wedge tibial osteotomy offers the advantage of correcting angular deformity while restoring tension to the collateral ligaments. Metallic fixation is usually unnecessary. In supracondylar corrections of posttraumatic deformities, prior operations very often make it necessary to plan and perform the osteotomy from the lateral approach, even in the presence of valgus angulation.

The success of a posttraumatic corrective osteotomy depends not only on the nature and degree of the injury but also on the age of the patient and the setting of realistic goals. The surgeon has an obligation to understand the biomechanical principles of angular deformities about the knee and to simulate the proposed operation on preoperative drawings.

References

1. Cotta H, Paul W (1976) Pathophysiologie des Knorpelschadens. Hefte Unfallheilkd 127:1–22
2. Debrunner Am (1970) Die operative Behandlung von Gonarthrosen. In: Nicod L (Hrsg) Die Gonarthrosen. Huber, Bern Stuttgart Wien
3. Dolanc B (1973) Die Behandlung des instabilen Kniegelenkes mit Achsenfehlstellung durch intraligamentäre Anhebe–Tibiaosteotomie. Arch Orthop Unfallchir 76:280–289
4. Frank W, Oest O, Rettig H (1974) Die Röntgenganzaufnahme in der Operationsplanung von Korrekturosteotomien der Beine. Z Orthop 112:344–347
5. Haas N, Behrens S, Jacobity J (1978) Technik und Ergebnisse der kniegelenknahen Osteotomien. Unfallheilkunde 81:634–641
6. Hagemann H, Schauwecker HH (1979) Möglichkeiten, Technik und Ergebnisse kniegelenknaher Osteotomien. Arch Orthop Trauma Surg 93:117–123
7. Kummer B (1977) Biomechanische Grundlagen "beanspruchungsändernder" Osteotomien im Bereich des Kniegelenkes. Z Orthop 115:923–928
8. Maquet P (1976) Biomechnics of the knee. Springer, Berlin Heidelberg New York
9. Maquet P (1979) Korrekturosteotomien in der Behandlung der Kniearthrose. Orthopäde 8:296–308
10. Müller KH (1979) Prinzipien kniegelenknaher Umstellungsosteotomien gestern und heute. Aktuel Traumatol 9:127–133
11. Müller KH (1981) Exogene Osteomyelitis von Becken und unteren Gliedmaßen. Springer, Berlin Heidelberg New York
12. Müller KH, Biebrach M (1977) Korrekturosteotomien und ihre Ergebnisse bei kniegelenknahen posttraumatischen Fehlstellungen. Unfallheilkunde 80:359–367

13. Müller KH, Biebrach M (1977) Korrekturosteotomien und ihre Ergebnisse bei idiopathischen kniegelenknahen Achsenfehlstellungen. Unfallheilkunde 80:457–464
14. Müller ME (1970) Posttraumatische Achsenfehlstellungen an der unteren Extremität. Huber, Bern
15. Müller W (1976) Die Tibia-Osteotomie in der Therapie posttraumatischer Arthrosen am Kniegelenk. Hefte Unfallheilkd 128:175–181
16. Muggler E, Huber D, Burri C (1975) Ergebnisse nach operativer Versorgung von 225 Tibiakopffrakturen. Chirurg 46:348–352
17. Oest O (1978) Die Achsenfehlstellung als präarthrotische Deformität für das Kniegelenk und die röntgenologische Beinachsenbeurteilung. Unfallheilkunde 81:629–633
18. Pauwels F (1973) Kurzer Überblick über die mechanische Beanspruchung des Knochens und ihre Bedeutung für die funktionelle Anpassung. Z Orthop 111:681–705
19. Rahmanzadeh R, Faensen M (1979) Zur operativen Behandlung der kniegelenknahen Fehlstellungen. Aktuel Traumatol 9:149–157
20. Rettig H (1973) Die Behandlung der Gonarthrose unter biomechanischen Gesichtspunkten. Arch Orthop Unfallchir 74:281–290
21. Skuginna A, Ludolph E, Hierholzer G (1979) Wahl des Operationsverfahrens bei der Umstellungsosteotomie im Tibiakopfbereich. Aktuel Traumatol 9:121–126
22. Trentz O, Tscherne H, Oestern HJ (1977) Operationstechnik und Ergebnisse bei distalen Femurfrakturen. Unfallheilkunde 80:441–448
23. Wagner H (1976) Indikation und Technik der Korrekturosteotomien bei der posttraumatischen Kniegelenkarthrose. Hefte Unfallheilkd 128:155–174
24. Zilch H, Adlkofer M, Groher W, Friedebold G (1978) Umstellungsosteotomien am Schienbeinkopf (Indikation, Technik und Ergebnisse). Unfallheilkunde 81:642–648

Forms and Techniques of the Supracondylar Femoral Osteotomy

U. Holz

Osteoarthritis is the result of a highly complex biomechanical and biochemical derangement. Despite improved insights into the metabolism and morphology of the hyaline cartilage, we are not yet able to intervent therapeutically at this level, and so we must direct our efforts toward the elimination of other factors involved in the pathophysiology of osteoarthritis. The major problem in this regard is incongruity of the articular surfaces, which is caused by damage to the joint surfaces, angular limb deformities, and laxity of capsular and ligamentous tissues.

Thus, the extraarticular correction of angular deformities, which contribute to both the etiology and progression of osteoarthritis, is a highly promising approach to the treatment of this disease, for it helps to restore physiologic loads even in joints that are already affected by degenerative change. Clinical experience has shown this to be effective in halting the further progression of disease. Improvements in the structure of the subchondral bone demonstrate the validity of these concepts.

The supracondylar femoral osteotomy is performed at the junction of the condyles with the flared metaphysis of the femur and permits correction of the following deformities:

- varus
- valgus
- rotation
- flexion (of the knee)
- recurvatum

A successful supracondylar osteotomy depends on an accurate evaluation of the deformity. Besides conventional measurements of intermalleolar distance in genu valgum and intercondylar distance in genu varum, standard roentgenograms of the knee joint are obtained in two planes with the patient standing and bearing weight [1].

With all corrective osteotomies, care must be taken that the knee joint line is level after surgery, for any deviation in this regard will expose the knee joint to potentially damaging shear forces. The goal is to achieve physiologic relations with an angle of 82° between the long axis of the femur and the knee joint line and a 92° angle between the knee joint line and tibial axis. These figures pertain to the lateral side [2].

In planning criteria favor a supracondylar osteotomy, it must be decided whether an *open wedge osteotomy* or *closed wedge osteotomy* is more

Corrective Osteotomies of the Lower Extremity
Edited by G. Hierholzer, K. H. Müller

appropriate. In the open wedge procedure a wedge of bone is interposed between the osteotomy surfaces to align the limb axis. In the closed wedge procedure a full or partial wedge of bone is resected. A varus or valgus osteotomy can be performed using either method. Virtually all recurvatum deformities are corrected by the closed wedge technique.

Unlike the interligamentous open wedge osteotomy of the proximal tibia, the supracondylar femoral osteotomy is unable to restore ligamentous tension. Nevertheless, the restoration of axial alignment with this procedure helps to stabilize the knee joint by re-establishing the muscular balance. The supracondylar osteotomy in adults must be securely stabilized so that postoperative physical therapy can be instituted without delay. This may be accomplished by internal or external skeletal fixation.

External fixation using a one-dimensional frame mounted on Steinmann pins or threaded half-pins (Schanz screws) is less stable than internal fixation. A biplane frame provides greater stability. However, a frame of this type can be cumbersome in the supracondylar area and may interfere with necessary postoperative physical therapy.

For these reasons we reserve external skeletal fixation for exceptional cases such as corrections in the presence of infection.

Internal fixation with osteotomy plates and condylar plates is the method of choice. These implants provide a high degree of stability that allows bone healing to progress undisturbed during postoperative exercise.

Because of the shape of the distal femur, the condylar plate is best for stabilizing an osteotomy performed on the lateral aspect of the bone. For medial corrections, the prominence of the medial femoral condyle favors use of the osteotomy plate, whose bend is offset by 1.5 to 2 cm. With both plates, care must be taken not to penetrate the opposite cortex when inserting the blade through the condyles. Blade lengths of 60 mm generally are sufficient. When checking the blade length on AP films, one should keep in mind that the condyles converge anteriorly, and that this might cause a perforating blade to be missed in the AP projection.

When a condylar plate is used on the lateral aspect of the femur, it is advantageous to insert one or two cancellous screws into the distal fragment to enhance the fixation. For medial corrections using an osteotomy plate, only one supplementary screw can be driven into the distal fragment.

Lateral Supracondylar Osteotomy

Closed Wedge Valgus Osteotomy

A varus deformity whose vertex is in the distal femur is most easily corrected by the resection of a bone wedge. The wedge is based laterally, and the opposite cortex is left intact. When the bone is realigned, this cortical bridge often will bend without breaking. If the transverse osteotomy is performed at a higher level, the intact cortex will almost always fracture when the bone is realigned. This closed wedge osteotomy causes some shortening of the limb, the exact amount depending on the level and width of the resected wedge. For

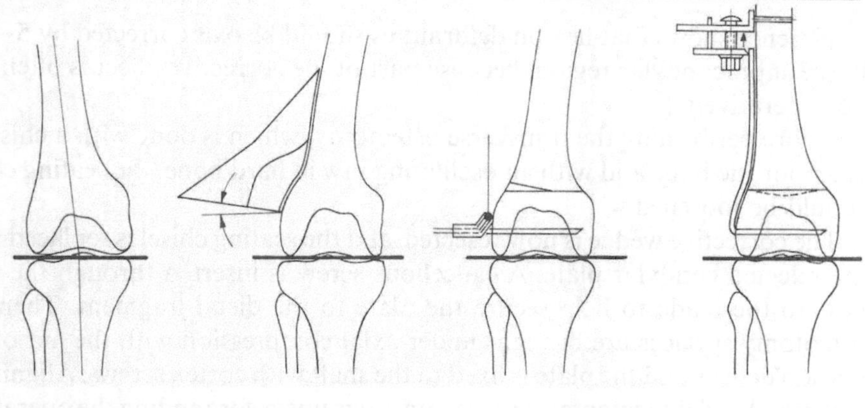

Fig. 1. Supracondylar valgus osteotomy

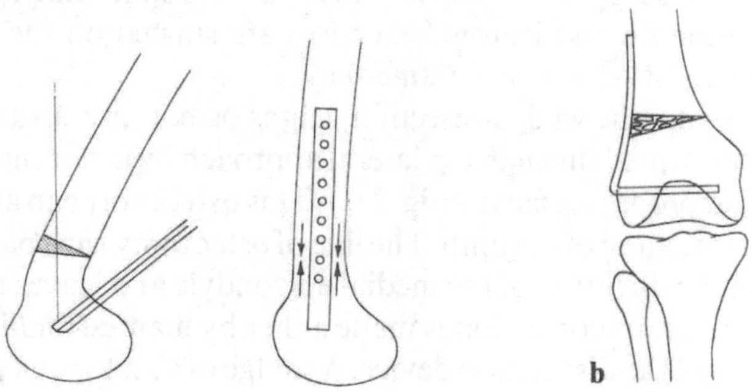

Fig. 2. a Extension osteotomy. **b** Varus open wedge osteotomy from the lateral approach

corrections in osteoporotic or atrophic bone, it is generally sufficient to resect a half-wedge. Hard bone, including bone that is sclerosed after trauma, require the resection of a full wedge that encompasses the entire cross-section of the femur.

Technique: The lateral aspect of the distal femur is approach through a longitudinal incision that is straight on an imaginary line connecting the greater trochanter and lateral femoral condyle, and then curves slightly from the lateral condyle toward the tibial tubercle. The vastus lateralis is released and retracted anteriorly with Hohmann retractors to expose the lateral cortex of the femur. The condylar plate guide is applied to the lateral cortex, and a triangular angle guide is placed against its lower edge to mark the desired angle of correction. A Kirschner wire is then twisted into the femoral condyles parallel to the lower edge of the angle guide. Normally this wire will be parallel to the joint line of the knee. It is helpful to mark the joint line with a second Kirschner wire inserted through the anterior part of the joint. The seating chisel for the angled blade plate is driven into the condyles parallel to the guide wires. The chisel guide that is attached to the seating chisel is aligned on the shaft axis (Fig. 1). If a flexion or recurvatum deformity must be corrected concurrently with the varus deformity, the chisel guide should diverge anteriorly or posteriorly by the desired angle of correction (Fig. 2 a).

Experience shows that flexion deformities should be overcorrected by 5 – 10° in the supracondylar region, because part of the corrective effect is often lost postoperatively [3].

Before performing the transverse osteotomy, which is done with a chisel in osteoporotic bone and with an oscillating saw in hard bone, the seating chisel should be loosened.

The corrective wedge is now resected, and the seating chisel is replaced with the selected condylar plate. A cancellous screw is inserted through the hole next to the blade to help secure the plate to the distal fragment. Then the osteotomy surfaces are brought under axial compression with the aid of the tension device, and the plate is fixed to the shaft with cortex screws. Alignment is checked and documented with roentgenograms before ending the operation. After surgery the leg is placed on a splint that is angled almost 90°, and isometric and isotonic exercises are started on the first postoperative day.

Open Wedge Varus Osteotomy

Besides the wedge-resection valgus osteotomy, a varus osteotomy can also be performed through the lateral approach by inserting a wedge graft between the osteotomy surfaces (Fig. 2 b). This osteotomy can also be used to correct mild shortening of the limb. The line of osteotomy runs parallel to the knee joint line in the direction of the medial epicondyle and leaves the opposite cortex intact. The varus correction is made either by manual manipulation of the limb or by use of the distraction device. A wedge of autologous or homologous cancellous bone is inserted into the resulting defect. The amount of length gained by this type of osteotomy is 1 – 2.5 cm.

Shortening Osteotomy with and without Concurrent Axial Correction

A step-out supracondylar osteotomy can also be performed through the lateral approach. To enhance stability following internal fixation of the shortening osteotomy, it is important to leave a tab of bone on the medial side that will abut against the femoral shaft impacted into the condyle. When aligning the shaft on the condyle, one should avoid creating an anterior "step" that would block patellar gliding. The trapezoidal bone segment that is removed to effect the shortening can be sloped upward medially to correct for varus angulation, the amount of the bevel depending on the amount of corrective valgus that is desired. Since the shortening may cause a marked prominence of the lateral condyle relative to the shaft, it is sometimes advantageous to fix the osteotomy with an angled blade plate that has a 1- to 1.5-cm offset at the bend.

Medial Supracondylar Osteotomy

Medial osteotomies of the distal femur are mostly wedge resections done to correct valgus deformity secondary to trauma or idiopathic osteoarthritis. Varus osteotomies of the medial side may also be indicated in children and adolescents who have incapacitating skeletal deformities secondary to metabolic disease. Details on the osteotomy technique in skeletally immature patients are discussed in Chapter VI.

Technique: The medial approach to the distal femur demands particular caution due to the proximity of nerves and vessels. The skin incision extends straight along the distal femur to the femoral epicondyle, where it curves slightly toward the tibial tubercle. The thick subcutaneous tissue layers at that location are divided, taking care to spare the branches of the anterior femoral cutaneous nerve and the infrapatellar ramus of the saphenous nerve, and the fascia of the adductor muscles is exposed. The sartorius muscle is then retracted posteriorly and the vastus medialis anteriorly to expose the medial aspect of the femur and the epicondylar region. The plexus-like blood vessels of the periosteum are coagulated. Retraction of the vastus and sartorius muscles is maintained with Hohmann retractors. Little pressure should be exerted on the posterior retractor to avoid injury to the neurovascular bundle and saphenous nerve that course deep to the sartorius.

The quadrangular positioning plate for varus osteotomies is now placed against the femoral shaft, the appropriate triangular guide is used to mark the calculated angle of correction, and a Kirschner wire is inserted parallel to the lower edge of the guide. The goal of this operation is to normalize the limb axis and obtain a level knee joint line (Fig. 3). The seating chisel with attached chisel guide is driven into the condyles parallel to the Kirschner wire. The chisel guide should be aligned with the long axis of the femoral shaft. The guide should deviate anteriorly from the shaft axis if both varus correction and anterior angulation are desired (Fig. 2 a); recurvatum deformity is corrected by moving the guide posteriorly.

The seating chisel is driven into the condyles an average blade length of 60 mm and then loosened slightly. The osteotomy is marked at the level of the bend of the plate, and it is carried out with a chisel or oscillating saw. A hald-wedge resection is sufficient in osteoporotic bone, whereas hard bone may require the excision of a full-diameter wedge. The seating chisel is replaced with a 90° osteotomy plate with a 1.5- to 2-cm offset, depending on the bone contour, and a screw is driven into the distal fragment through the offset of the plate. Then the osteotomy is brought under axial compression with the tension device, and the plate is secured to the shaft with cortex screws (Fig. 4).

Wound closure following a medial osteotomy is straightforward, for the sartorius and vastus muscles will appose neatly over the osteotomy plate once

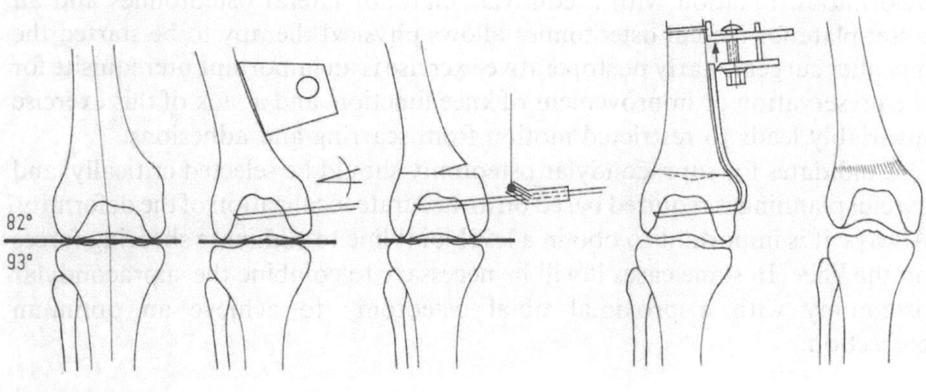

Fig. 3. Supracondylar varus osteotomy

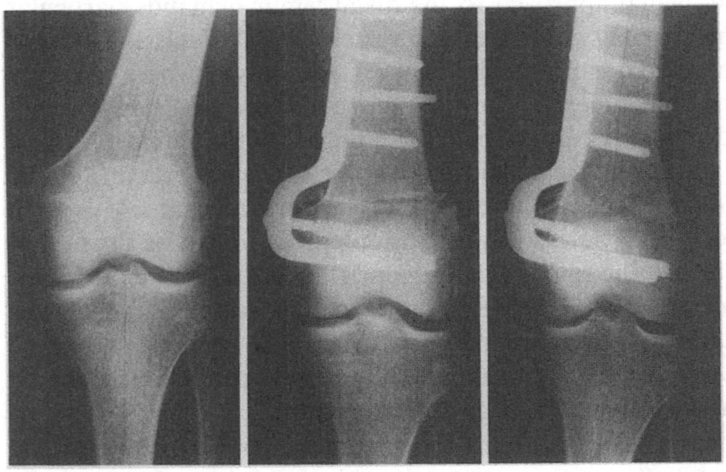

Fig. 4. Varus osteotomy with resection and transposition of a half-wedge to the lateral side

the Hohmann retractors are removed. Only a skin suture and occasionally a subcutaneous suture are required.

As before, the operated limb is placed on a right-angle splint, and exercises are initiated on the first postoperative day.

Supracondylar Rotational Osteotomies

Rotational alignment of the femur is easily corrected during supracondylar osteotomies for other deformities. The planned correction angle is marked with Kirschner wires inserted above and below the plane of the osteotomy. Rotational realignment is always the first step in combined corrections. Rotational corrections in the supracondylar region have a limit of approximately 45°; greater amounts of rotation will cause muscular imbalance and incongruity of the femoropatellar articulation [3].

The supracondylar femoral osteotomy enables the correction of various deformities. Fixation with a condylar plate for lateral osteotomies and an offset plate for medial osteotomies allows physical therapy to be started the day after surgery. Early postoperative exercise is an important prerequisite for the preservation or improvement of knee function, and a lack of this exercise invariably leads to restricted motion from scarring and adhesions.

Candidates for supracondylar osteotomy should be selected critically, and careful planning is required based on an accurate localization of the deformity. Always, it is important to obtain a level joint line to eliminate shearing forces on the knee. In some cases it will be necessary to combine the supracondylar osteotomy with a proximal tibial osteotomy to achieve an optimum correction.

References

1. Frank W, Oest O, Rettig H (1974) Die Röntgenaufnahme in der Operationsplanung von Korrekturosteotomien der Beine. Z Orthop 112:344–347
2. Rettig H (1973) Die Behandlung der Gonarthrose unter biomechanischen Gesichtspunkten. Arch Orthop Unfallchir 74:281–290
3. Wagner H (1977) Korrekturosteotomien am Bein. Orthopäde 6:145–177

Intraligamentous Elevating Osteotomies for Posttraumatic Deformities about the Knee

R. Kleining and P. M. Hax

Today much is known about human gait, joint mechanics, and the functional adaptation of bone and cartilage. With this knowledge we are able to analyze the pathologic sequelae of trauma and their effects on joint function and derive corrective measures from the result of this analysis. Arthroplasty appears to be justified only if other types of corrective surgery have no prospect of success. This particularly applies to the knee joint.

Mechanics of the Knee Joint

Active and passive stabilizers of the knee work together to ensure that only pressure is transferred from one part of the joint to the other. The vectors of the body weight and muscular force combine to produce a vector sum R (also called the resultant pressure load), which passes through the center of the knee joint (Fig. 1).

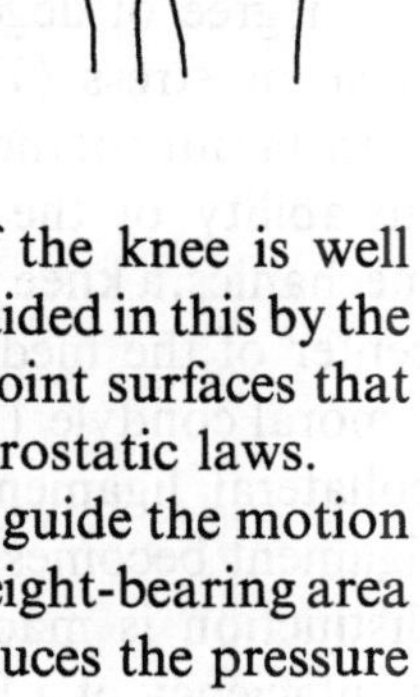

Fig. 1. Diagram of the load vectors at the knee. **KG** Body weight, **M** muscular force, **R** resultant pressure load, **a,b** lever arms

The hyaline cartilage covering the articular surfaces of the knee is well equipped structurally to handle this compressive stress. It is aided in this by the synovial fluid, which forms a lubricating film between the joint surfaces that helps to distribute pressure evenly in accordance with hydrostatic laws.

The fibrous and cartilaginous menisci of the knee help to guide the motion of the femoral condyles, and they significantly increase the weight-bearing area of the tibial plateau. This increased area of articulation reduces the pressure per unit area that is exerted on the cartilage.

Corrective Osteotomies of the Lower Extremity
Edited by G. Hierholzer, K. H. Müller

Pathomechanics

Intraarticular fractures disrupt the distribution of pressure in the joint. A step-like incongruity in the joint decreases the area of contact between the articular surfaces. This creates a concentration of compressive stresses that may exceed the tolerance of the cartilage (Fig. 2). The same effect is produced by angular deformities. Angulation of the limb displaces the resultant pressure load R away from the center of the knee. The eccentric pressure load decreases the load-bearing area of the joint and produces a local concentration of compressive stresses (Fig. 3).

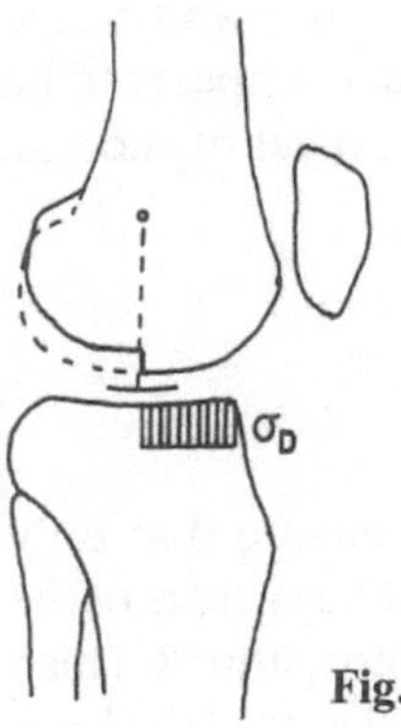

Fig. 2

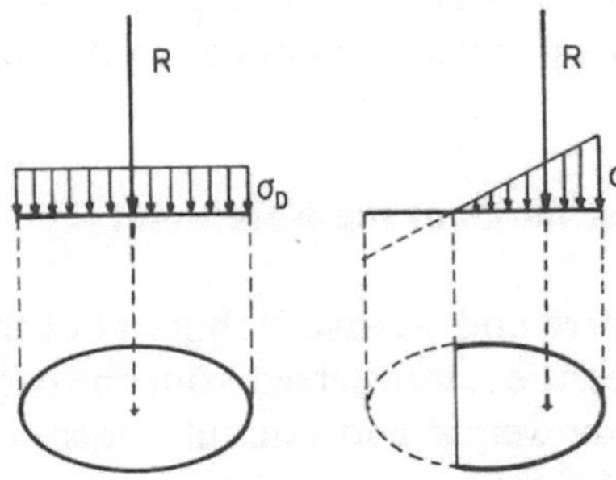

Fig. 3

Fig. 2. A step-like incongruity in the joint reduces the area of contact between the cartilaginous surfaces; σ_D compressive stress

Fig. 3. An eccentric shift of the pressure load **R** leads to a reduction of load-bearing area; σ_D compressive stress

Varus and valgus deformities are the most serious angular deformities from a biomechanical standpoint. When pronounced, they amplify the shear component of the resultant load R, causing shearing stresses to be exerted on the cartilage. The greater the traumatic damage to the cartilage or the greater the degree of degenerative disease, the more serious are the effects of this shearing stress (Fig. 4).

Instability of the knee joint is significant in this regard. The literature defines instability of the knee joint in various ways. According to the laws of mechanics, a knee joint is unstable only if the vector sum R passes medial to the center of the medial femoral condyle or lateral to the center of the lateral femoral condyle (Fig. 5). In such cases the checkrein capacity of the medial collateral ligament or iliotibial tract becomes inadequate. The collateral ligament becomes stretched, or the iliotibial tract becomes fatigued. A basic distinction is made between the stretching of a ligament and the relative insufficiency of a ligament. Relative ligamentous insufficiency is a positional laxity ("pseudolaxity") resulting from caudal displacement of the tibial plateau and does not necessarily cause knee instability (Fig. 6). Relative ligamentous insufficiency also occurs in association with shear fractures of the

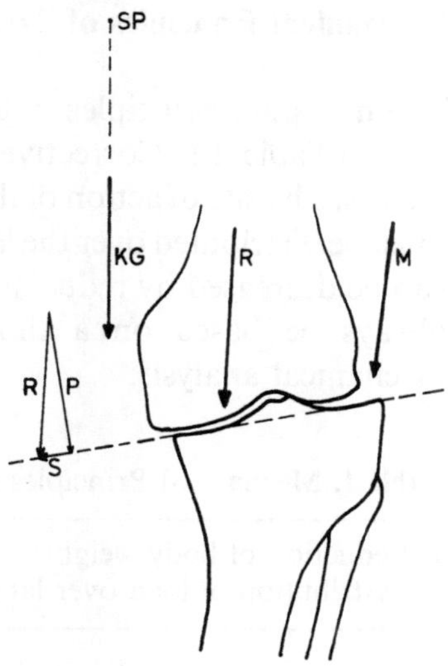

Fig. 4. Vector diagram for an eccentric vector sum **R. P** Pressure load perpendicular to the cartilage surface, **S**, shear force perpendicular to the pressure load **P**, **KG** body weight, **SP** center of body gravity, **M** muscular force

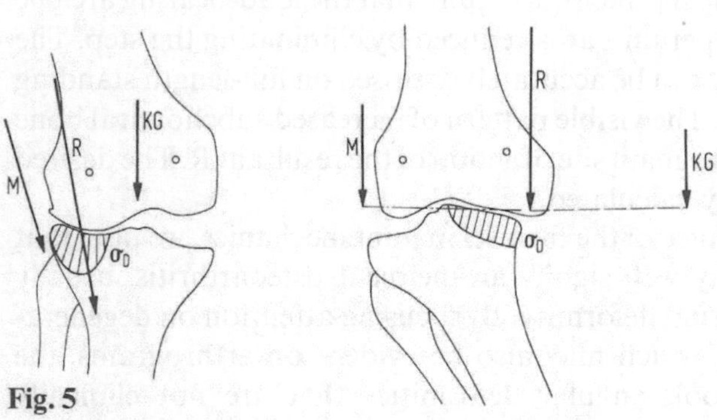

Fig. 5

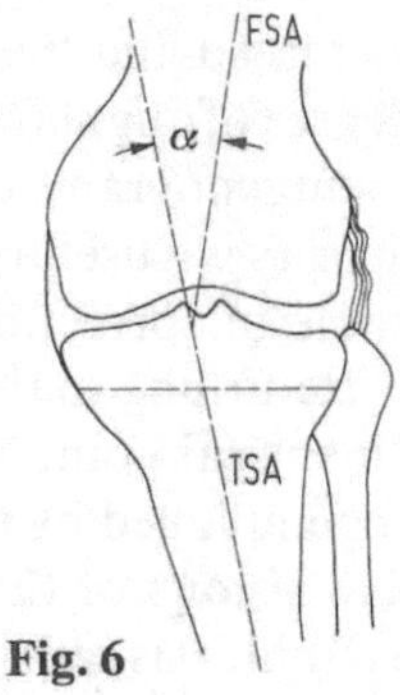

Fig. 6

Fig. 5. Knee joint instability in the presence of valgus (*left*) and varus deformity (*right*). With valgus deformity the vector sum **R** passes lateral to the center of the lateral femoral condyle, and the compressive stress σ_D is concentrated on the lateral tibial plateau. With varus deformity, the vector sum **R** passes medial to the center of the medial femoral condyle, and compressive stress σ_D is concentrated on the medial plateau (abbreviations as in Fig. 4)

Fig. 6. Relative ligamentous insufficiency in genu valgum resulting from caudal displacement of the lateral tibial plateau. **FSA** Femoral shaft axis, **TSA** tibial shaft axis, α angle between **FSA** and **TSA**

medial or lateral femoral condyle. These mostly posterior fractures are manifested clinically by marked medial or lateral joint opening in certain positions of flexion. With a shear fracture that has healed with proximal displacement, the displaced part of the femoral condyle will articulate with the tibial plateau when the knee is flexed beyond a certain point. In this situation the collateral ligament is intact but is too long, creating a condition of relative ligamentous insufficiency.

Mechanical Principles of Treatment

The necessary principles of treatment follow logically from the pathomechanics (Table 1). Corrective surgery must eliminate two pathomechanical factors. The site of action of the vector sum R must be optimized, and the load must be distributed over the largest possible area of joint surface. The vector R can be decreased by reducing the body weight. Planning of the surgery must always be based on a thorough clinical examination and an accurate mechanical analysis.

Table 1. Mechanical Principles of Treatment

1. Reduction of body weight
2. Distribution of load over largest possible area

The presence of a step in the joint surface presents the least difficulties in terms of planning. Mechanical principles require that the load-bearing area be increased and the pressure per unit area reduced by eliminating the step. The degree of angular deformity can be accurately assessed on full-length standing roentgenograms of the legs. The visible pattern of increased subchondral bone density is a useful guide to the main site of action of the resultant R. The desired angle of correction is easily calculated.

Returning to the importance of the menisci in joint mechanics, we note that "meniscal complaints" may well signify an incipient osteoarthritis, usually accompanied by a genu varum deformity. By focusing attention on degenerative lesions of the menisci, which may also be evident on arthrograms, the examiner is apt to overlook angular deformities that are not clinically apparent. Radionuclide bone scans are useful in identifying the true cause of the complaints. Before bone changes become evident on x-rays, bone scans will reveal an increase of activity in the affected compartment. Surgery to correct angular deformity can improve clinical symptoms without the need for meniscectomy.

Indications

From our knowledge of biomechanics we can derive two main indications for corrective osteotomies after trauma:
1. Step-like joint incongruity and
2. angular deformity.

Types of Corrective Procedure

The type of corrective procedure used depends in part on the stability of the knee and the condition of the articular cartilage (Table 2). Unstable joints will additionally require ligament reconstruction. Both relative ligamentous

Table 2. Preoperative Findings

I. Angular deformity without compartmental disease
a) With stable knee
b) With unstable knee

II. Angular deformity with compartmental disease
a) With stable knee
b) With unstable knee

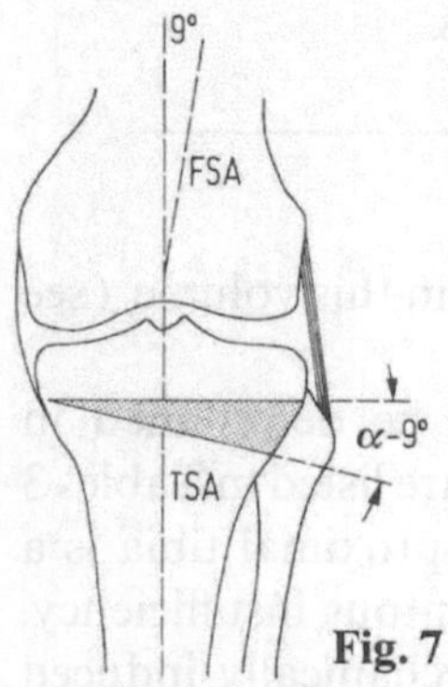

Fig. 7

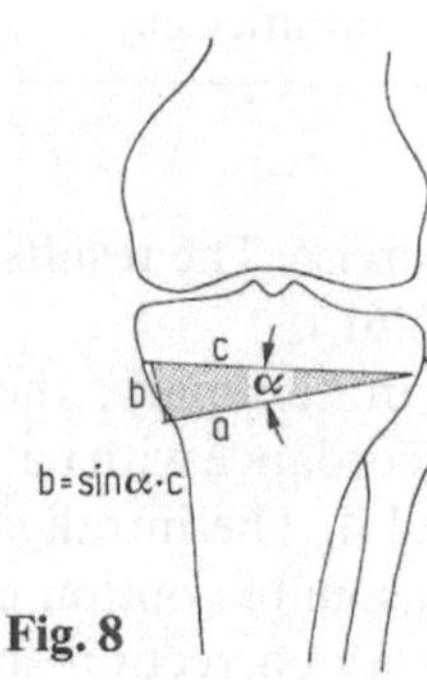

Fig. 8

Fig. 7. An open wedge osteotomy of the proximal tibia elevates the plateau and restores tension to the lateral collateral ligament. **FSA** Femoral shaft axis, **TSA** tibial shaft axis, angle of correction $=\alpha-9°$ (physiologic angle between **FSA** and **TSA** is 9°)

Fig. 8. Elevating osteotomy of the proximal tibia. Formula for determining the height of the base (**b**) of the corticocancellous wedge graft; **a** and **c** are the distal and proximal sides of the wedge

insufficiency and angular deformity are relieved by an intraligamentous elevating osteotomy of the proximal tibia (Figs. 6 and 7). A formula is available for calculating the height of the base of the corticocancellous wedge grat when the angle of correction is known (Fig. 8).

We immobilize the elevating osteotomy with a T-plate to prevent secondary loss of alignment and create the stability necessary for early postoperative

Table 3. Options Available for the Surgical Correction of Angular Deformities

Pathologic findings Angular deformity (varus, valgus)	Mechanical treatment principle Type of surgical correction
With stable ligaments	Corrective osteotomy with anatomic restoration
With unstable ligaments	Corrective osteotomy with anatomic restoration
a) Decompensation	*and* reefing of ligament
b) Relative ligamentous insufficiency	Intraligamentous elevating osteotomy with anatomic restoration

Table 4. Options Available for the Surgical Correction of Angular Deformities with Compartmental Disease

Pathologic findings Angular deformity (varus, valgus) Compartmental disease	Mechanical treatment principle Type of surgical correction
With stable ligaments	Overcorrecting osteotomy
With unstable ligaments a) Decompensation	Overcorrecting osteotomy *and* reefing of ligament
b) Relative ligamentous insufficiency	Overcorrecting intraligamentous elevating osteotomy

exercise. The results are described by Skuginna elsewhere in this volume (see p. 261).

In summary, the type of corrective procedure must be determined in accordance with pathologic findings. The various options are listed in Tables 3 and 4. The intraligamentous elevating osteotomy of the proximal tibia is a reasonable option only in the presence of relative ligamentous insufficiency. Every correction should protect the knee joint from mechanically induced damage and therefore should be based on mechanical principles.

Proximal Tibial Osteotomies: Forms and Techniques

G. Friedebold and R. Wolff

Diseases of the hip and knee joints occupy an important place in clinical orthopedics. On the one hand they are relatively frequent, and on the other they can severely limit the scope of human activities and thus lessen the quality of life. Unphysiologic loads associated with primary or secondary changes in the axis of the lower extremity are a major factor in the pathogenesis of early osteoarthritis. Based on present knowledge of biomechanics, the correction of posttraumatic, preosteoarthritic limb deformities by a suitable osteotomy is practically the only and certainly the most successful means of preventing impending osteoarthritis, delaying its onset, or arresting the progress of established disease and improving subjective symptoms through elimination of the mechanical factor.

Procedures of this kind are of particular importance in the knee, considering that the long-term results of total replacements of that joint have been far less encouraging than in the hip [31]. The goal of surgical intervention is to correct the axial alignment of the limb, thereby reducing the pressure in the joint to a level that can be tolerated by the involved tissue.

Biomechanical Principles

The major studies dealing with the biomechanics of the knee [14,15,28,29,32] were reviewed, and some critically evaluated, by Maquet [19]. Building on Pauwels' studies of the hip [30], Maquet analyzed the forces exerted on the knee. To aid the reader in understanding the pathomechanics of osteoarthritis of the knee, we shall review Maquet's discussion of this topic [19]:

In the normal knee the line of action of force p, caused by the body weight minus the weight of the supporting lower leg and foot, passes medial to the knee (Fig. 1). It is balanced by the lateral muscular force L. The resultant force R (calculated from the parallelogram of forces) normally crosses the center of gravity of the weight-bearing surface of the knee. The line of action of L is known, and that of P can be closely estimated for each phase of stance (the origin of P is at the center of body gravity, which was determined by Braune and Fischer [3] in 1889 for various phases of stance). From this we can calculate the resultant force R.

A decrease in the magnitude of force L (muscular force) or an increase in P (body weight) that is not offset by a corresponding increase in L causes the resultant to be displaced medially, bringing it closer to the vertical. If L is

Corrective Osteotomies of the Lower Extremity
Edited by G. Hierholzer, K. H. Müller

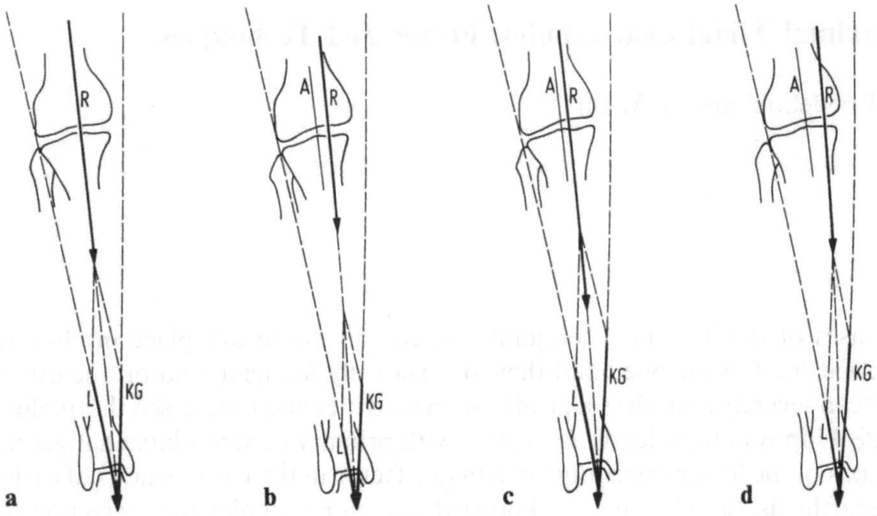

Fig. 1 a–d. Forces exerted on the knee joint. **a** Normal; **b** decrease of lateral muscular force (**L**); **c** increase of body weight (**KG**); **d** increase of body weight (**KG**) and decrease of muscular force (**L**); **R** resultant force, **A** mechanical limb axis (after Maquet [19])

decreased while body weight is increased, as in postmenopausal women, for example, an even greater medial displacement of R will occur.

A varus deformity of the knee alters the direction of pull of the vector L, increasing the distance between the line of action of P and the knee. This causes a medial shift of the resultant force R, which increases the stresses on the medial compartment of the knee.

A valgus deformity of the knee has the opposite effect. If the resultant force R passes through the center of gravity of the weight-bearing surfaces, this force is smaller than in the normal knee, and so the forces exerted on the knee joint are also smaller. Thus, a valgus deformity of the knee does not necessarily lead to osteoarthritis. Nevertheless, degeneration can still occur in the lateral compartment even with a valgus deformity.

These biomechanical principles, which were only touched upon here, have important implications with regard to the planning of proximal tibial osteotomies and the determination of optimum correction angles. A valgus deformity generally should be corrected to a normal alignment, while a varus deformity should be slightly overcorrected [19].

A flexion contracture of the knee shifts the zone of greatest weight bearing posteriorly and causes loads to be transmitted over a smaller area of joint surface, resulting in an increase of compressive stress (the radius of curvature of the femoral condyles diminishes posteriorly).

Thus, mechanical osteoarthritis of the knee is caused either by an abnormal distribution of the forces exerted on the joint, or by a pathologic increase of these forces in a localized region of the joint.

Historical Review

Corrective osteotomies of the proximal tibia have been known for over a century. As early as 1854 the German orthopedist Mayer of Würzburg corrected genu valgum by resecting a bony wedge with a saw. Billroth described an upper tibial osteotomy with a chisel in 1874. Schede added a fibular osteotomy in 1877 (performed below the fibular head, hence the danger of peroneal nerve injury). The form of the tibial osteotomy was frequently varied. Mayer and Schede removed a wedge with a medial base (leaving the lateral cortex intact!), while Perthes resected a curved, concave – convex fragment to obtain a greater area of bone contact (quoted in [17,37]). Lexer used a wedge – resection osteotomy to straighten the upper tibia in genu recurvatum. For correction of genu varum Lange [17] described the inverted – V tibial osteotomy, combined if necessary with the insertion of a wedge graft to elevate the medial tibial plateau (Fig. 2 a,b). The limb was immobilized postoperatively in plaster, and Blount clamps or Kirschner wires were used to supplement the fixation.

Today, most proximal tibial osteotomies are of the wedge or barrel – vault type (Fig. 2 c). The osteotomy is made stable for exercise by plating it internally or by applying an external frame. Kirschner wires and plaster are used only in exceptional cases.

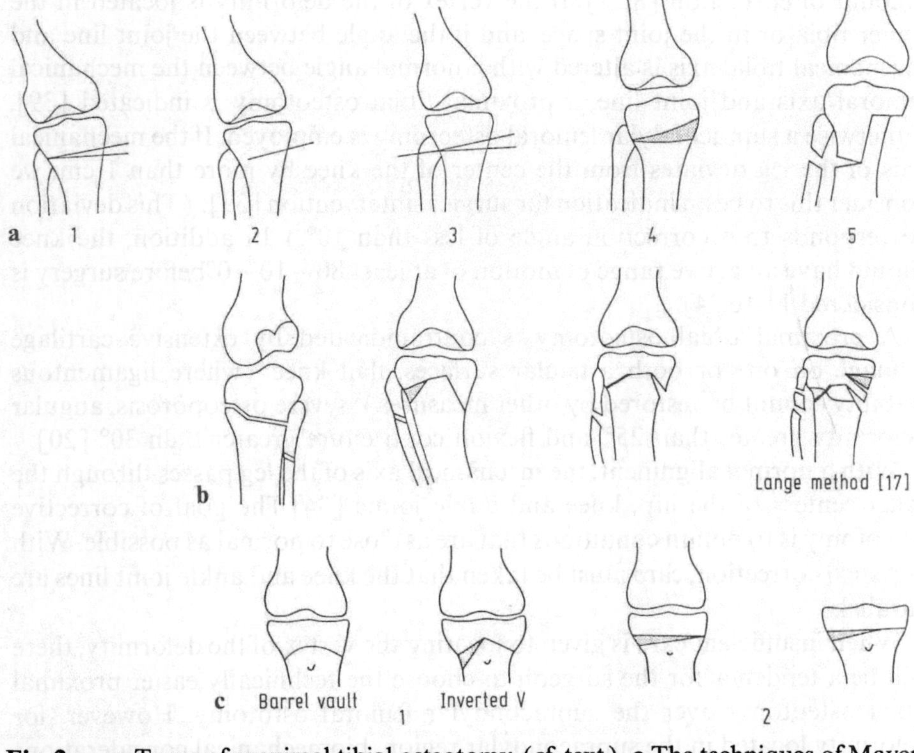

Fig. 2 a – c. Types of proximal tibial osteotomy (cf. text). **a** The techniques of Mayer, 1854 (**1**); Billroth, 1874 (**2**); Schede, 1877 (**3**); Perthes (**4**) [quoted in 17,37]; and Schanz (**5**). **b** The technique of Lange [17]. **c** Pendulum osteotomies (**1**) and wedge osteotomy (**2**)

Indication for Proximal Tibial Osteotomies

The main indication for a proximal tibial osteotomy is unilateral osteoarthritis of the knee associated with genu varum or genu valgum [1,5,38,39]. It is also indicated for posttraumatic deformities about the knee that might be precursors of osteoarthritis [11, 16, 38]. The need for osteotomy is controversial in unilateral osteoarthritis with a normal mechanical axis [39]. Here the plane of the joint line is the decisive factor: If it is oblique, a supra– and infracondylar correction is indicated.

Accurate planning of the osteotomy relies on full–length roentgenograms of the leg during stance with the knee frontalized. (Oest [27] states that a solitary flexion deformity up to 20° or a mild rotational deformity of 20° or less with the knee extended does not alter the position of the mechanical axis, in contrast to a 20° flexion deformity that is accompanied by an equal amount of internal or external rotation. This is why the knee joint must be frontalized when the films are taken.) The extent of the genu valgum or varum as well as the location of the angular deformity and thus the site of the axial correction can be accurately determined.

Maquet [19] stresses the need for additional roentgenograms in the one–legged stance as well as tangential views of the femoropatellar groove. These films are used to ascertain the level ot the osteotomy and the necessary amount of correction [8,27]. If the vertex of the deformity is located in the upper tibia or in the joint space, and if the angle between the joint line and mechanical tibial axis is altered with a normal angle between the mechanical femoral axis and joint line, a proximal tibial osteotomy is indicated [39]. Otherwise a supracondylar femoral osteotomy is employed. If the mechanical axis of the leg deviates from the center of the knee by more than 1 cm, we consider this to be an indication for surgical intervention [39]. (This deviation corresponds to a correction angle of less than 10°.) In addition, the knee should have an active range of motion of at least 80–10–0°before surgery is considered [1,16,24].

A proximal tibial osteotomy is contraindicated by extensive cartilage damage on one or both articular surfaces, flail knee (where ligamentous stability cannot be restored by other measures), severe osteoporosis, angular deformity greater than 25°, and flexion contracture greater than 30° [20].

With a normal alignment, the mechanical axis of the leg passes through the exact centers of the hip, knee and ankle joints [34].The goal of corrective osteotomy is to obtain conditions that are as close to normal as possible. With any such correction, care must be taken that the knee and ankle joint lines are parallel.

When insufficient care is given to locating the vertex of the deformity, there will be a tendency for the surgeon to choose the technically easier proximal tibial osteotomy over the supracondylar femoral ostotomy. However, for deformity located in the supracondylar region, biomechanical considerations require that the femoral osteotomy be used [21,22].

A genu valgum or genu varum that is unaccompanied by osteoarthritis or subjective complaints should be corrected only if the deformity exceeds about

10 – 15°, for not every varus or valgus deformity will lead to osteoarthritis [39]. Surgery for aesthetic reasons alone demands thorough preoperative counseling that includes an explanation of risks.

Indications and Technique of the Intraligamentous Tibial Osteotomy

The principal indications are [7,35]:

1. posttraumatic instability with angular deformity caused by depression of the tibial plateau;
2. genu varum or genu valgum with collateral ligament insufficiency, including cases secondary to premature, unilateral epiphyseal plate closure; and
3. certain cases of osteoarthritic instability with angular deformity in which at least some articular cartilage is preserved.

The technique of the osteotomy presents no major difficulties. The knee joint itself does not have to be opened, although the position of the joint space should be marked with Kirschner wires. The osteotomy should be performed as far from the joint as possible so that the plateau will not fracture when the prepared autologous cancellous graft from the iliac crest is screwed into place (this cannot always be avoided in severely osteoporotic bone). The opposite cortex is left intact. The posterior cortex should be osteotomized with a chisel while the knee is flexed to protect the posterior blood vessels (tibial artery). Usually the fibula does not have to be sectioned. Postoperative immobilization in plaster is unnecessary owing to the chekrein effect of the patellar tendon and collateral ligament (Fig. 3 a – c).

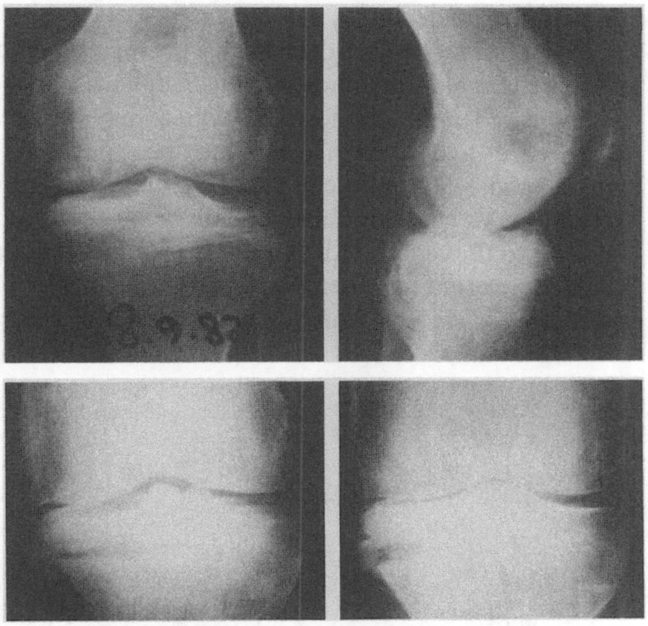

Fig. 3. a W. R., intraligamentous open wedge osteotomy with insertion of homologous graft. **b** Resorption of the homologous graft after 4 months. **c** Repeat intraligamentous open wedge osteotomy with insertion of autologous graft from the iliac crest

Wedge and Pendulum Osteotomies

If collateral ligament insufficiency is absent or mild, the tibia is osteotomized just proximal to the insertion of the patellar tendon [21,22]. This may be done using either a wedge osteotomy or a "pendulum" osteotomy. If the leg is already shortened, a transverse osteotomy combined with the insertion of a wedge graft on the concave side can prevent further shortening [39]. Again, the opposite cortex is not divided (Fig. 4).

The true pendulum osteotomy has two forms: the "barrel vault" and the inverted V, the latter involving the resection of a wedge. The vertex of the pendulum or wedge osteotomy is on the tibial side in genu valgum and on the fibular side in genu varum [39]. Opinions differ as to the amount of correction needed. Huggler [12] and Mohing [20] recommend a slight overcorrection, and Müller [24] and Thiel [36] recommend an exact correction or possibly a slight overcorrection. Breitenfelder [5] also favors correction to a normal alignment, taking care that the ankle joint is correctly positioned. Maquet [19] states that varus deformity should be slightly overcorrected by about 2–4°, noting that correction to a normal alignment would be insufficient to recenter the resultant force. Particularly if the varus deformity is secondary to osteoarthritis, an exact correction would only restore the original situation that precipitated the deformity. Since it is often difficult to tell whether a varus deformity is primary or secondary, a slight overcorrection is the most reasonable course of action, as it compensates for a decrease in lateral muscle power. Kettelkamp and Chao [14] and Blaimont et al. [2] tried to calculate the most favorable amount of correction. However, there are basic reasons (such as the unknown potential strength of the lateral femoral muscles) why only approximate values can be stated.

With a primary valgus deformity, a postoperative varus position generally is undesired for biomechanical reasons. But if the valgus deformity is the result of an increased muscular force L, which may be necessary to keep the hip balanced, a slight overcorrection may be warranted [19]. The correction of a severe valgus deformity can cause significant obliquity of the tibial plateau, giving rise to shearing forces. In this case the resultant force vector is not brought to the center of the knee. This is why the supracondylar osteotomy is usually preferred in patients with valgus deformity [19]. The proximal tibial osteotomy is suitable only for mild degrees of valgus angulation (less than

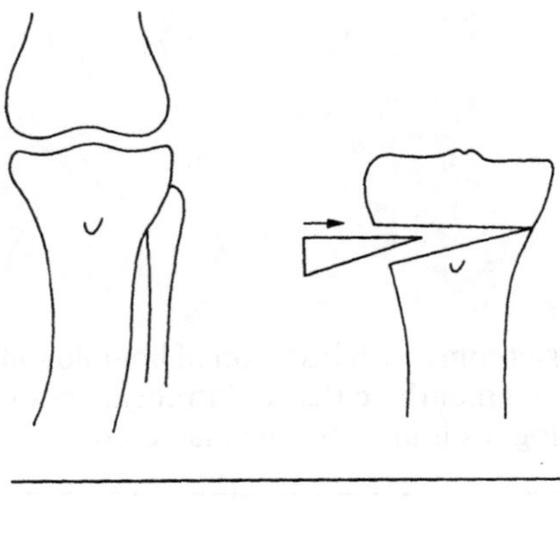

Fig. 4. Principle of the open wedge osteotomy. With limb shortening, the plateau on the concave side of the deformity is elevated and supported by an autologous graft

15°) and for valgus caused by deformity of the upper tibia. On the whole, however, this type of operation is more difficult, and an imperfect osteotomy can easily increase the mechanical stresses on the knee.

Osteotomies distal to the insertion of the patellar tendon are mainly performed in adults with posttraumatic deformity in which the vertex of the deformity is located below the patellar tendon in the proximal tibia. This osteotomy may also be considered in cases of crus varum. In children we perform all osteotomies in the metaphysis due to the proximity of the epiphyseal plate [39].

Technique of the Wedge Osteotomy

The fibula is osteotomized first so that it will not interfere with the correction. This is done at the junction of the proximal and middle thirds to protect the peroneal nerve. A simple osteotomy is sufficient when a varus correction is proposed. For a valgus correction, approximately 1 cm of fibula is resected or an oblique osteotomy is performed so that the fragments can override. Maquet [19] states a fibular osteotomy is not necessary for the correction of valgus deformities of less than 15°. We usually approach the tibia through an anterior S-shaped incision over the knee joint and upper tibia. The tibial metaphysis is exposed, and the patellar tendon is undermined. On the medial side, a Hohmann retractor is passed subperiosteally around the medial surface of the tibial metaphysis. On the lateral side, a heavy prying action would jeopardize neurovascular structures, and so a simple blunt retractor is used. The line of the knee joint is marked with a Kirschner wire, and a bone wedge is resected with a chisel or oscillating saw. The size of the wedge and the location of its base will depend on the nature and amount of angular correction required (lateral base for a valgus osteotomy, medial base for a varus osteotomy). The opposite cortex should be left intact to provide a tension-band effect when the bone is plated. If the osteotomy is to be compressed with Steinmann pins and an external frame, the angle of correction is defined by inserting the distal Steinmann pin perpendicular to the tibial axis. The proximal pin is inserted about 1 cm distal to the knee joint and parallel to it. Accurate placement of the pins can be verified by intraoperative roentgenograms. Both pins will be parallel after the limb is realigned. Up to 1 cm of AP adjustment can be obtained at this time by displacing the distal pin, in which case the opposite cortex must be divided. The use of external fixation will permit interfragmental compression to be increased as needed postoperatively; rotational corrections also can be carried out. A margin of at least 1–2 cm should be allowed between the Steinmann pins and the planned osteotomy, and more in osteoporotic bone [9]. When Steinmann pins are used, they should be inserted in a lateral-to-medial direction to avoid peroneal nerve injury (pilot holes are predrilled with a bit, and the pins are inserted with a hand chuck to avoid thermal necrosis).

We prefer to fix wedge osteotomies with a T-plate or buttress plate. (Occasionally we use Kirschner wires followed by plaster immobilization in

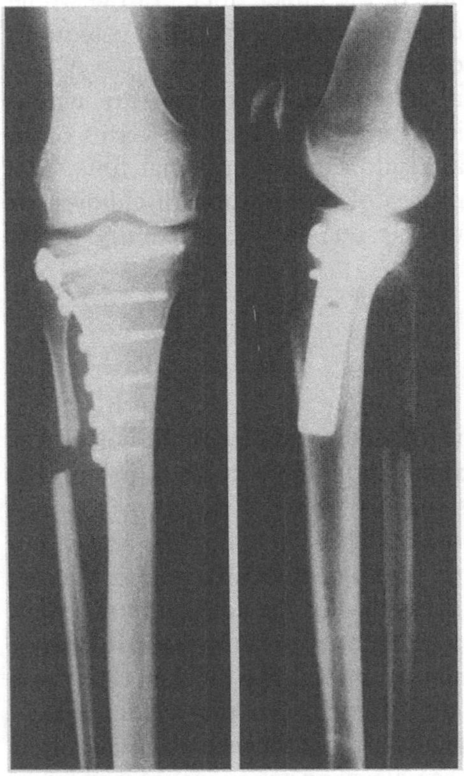

Fig. 5. Valgus wedge osteotomy fixed with a lateral T plate

children and adolescents.) Generally the plate is attached to the lateral side (Fig. 5), especially after a valgus osteotomy [39]. Lateral plating requires less dissection of muscles and ligaments and is advantageous biomechanically. If a varus osteotomy is plated laterally, the fixation should be reinforced with a small tension-band plate on the medial side.

Technique of the Pendulum Osteotomy

The barrel-vault osteotomy is the more commonly used form and permits even large angular corrections to be carried out when combined with external skeletal fixation (Fig. 6). The surgical procedure (exposing the bone,

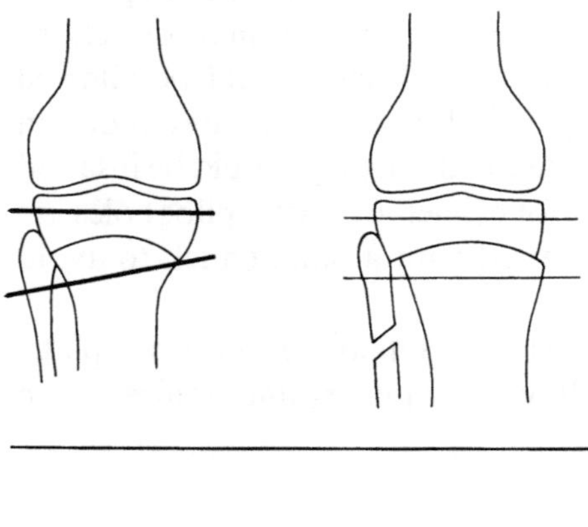

Fig. 6. Principle of the barrel-vault osteotomy. The distal Steinmann pin defines the angle of correction

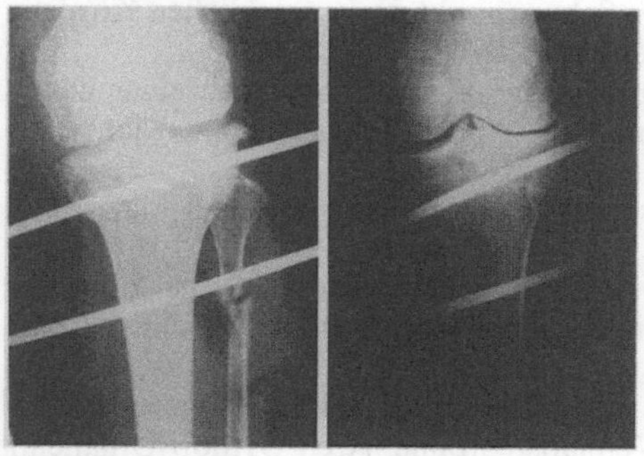

Fig. 7

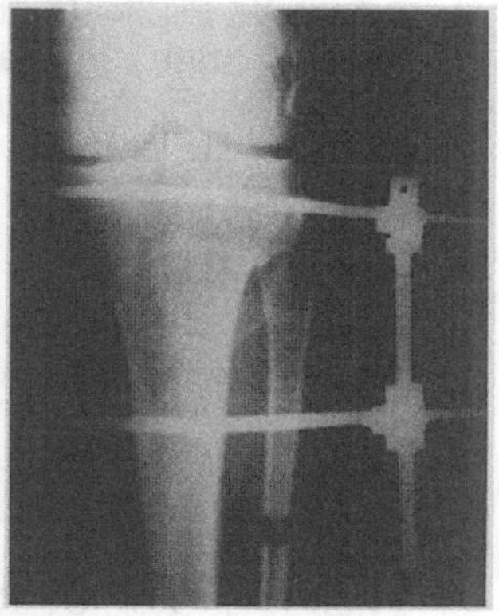

Fig. 8

Fig. 7. The poximal Steinmann pin was placed too close to the osteotomy and broke loose 2 weeks after surgery. Note the high fibular osteotomy, which endangers the peroneal nerve

Fig. 8. The Steinmann pins are correctly placed in this inverted-V osteotomy

marking the angle of correction) is like that of the wedge-resection osteotomy. Care must be taken to obtain an accurate placement of the Steinmann pins (Figs. 7 and 8). If the pins are placed too close to the osteotomy, they may break loose (Fig. 7). The proximal pin should pass about 1 cm distal to the articular surface, parallel to the joint line. The osteotomy is performed with a narrow chisel, which must be held level while the bone is sectioned. With retropatellar chondromalacia as evidence of early osteoarthritis of the femoropatellar joint, the distal tibial fragment is displaced anteriorly to alleviate pressure in the femoropatellar groove.

Summary

Corrective osteotomies of the proximal tibia have been performed for more than a century. Unilateral osteoarthritis associated with genu valgum or genu varum and posttraumatic deformities of the knee joint are the principal indications. The goal of surgery is to reduce joint pressure to a level that can be tolerated by the involved joint and will not damage the healthy joint. Three main procedures are used in the proximal tibia: the pendulum osteotomy, the wedge osteotomy, and the intraligamentous elevating osteotomy. The biomechanical principles and technical details of the operation are described.

References

1. Baacke M, Seidel K (1975) Wege zur Indikation operativer Gonarthrosebehandlung im Alter. Orthopäde 4:165
2. Blaimont P, Burnotte J, Baillon JM, Duby P (1971) Contribution biomécanique à l'étude des conditions d'équilibre dans le genou normal et pathologique. Acta Orthop Belg 37–573

3. Braune W, Fischer O (1889) Über den Schwerpunkt des menschlichen Körpers. Abhandl Math Phys Sächs Ges Wissensch 15:561
4. Braune W, Fischer O (1891) Bewegungen des Kniegelenks nach einer neuen Methode an lebenden Menschen gemessen. Abhandl Math Phys Sächs Ges Wissensch 17:75
5. Breitenfelder J (1973) Rundtischgespräch: Die Osteotomie am Tibiakopf. Z Orthop 111:543
6. Coventry MB (1965) Osteotomy of the upper portion of the tibia for degenerative arthritis of the knee: A preliminary report. J Bone Joint Surg [Am] 47:984
7. Dolanc B (1973) Die Behandlung des instabilen Kniegelenks mit Achsenfehlstellung durch intraligamentäre Anhebe-Tibiaosteotomie. Arch Orthop Unfallchir 76:280
8. Frank W, Oest O, Retting H (1974) Die Röntgenganzaufnahme in der Operationsplanung von Korrekturosteotomien der Beine. Z Orthop 112:344
9. Goerttler TP, Debrunner AM (1969) Die Tibiakopfosteotomien bei der Behandlung der Gonarthrose. Z Orthop 106–551
10. Hanslik L, Saydo M (1971) Der gegenwärtige Stand der chirurgischen Behandlung schwerer Kniegelenkschäden. Monatsschr Unfallheilkd 74:397
11. Hierholzer G, Voorhoeve A, Kleining R, Kehr H (1975) Reinterventionen nach Schienbeinkopfbrüchen. Chirurg 46:352
12. Huggler AH (1973) Rundtischgespräch: Die Osteotomien am Tibiakopf. Z Orthop 111:543
13. Jonasch E (1959) Zur Klassifizierung der Arthrose im Röntgenbild (Kongreßbericht). Z Orthop 91:579
14. Kettelkamp DB, Chao EY (1972) A method for quantitative analysis of medial and lateral compression forces at the knee during standing. Clin Orthop 83:202
15. Kettelkamp DB, Jacobs AW (1972) Tibiofemoral contact area: Determination and implications. J Bone Joint Surg [Am] 54:349
16. Klems H (1976) Infrakondyläre Tibiaosteotomie-Stabilisierung mit äußerem Spanner – Indikation, Technik, Komplikationen. Z Orthop 114:26
17. Lange M (1951) Orthopädisch-chirurgische Operationslehre. Bergmann, München, S 660.
18. MacIntosh PL (1970) The surgical treatment of osteoarthritis of the knee. S. I. C. O. T., XIè Congrès, Mexico, 1969. Imprimerie des Sciences, Bruxelles, p 400
19. Maquet PGJ (1976) Biomechanics of the knee. Springer, Berlin Heidelberg New York
20. Mohing W (1973) Osteotomien. Orthopäde 2:94
21. Müller KH, Bierbach M (1977) Korrekturosteotomien und ihre Ergebnisse bei kniegelenknahen posttraumatischen Fehlstellungen. Unfallheilkunde 80:359
22. Müller KH, Bierbach M (1977) Korrekturosteotomien und ihre Ergebnisse bei idiopathischen kniegelenknahen Achsenfehlstellungen. Unfallheilkunde 80:457
23. Müller ME, Allgöwer M, Schneider R, Willenegger H (1977) Manual der Osteosynthese. Springer, Berlin Heidelberg New York
24. Müller W (1973) Rundtischgespräch: Die Osteotomie am Tibiakopf. Z Orthop 111:543
25. Müller W (1976) Die Tibia-Osteotomie in der Therapie posttraumatischer Arthrosen am Kniegelenk. Hefte Unfallheilkd 128:175
26. Neurath F (1973) Rundtischgespräch: Die Osteotomie am Tibiakopf. Z Orthop 111:543
27. Oest O (1973) Röntgenologische Beinachsenbestimmung. Z Orthop 111:497
28. Paul JP (1965) Bioengineering studies of the forces transmitted by joints. In: Kenedi RP (ed) Biomechanics and related bioengineering topics. Pergamon Press, Oxford p 369
29. Paul JP (1966–67) Forces transmitted by joints in the human body. Proc Inst Mech Eng 181:8

30. Pauwels F (1973) Atlas zur Biomechanik der gesunden und kranken Hüfte. Prinzipien, Technik und Resultate einer kausalen Therapie. Springer, Berlin Heidelberg New York
31. Pauwels F (1976) Im Vorwort zu: In: Maquet PGJ (ed) Biomechanics of the knee. Springer, Berlin Heidelberg New York
32. Rabischong P, Courvoisier E, Bonnel F, Peruchon E, Devaud G (1970) Etude biomécanique de la répartition des forces au niveau des condyles fémoraux en charge statique. In: Nicod L (Hrsg) Die Gonarthrose. Huber, Bern Stuttgart Wien, S 36
33. Rettig H (1973) Rundtischgespräch: Die Osteotomie am Tibiakopf (Kongreßbericht). Z Orthop 111:543
34. Rettig H (1973) Die Behandlung der Gonarthrose unter biomechanischen Gesichtspunkten. Arch Orthop Unfallchir 74:281
35. Talke M, Friedebold G (1977) Indikation und Technik der intraligamentären Tibiaosteotomie bei Kniegelenkinstabilität. Hefte Unfallheilkd 129:182
36. Thiel A (1973) Rundtischgespräch: Die Osteotomie am Tibiakopf. Z Orthop 111:543
37. Vulpius O, Stoffel A (1920) Orthopädische Operationslehre. Enke, Stuttgart
38. Wagner H (1976) Indikation und Technik der Korrekturosteotomien bei der posttraumatischen Kniegelenkarthrose. Hefte Unfallheilkd 128:155
39. Zilch H, Adlkofer M, Groher W, Friedebold G (1978) Umstellungsosteotomien am Schienbeinkopf. Unfallheilkunde 81:642

Results of Corrective Osteotomies of the Proximal Tibia

H. Zilch and D. Rogmans

Patient Population

From September 1, 1969, through December 31, 1981, a total of 196 corrective osteotomies of the proximal tibia were performed in 155 patients at the Orthopedic Clinic (Oskar-Helene-Heim) of the Free University of Berlin. One hundred-nine patients who underwent 136 osteotomies (70%) were followed. The follow-up examinations were conducted in two series: Series 1, consisting of patients who had been operated from September 1, 1969, through September 30, 1977, in whom an average interval of 3.5 years (8 months to 5.5 years) passed between surgery and follow-up; and Series 2, comprising patients operated between October 1, 1977, and December 31, 1981, in whom the average interval was 2.9 years (13 months to 5.3 years). The patients ranged in age from 3 to 76 years. Ten of the patients were children; 71% of the adults were between 55 and 70 years of age at the time of surgery. Only adults were followed.

The preoperative deformity consisted of varus angulation in 119 cases and valgus angulation in 73. The ratio of males to females with varus deformity was 56 to 63. The valgus deformities showed a significant predominance of females (55 to 14).

Complications

In the 196 proximal tibial osteotomies that were performed, there were 14 instances (7.1%) of wound healing difficulties. A T plate had been used in 11 of these cases, and external skeletal fixation in 3. The 14 cases of impaired wound healing included 4 seromas (2%), 5 cases of marginal wound necrosis (2.5%), 4 soft-tissue infections (2%), and 1 osseous infection (0.5%). Thirteen patients showed signs of postoperative peroneal nerve irritation, which was transient in 10 patients and caused permanent weakness of toe extension in the remaining 3 (1.5%). Nine of the peroneal nerve injuries occurred in patients treated for valgus deformity, and four in patients treated for varus.

Results

Because improvement of pre-existing osteoarthritis is difficult to demonstrate objectively, the success of surgery must be judged largely on the basis of

Corrective Osteotomies of the Lower Extremity
Edited by G. Hierholzer, K. H. Müller

subjective ratings. We selected relief of pain and improvement of walking ability as our criteria. Many patients reported that 6–8 months passed before significant improvement or complete relief of pain was noted.

Based on these two criteria, 110 patients (81%) rated the outcome as positive, 12 patients (9%) reported no change in pain or walking ability, and 14 patients (10%) rated the outcome as poor (Table 1).

These patients were assigned respectively to Groups 1, 2, and 3 so that the characteristics of the different groups could be compared.

We first noted the types of deformity (varus or valgus) that were present in the different groups (Table 2). We found that 89% of the varus deformities were in Group 1 while only 7% were in Group 3. However, the latter group accounted for 21% of the valgus deformities. Thus, valgus deformity appears to imply a less favorable prognosis for subjective improvement after surgery.

When we studied the grade of severity of osteoarthritis that existed in the different groups at the time of surgery (according to the Jonasch scale), we found that all patients without osteoarthritis belonged to Group 1, while half the patients in Group 3 already had grade 4 osteoarthritis at the time of surgery (Table 3). Roentgenograms were also used to monitor the postoperative course of osteoarthritic disease. At follow-up they showed a progression of disease in 60%, no change in 34%, and improvement of disease in 6%. However, this improvement was based solely on a decrease in the density of the

Table 1. Subjective Evaluation of Results (Pain, Ambulation)

Improved	110 patients (81%)	(Group 1)
No change	12 patients (9%)	(Group 2)
Worse	14 patients (10%)	(Group 3)

Table 2. Results by Type of Deformity

	Varus n (%)	Valgus n (%)
Group 1	75 (89)	33 (63)
Group 2	3 (4)	8 (16)
Group 3	6 (7)	11 (21)
Total	84 patients	52 patients

Table 3. Results by Grade of Severity of Osteoarthritis at Operation

Grade of osteoarthritis	0 n (%)	1 n (%)	2 n (%)	3 n (%)	4 n (%)
Group 1	8 (7)	15 (14)	41 (37)	33 (30)	13 (12)
Group 2			2 (15)	7 (60)	3 (25)
Group 3			2 (14)	5 (36)	7 (50)

Table. 4. Roentgenographic Evaluation of Osteoarthritis as a Function of Lateral Ligamentous Stability

Osteoarthritis	Lateral ligamentous stability		
	Moderate laxity	Slight laxity	No laxity
60% progressive	46 patients	32 patients	4 patients
34% unchanged	10 patients	30 patients	6 patients
6% improved (sclerotic margin)	–	–	8 patients

sclerotic layer. A strong correlation was noted between the progression of osteoarthritis and the condition of the collateral ligaments. Progression of the disease was almost invariably associated with slight to moderate laxity of a collateral ligament (Table 4).

Range of joint motion was improved in 40% of the patients who were followed after surgery. Average improvement was 10–15°, with a maximum of 25°. Range of motion was unchanged in 42 patients, and it was diminished in 39. Of the 55 patients with improved motion, 47 had undergone surgery for

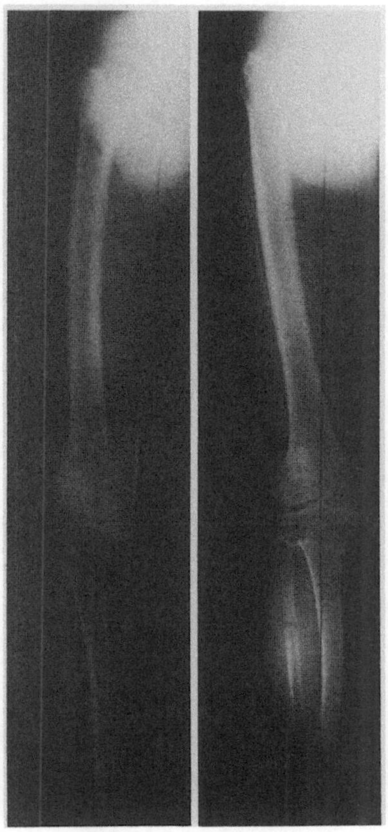

Fig. 1. Predominantly medial osteoarthritis of the knee with marked varus deformity. The mechanical axis passes medial to the center of the knee (*left*). After surgery (*right*) the mechanical axis is centered on the knee

varus deformity. Thirty of the 39 patients with decreased motion had been treated for valgus deformity.

Proximal tibial osteotomies yield a good result in approximately 80° of cases, provided the operation is technically precise and is able to center the mechanical axis of the leg on the knee joint (Fig. 1). It is apparent, however, that the surgical correction of varus deformities has a higher overall success rate than the correction of valgus deformities.

References

1. Zilch H, Adlkofer M, Groher W, Friedebold G (1978) Umstellungsosteotomien am Schienbeinkopf (Indikation, Technik und Ergebnisse). Unfallheilkunde 81:642

Results of the Intraligamentous Open Wedge Osteotomy of the Proximal Tibia (Elevating Osteotomy)

E. Walter and U. Holz

We consider the intraligamentous open wedge osteotomy of the proximal tibia as described by Debyere [2] and Dolanc [3] to be the treatment of choice for genu varum and genu valgum deformities with associated ligamentous instability. In addition to realigning the limb, this operation also restores tension to lax ligaments and obviates the need for a separate ligament-tightening procedure like that necessary after the wedge osteotomy of Coventry [1]. Compared with the lateral side of the knee, where the collateral ligament inserts into the fibular head no more than 2 cm from the joint line, the medial tibial condyle offers a "clearance" of 4–6 cm for performing the osteotomy [4].

In this article we report the results of follow-up examinations conducted at our trauma clinic in Tübingen. A total of 83 patients were operated on between 1975 and 1980. It is still too early to review 11 other patients who underwent surgery at our Stuttgart facility after 1980. Of the 83 patients who were followed, 42 were women (50.7%) and 41 were men (49.3%).

Posttraumatic deformities were twice as frequent in the men as in the women, while the women had a three times higher incidence of idiopathic osteoarthritis than the men (Table 1).

Varus deformities were far more prevalent than valgus deformities (73 versus 10). All prophylactic osteotomies were performed for posttraumatic angular deformities that were uncomplicated by osteoarthritis (Table 2). Of the 69 varus deformities in which osteoarthritis was present, 55 patients showed less than 10° of angulation. The small number of valgus deformities (10) showed a more even distribution (Tables 3 and 4).

Complaints relating to pain, walking distance, and reliance on ambulatory aids were elicited with questionnaires and then evaluated according to a point scoring system (Table 5).

Table 1. Conditions Necessitating Corrective Osteotomy

	Men	Women	Percentage
Idiopathic osteo-arthritis of the knee	9	26	42
Posttraumatic deformity	20	10	36
Prior meniscectomy	11	6	20
Other causes (e.g., tuberculosis)	1		2

Corrective Osteotomies of the Lower Extremity
Edited by G. Hierholzer, K. H. Müller

Table 2. Distribution of Cases by Type of Deformity and Patient Age and Gender

Type of deformity	Varus			Valgus			Total
Gender	Total	M	F	Total	M	F	
Number	73	34	39	10	7	3	83
Age (average)							53.6
Youngest patient	27	27	33	19	19	45	19
Oldest patient	76	76	75	71	53	71	76
Prophylactic	4	3	1	5	3	2	9
Joint-preserving	69	31	38	5	4	1	74

Table 3. Distribution of Cases by Amount of Varus Angulation

Varus angulation	Up to 5°	Up to 10°	Up to 15°	<15°	Total
Without osteo-arthritis	2	1	1	0	4
With osteoarthritis	17	38	8	6	69
Total	19	39	9	6	73

Table 4. Distribution of Cases by Amount of Valgus Angulation

Valgus angulation	Up to 5°	Up to 10°	Up to 15°	<15°	Total
Without osteo-arthritis	0	2	0	3	5
With osteoarthritis	1	2	1	1	5
Total	1	4	1	4	10

In 96% of the patients pain was the chief presenting complaint, with 70% reporting pain of moderate to severe intensity. After surgery, almost 80% of the patients reported that pain was absent or significantly improved (Table 6).

The goal of surgery was to restore the 87° anatomic angle between the plane of the femoral condyles and the tibial shaft axis to an accuracy of ±2°. Fifty-nine percent of the valgus and varus deformities were corrected to nominal accuracy, 31% were overcorrected, and 10% were undercorrected.

Surgery increased the range of knee flexion by up to 15° in 37% of cases, and it increased extension by up to 5° in 28% of cases (Table 7).

The effect of the surgery on the progression of osteoarthritis is shown in Table 8. We see that a nominal correction produced a stabilization of disease in 80% of cases, while undercorrection was followed by exacerbation of disease in 50%. In treating osteoarthritis with varus deformity, Richter [6]

Table 5. Scoring System for Evaluation of Complaints

Complaints relating to pain, walking distance, and reliance on ambulatory aids were elicited in questionnaires and scored on a four-point scale:

1. Pain:	
No pain	0 Points
Mild, constant pain or pain only on weight bearing	1 Point
Pain with any movement	2 Points
Severe pain at rest or sleep disturbance due to pain	3 Points
2. Walking distance:	
More than 1 km	0 Points
Up to 1 km	1 Point
Up to about 100 m	2 Points
Around the house only	3 Points
1. Ambulatory aids:	
None	0 Points
1 cane outside the house	1 Point
1 cane at all times	2 Points
2 canes or crutches at all times	3 Points

Table 6. Results of Follow-Up Examinations Regarding Preoperative and Postoperative Complaints

Preoperative / Postoperative	3 Points [%]	2 points [%]	1 Point [%]	0 Points [%]
Pain	56 / 12	14 / 9	26 / 61	4 / 18
Walking distance	12 / 3	21 / 4	30 / 35	37 / 58
Ambulatory aids	5 / 9	9 / 4	25 / 18	61 / 69

Table 7. Effect of Osteotomy on Range of Motion

	Flexion	Extention	
Gain ≧15°	37%	28%	Gain ≧5°
No change	60%	65%	No change
Loss	3%	7%	Loss

Table 8. Amount of Correction versus Osteoarthritis

Correction	Stabilized [%]	Worsening of osteoarthritis [%]
Nominal	80	20
Over	75	25
Under	50	50

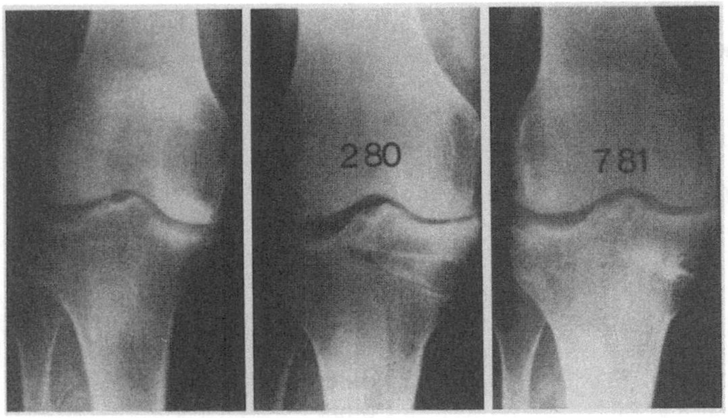

Fig. 1. Infraction of the tibial articular surface that occurred during the osteotomy

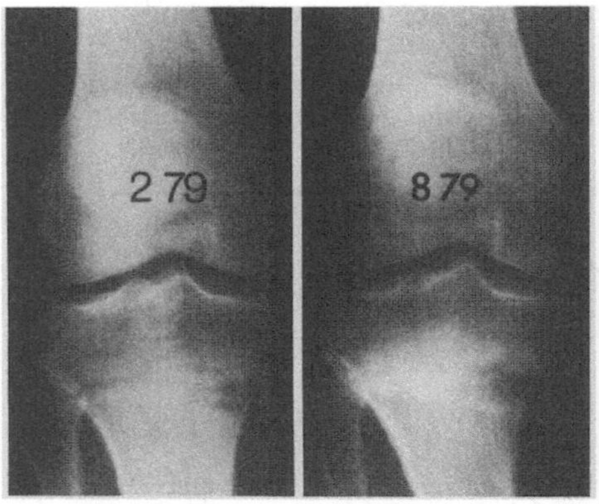

Fig. 2. Loss of correction after insertion of an homologous wedge graft

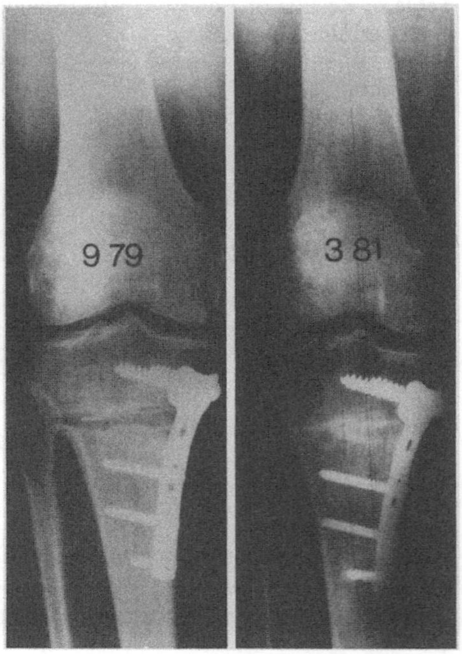

Fig. 3. Penetration of the opposite cortex and stabilization with a T-plate

considers the "ideal correction" to be a slight overcorrection into physiologic valgus. This is also advocated by Maquet [5] and Zilch [8]. Wagner [7] stresses the value of overcorrection in the operative treatment of flexion contractures of the knee. Corrections greater than 20° are technically difficult to achieve with an intraligamentous elevating osteotomy of the tibia [8].

The only significant complications in this series were nine infractions of the tibial articular surface that occurred when the osteotomy was carried out (Fig. 1). No problems of consolidation were encountered.

We used 70 homologous wedge grafts and 13 autologous grafts to elevate the tibial plateau. We found that homologous grafts may collapse and cause a loss of correction that necessitates reoperation (Fig. 2). This did not occur with any of the autologous grafts. If the cortex opposite the wedge is penetrated, supplementary internal fixation is required. This was necessary in 12 cases (Fig. 3).

References

1. Coventry MB (1973) Osteotomy about the knee for degenerative and rheumatoid arthritis. J Bone Joint Surg [Am] 55/1:23
2. Debeyre J, Artigou JM (1972) Résultat à distance de 260 ostéotomies tibiales pour deviation frontale du genou, Ref Chir Orthop 58:355
3. Dolanc B (1973) Die Behandlung des instabilen Kniegelenks mit Achsenfehlstellung durch die intraligamentäre Anhebe-Tibiaosteotomie. Arch Orthop Unfallchir 76:280
4. Hattab A, Lauttamus L (1976) Die proximale Tibiaosteotomie bei Behandlung der Arthrosis deformans des Kniegelenks. Z Orthop 114:773
5. Maquet P (1979) Korrekturosteotomien in der Behandlung der Kniegelenksarthrose. Orthopäde 8:296
6. Richter R (1974) Erfahrungen mit der Tibiakopfosteotomie bei Gonarthrosen. Arch Orthop Unfallchir 80:107
7. Wagner h (1976) Indikation und Technik der Korrekturosteotomien bei der posttraumatischen Kniegelenksarthrose. Hefte Unfallheilk 128:155
8. Zilch H, Adlkofer M, Groher W, Friedebold G (1978) Umstellungsosteotomien am Schienbeinkopf (Indikation, Technik und Ergebnisse). Unfallheilkunde 81:642

Results of Proximal Tibial Osteotomies Stabilized with the T-Plate for Correction of Posttraumatic Deformity

A. Skuginna, P. M. Hax and G. Schneppendahl

Corrctive osteotomies of the proximal tibia will consolidate in due time even when simple plaster immobilization is used [1,5]. However, we prefer a secure fixation that will permit the limb to be exercised after surgery [4]. In the plateau-elevating osteotomy without metallic fixation, the necessary stability is provided by the taut collateral ligaments [2]. For reasons that will become clear, we prefer to supplement this physiologic stabilization with a T plate. A T plate applied to the osteotomized upper tibia provides excellent exercise stability. Follow-ups of patients treated by this method have been conducted in an effort to identify potential problems that could compromise the clinical result.

In planning the corrective osteotomy and T-plate fixation, we followed recognized principles in establishing the site of the osteotomy and the amount of correction required. In all cases whole-leg roentgenograms were used to determine the optimum angle of correction. We performed the osteotomy either in the intraligamentous region of the tibia or below the distal attachments of the collateral ligaments, depending on ligament tension. As a rule, we angle the line of osteotomy gently upward toward the opposite cortex, leaving an intact bridge of bone to serve as a natural tension band. Of course, this is not possible in cases where rotational correction or anterior displacement is also carried out. In these cases the fixation may be enhanced by inserting a cancellous lag screw obliquely across the osteotomy or by

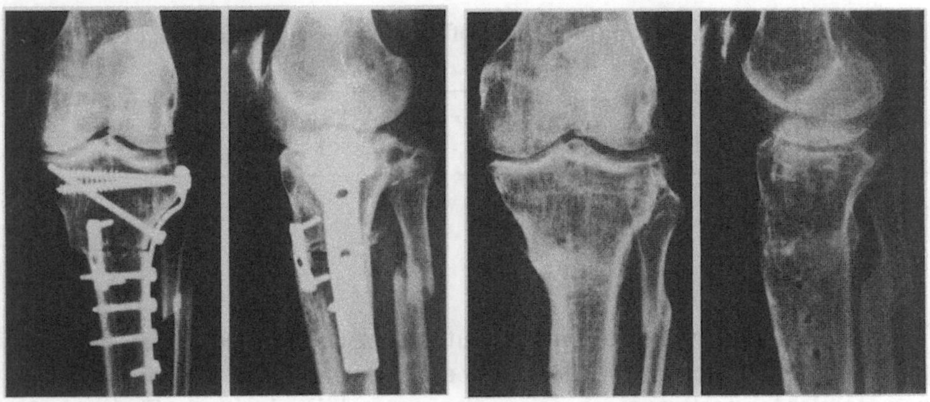

a b

Fig. 1 a,b. a F.-W. B., example of a small contralateral plate applied in the tension-band mode to maintain closure of the osteotomy. **b** Status after bony consolidation and removal of metal

Corrective Osteotomies of the Lower Extremity
Edited by G. Hierholzer, K. H. Müller

attaching a small tension-band plate (Fig. 1). In every case attention should be given to the treatment of coexisting lesions such as relative collateral ligament instability or femoropatellar osteoarthritis. The latter condition may respond favorably to incision of the retinaculum or anterior advancement of the tibial tuberosity, while relative collateral ligament instability is usually relieved by an elevating osteotomy. Coexisting deformities such as anterior or posterior angulation or malrotation are corrected concurrently with the principal deformity.

We feel that the comparison of preoperative and postoperative whole-leg roentgenograms is essential for an objective assessment of the operative result. For various reasons we were unable to obtain whole-leg roentgenograms in every follow-up examination. Such records are available for 17 of our patients, all of whom had undergone an elevating osteotomy of the upper tibia. Eight of these osteotomies were stabilized with a T plate, thus providing an opportunity to assess the potential benefit of the T-plate fixation in preventing secondary loss of correction. We used the slope of the tibial plateau as our main criterion for assessing the quality of the correction (Fig. 2). Additional criteria are listed in Table 1.

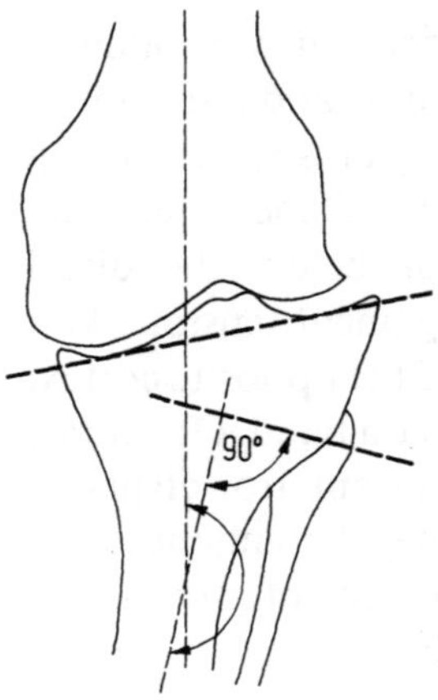

Fig. 2. Slope of the tibial plateau

Table 1. Criteria for Evaluating the Results of Elevating Osteotomies with or without a T plate

1. FSA-KB angle	3. FSA-TSA angle
2. TSA-KB angle (slope of plateau)	4. Angle of correction

Results

The sites of corrective osteotomies about the knee performed at our center for posttraumatic or degenertive deformity are shown in Table 2. Proximal tibial osteotomies for posttraumatic deformity were stabilized with the T plate in 38 cases, with an external frame in 15 cases, and with a different kind of metallic fixation in 2 cases. In 15 posttraumatic corrections no metallic fixation was used (Table 3).

Table 2. Corrective Osteotomies about the Knee (Duisburg-Buchholz Trauma Clinic, 1973–1981, n = 208, 196 patients)

	Proximal tibia n = 146	Supracondylar femur n = 62
Posttraumatic	48	19
	23	11
Degenerative	31	14
	44	18

Table 3. Corrective Operations of the Proximal Tibia, Fixation Methods, 1973–1981 (n = 146)

	T-plate	External frame	Other metallic fixation	No metallic fixation
Posttraumatic	38	15	2	15
Degenerative	14	58	–	4

Table 4. Corrective Operations of the Proximal Tibia Fixed with a T-Plate, 1973–1981 (n = 38)

	Varus	Valgus
Without coexisting lesions	12	8
With coexisting lesions	5	8
With coexisting deformity	3	2

Of the 38 patients whose tibial osteotomies were fixed with a T-plate, 28 were men and 10 were women (Table 4). Coexisting disorders and deformities were as follows:

– Coexisting disorders: Ligament laxity (8), femoropatellar osteoarthritis (3)

– Coexisting deformities: Malrotation, anterior or posterior angulation (6)

With regard to complications, wound healing difficulties arose in 5 patients whose osteotomies had been fixed with the T plate. These patients already had unfavorable preoperative scarring secondary to the previous internal fixation of proximal tibial fractures. In two cases the healing disturbances did not resolve until the metal implant was removed. We encountered three cases of postoperative peroneal nerve palsy, two of which were transient.

Based on the criteria in Table 5, we rated the result of the operation as good (+ + +) in 14 cases, fair (+ +) in 10 cases, and poor (+) in 5 cases. We used the criteria in Table 1 to assess the quality of the correction. The results are shown in Table 6. The preoperative angular deformity, the desired angle of correction, and the slope of the tibial plateau (preoperative and at follow-up)

Table 5. Proximal Tibial Osteotomy: Evaluation at Follow-Up

+ + +	Unimpeded gait Unlimited walking distance Unlimited extension Flexion to 120°
+ +	Slight limp Walking distance up to 1 km Up to 10° loss of extension Up to 100° flexion
+	Cane required Up to 20° loss of extension Up to 90° flexion

Table 6. Proximal Tibial Osteotomies Fixed with a T-plate: Results at Follow-Up (n=29)

+ + +	14
+ +	10
+	5

Table 7. Elevating Osteotomies of the Tibial Plateau: Preoperative Angular Deformity

∢	n
< 5°	2
> 5°	6
>10°	9

Table 8. Elevating Osteotomies of the Tibial Plateau: Angle of Correction

∢	n
< 5°	1
> 5°	4
>10°	12

Table 9. Elevating Osteotomies of the Tibial Plateau: Slope of the Plateau

∢	Preoperative n	At follow-up n
< 5°	2	14
> 5°	6	3
>10°	9	0

Table 10. Elevating Osteotomies of the Tibial Plateau: Loss of Correction at Follow-Up

∢	Without T-plate n	With T-plate n
> 5°	3	0
>10°	0	0

are indicated in Tables 7–9. These tables pertain to 17 patients who had had an elevating osteotomy for posttraumatic deformity of the upper tibia. In eight of these patients the osteotomy had been fixed with a T-plate; in nine patients metallic fixation was not employed.

Our measurements indicated tha overcorrection had been achieved in some cases. This was intentionally planned in order to remove stress from the involved compartment of the knee. We also noted a loss of correction in three patients whose elevating ostotomies had not been stabilized with a T plate (Table 10).

Discussion

The results of operations in which a high tibial osteotomy was fixed with a T plate demonstrate that this procedure provides a secure primary fixation that is stable enough to allow immediate exercise. Use of the T plate permits the correction of various angular deformities that require a complete transection of the bone, i.e., an osteotomy that includes the opposite cortex. In these cases we apply a supplementary plate to the tension side of the bone to prevent gaping of the osteotomy. We have not observed any loss of motion referrable to the operative procedure described. T-plate fixation appears to have a higher association with wound healing problems than external skeletal fixation in patients who have unfavorable pre-existing skin conditions or scarring. In these circumstances we recommend that T-plate fixation be used with caution (Fig. 1).

Of course, T-plate fixation lacks the advantage of allowing postoperative adjustments of alignment or rotation like that possible with an external frame. Consequently, the angle of correction must be determined with extremely high precision when this technique is used. Allowance must be made for possible compression and impaction of the osteotomy fragments, which may lead to overcorrection.

Evaluation of the result of the operation using the criteria listed above and full-length roentgenograms of the legs shows that the T plate protects against loss of correction in elevating osteotomies of the proximal tibia. The T plate thus exerts a favorable buttressing effect when combined with the insertion of a wedge graft (Fig. 3).

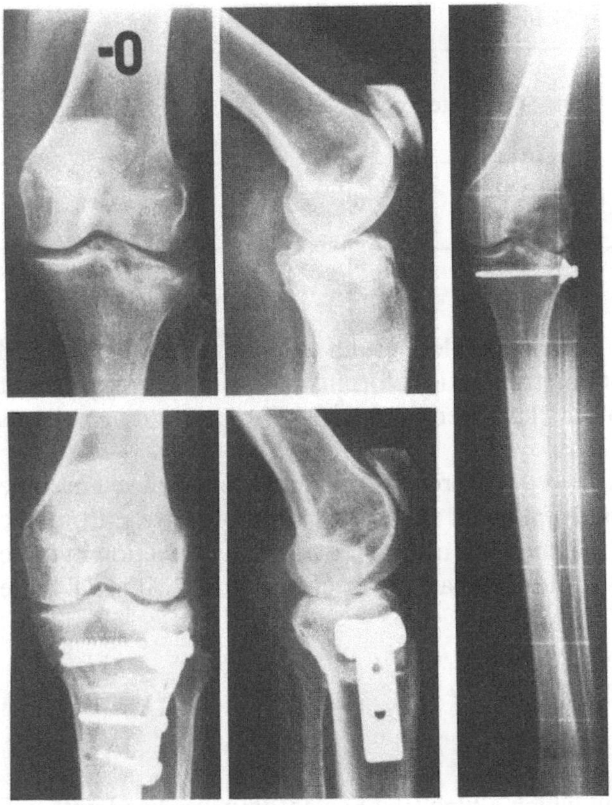

a c b

Fig. 3. a M. D., lateral tibial condyle fracture with depression of the plateau. **b** Primary treatment by inadequate internal fixation. **c** Correction with an elevating osteotomy and stabilization with a T plate

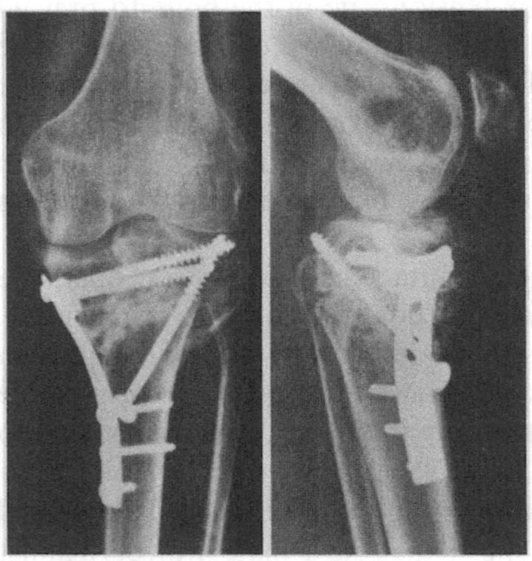

Fig. 4. J. H., valgus osteotomy with wedge insertion and correction of flexion deformity. Stabilization with a T plate and lag screw

The clinical results of the proximal tibial osteotomy with T plate fixation are somewhat difficult to evaluate. This is due in part to the diversity of presenting conditions that exist in patients who are selected for surgery. Some patients will have angular deformity that is accompanied by little or no degenerative disease, while others will have severe osteoarthritis of the tibial joint surface as a result of a previous trauma. Like other authors, we have been unable to confirm a regression of marked, pre-existing, secondary osteoarthritic changes in roentgenograms taken during follow-up examinations [3]. Also, we were not always able to draw a clear correlation between roentgenologic changes and subjective complaints.

In summary, we see the following advantages of T-plate fixation in corrective osteotomies of the proximal tibia:

It enables a biomechanically correct axial correction to be carried out.

Postoperative exercise is facilitated by stable internal fixation, and postoperative pain is reduced.

Bony consolidation is prompt.

Additional therapeutic measures such as the correction of flexion deformity, improvement of femoropatellar osteoarthritis, or the correction of coexisting malrotation are easily incorporated into the procedure.

Use of the T plate in conjunction with the elevating osteotomy protects against possible loss of correction (Fig. 4).

References

1. Aldinger G (1981) Mittelfristige Ergebnisse der kniegelenknahen Osteotomie in der Behandlung der Gonarthrose. Z Orthop 119:516–520
2. Dolanc B (1973) Die Behandlung des instabilen Kniegelenks mit Achsenfehlstellung durch die intraligamentäre Anhebetibiaosteotomie. Arch Orthop Unfallchir 76:280–289
3. Müller KH, Thelen E (1976) Ergebnisse und posttraumatische Arthrose nach operativ versorgten Tibiakopffrakturen. Aktuel Traumatol 6:55–60
4. Skuginna A, Ludolph E, Hierholzer G (1975) Wahl des Operationsverfahrens bei der Umstellungsosteotomie im Tibiakopfbereich. Aktuel Traumatol 9/3:121–126
5. Wagner H (1977) Prinzipien der Korrekturosteotomien am Bein. Orthopäde 6:145–177

Results of Proximal Tibial Osteotomies Stabilized by External Skeletal Fixation

J. D. Wolf and K. H. Müller

When an indication exists for a corrective osteotomy of the proximal tibia, the task remains to select an appropriate mode of fixation. In soft-tissue conditions about the knee are precarious, especially in patients who have had previous operations in that area, or if complications have already occurred or are anticipated, external skeletal fixation is the best solution.

From 1973 to 1982 a total of 51 corrective osteotomies of the proximal tibia for posttraumatic deformities were performed at the Bergmannsheil Clinic in Bochum. Eighteen of these osteotomies (35.2%) were stabilized by external skeletal fixation. In 11 patients the deformities were secondary to injuries sustained at work, in 5 patients they were secondary to accidents away from work, and 2 patients had deformities secondary to war injuries.

Seventeen of the 18 patients presented for follow-up examination an average of 31.4 months after their corrective surgery, with a range from 6 months to 10 years.

Ten of the patients had had previous surgical treatment for their injuries, and 8 had been treated conservatively. One of the surgical patients had been operated by us.

Males predominated in this series by a ratio of 15:3. Both sides of the body were equally represented (9:9). Two patients had injuries to both proximal tibiae, but in each case only one side required operative correction.

The shortest interval between injury and corrective osteotomy was five months, which is certainly the most favorable in terms of a good long-term result. The longest interval was 36 years and followed a gunshot fracture sustained during wartime (Fig. 1). The average interval between injury and corrective surgery was 12.8 years (disregarding the extreme cases of 30 and 36 years). The oldest patient was 63 years of age, the youngest 17.

The indications for surgery were varus deformity in 8 cases, valgus deformity in 9 cases, and a 25° internal rotation deformity in 1 case. Concomitant backward displacement of 10 – 15° had to be corrected in 2 patients (cf. Fig. 11, p. 214).

Ten patients were diagnosed as having tibial condylar fractures, and eight as having proximal tibial fractures. The tibial injury was solitary in only seven cases, and in five cases it was one of multiple injuries.

The osteotomies were stabilized either with the tubular external fixation system of the ASIF using 2, 3 or 4 Steinmann pins, or with the ASIF threaded-rod external fixator (cf. Fig. 12, p. 216).

The fixation material was left in place an average of 3.7 months, ranging from a minimum of 7 weeks to a maximum of 8 months.

Corrective Osteotomies of the Lower Extremity
Edited by G. Hierholzer, K. H. Müller

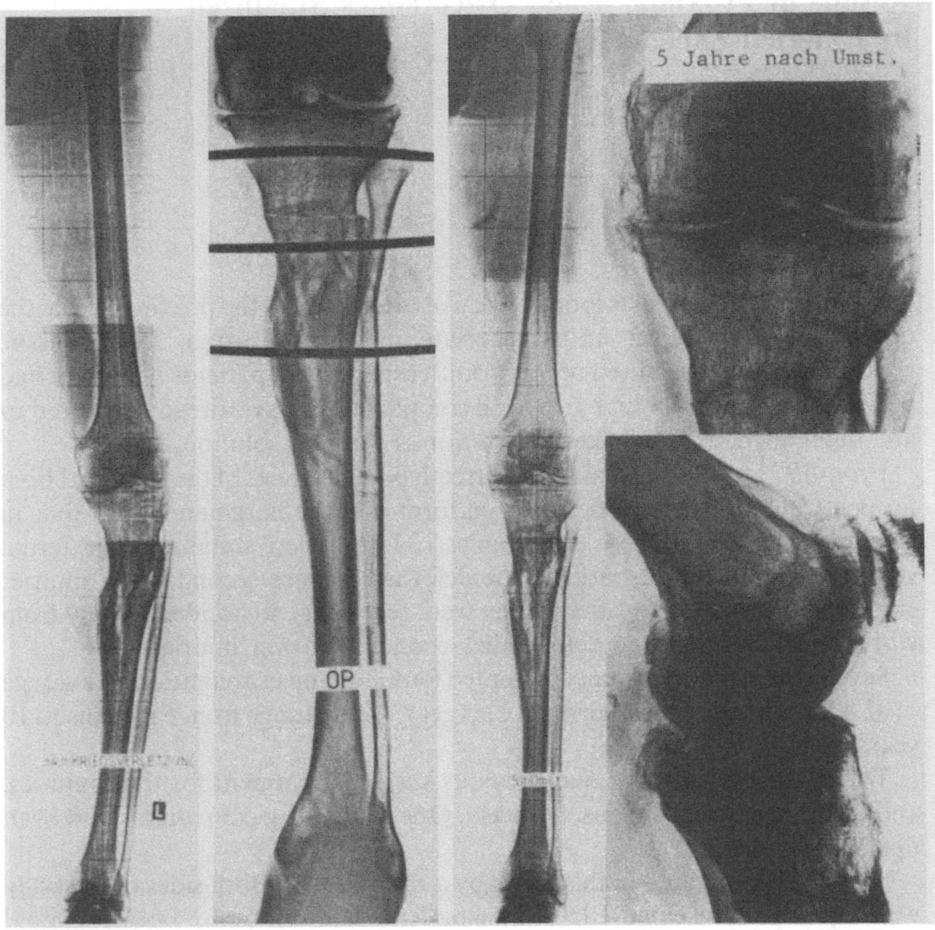

a b c

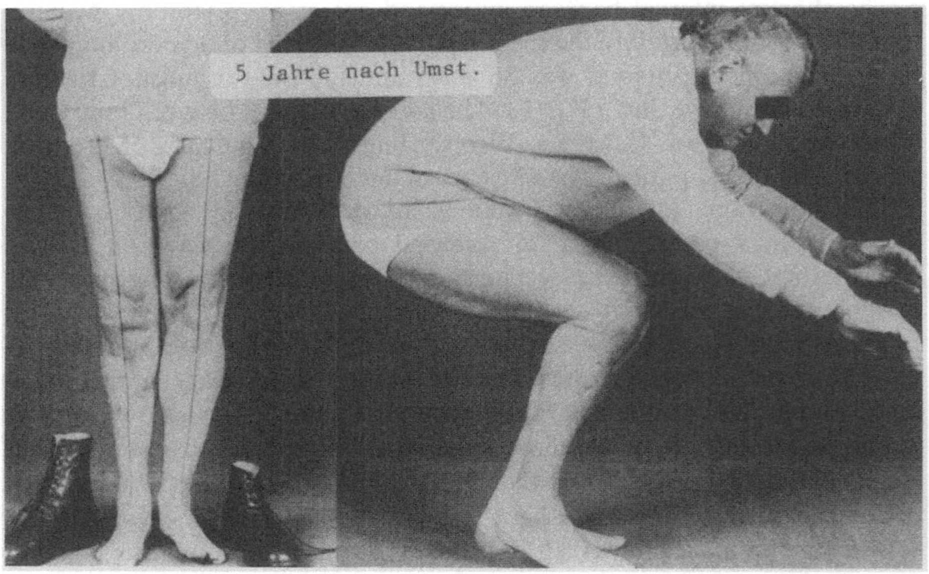

d

Preoperative complications included peroneal nerve injury in five cases, thrombosis in two cases, osteomyelitis in two cases, and one nonunion. One patient developed a controllable pulmonary embolism postoperatively despite early mobilization and weight bearing. In three cases a pin-track fistula developed after removal of the external frame and persisted for two to six weeks.

At follow-up we observed an average limb shortening of approximately 1.7 cm and an average loss of 1.0 cm muscle girth in the operated limb. Knee joint mobility was consistently good. The average range of knee motion was 0–0–110°; the poorest was 0–5–90°. There was no obvious evidence of knee joint irritation, although clear clinical and radiologic signs of osteoarthritis were noted in 15 cases.

Two patients showed cruciate ligament laxity that was not fully compensated by muscular activity, and three patients showed collateral ligament weakness. No documentation was available on the preoperative status of these patients.

Eight patients were dependent on aids such as an elevated heel or sole, peroneal splint, orthopedic footwear, elastic stocking, cane or crutch (two elderly patients).

Follow-up roentgenograms showed only 3 cases in which the mechanical axis of the limb deviated more than 2 cm from the center of the knee. Roentgenologic evidence of progression of osteoarthritis appears to contradict the relatively good clinical function of the knee joint observed after corrective surgery. This finding is consistent with general reports in the literature [1–10].

With regard to subjective outcome, 16 patients rated their condition following corrective osteotomy as good and improved. Only one patient rated the outcome as poor. Common complaints were sensitivity to weather changes and pain and swelling at the knee after prolonged exertion.

No patient reported disability or other problems from the external fixation device, even when questioned specifically about such problems. The three cases documented in Figs. 1–3 illustrate the value of external skeletal fixation in the correction of deformities when soft-tissue conditions, osseous injuries and the patient's history are amenable to that mode of fixation.

◄

Fig. 1 a–d. R. H., male, independent engineer, in 1944 sustained a gunshot fracture of the left tibia in addition to an olecranon fracture and eyelid injury. There was peroneal nerve damage and subsequent osteomyelitis. **a** Malunion with backward displacement and varus deformity. Knee motion was painful with a range of 0–0–100°. Arthrodesis was considered. **b** Thirty-six years after the trauma a corrective osteotomy was performed in 2 planes (15° valgus, 10° recurvation). **c** The osteotomy healed uneventfully and is solid at 5 years after surgery. **d** Range of knee motion at 5 years is 0–0–130°. The patient can walk 4–5 km without complaints and enjoys golf. At times an orthopedic shoe is worn (preexisting peroneal nerve damage)

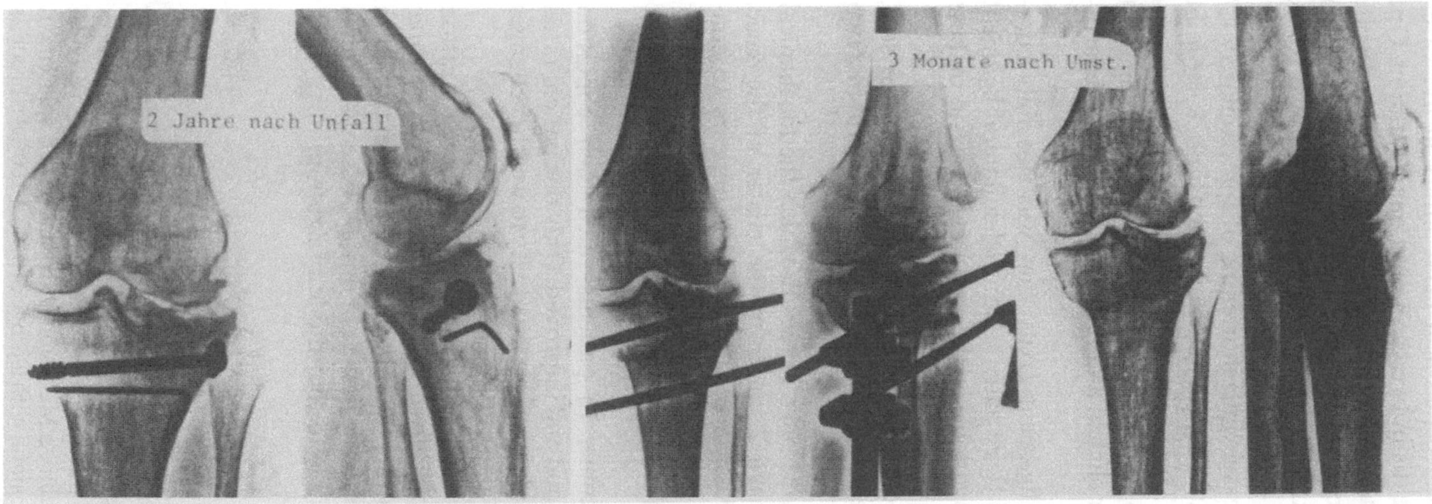

a b c

Fig. 2 a–d. A. W., female, independent innkeeper, sustained a left tibial condylar fracture on Oct. 27, 1975. **a** Operative treatment elsewhere, roentgenogram at 2 years postinjury; range of motion is 0°/10°/40°. **b** Varus osteotomy for 12° posttraumatic valgus with associated symptoms (III–IV), overweight. **c** Three months after osteotomy: excellent alignment. **d** Six years after osteotomy: range of knee motion 0–0–100°. The patient works a full 12-h day tending counter. Roentgenograms show only slightly increased evidence of joint wear ("healthy" right side is shown for comparison)

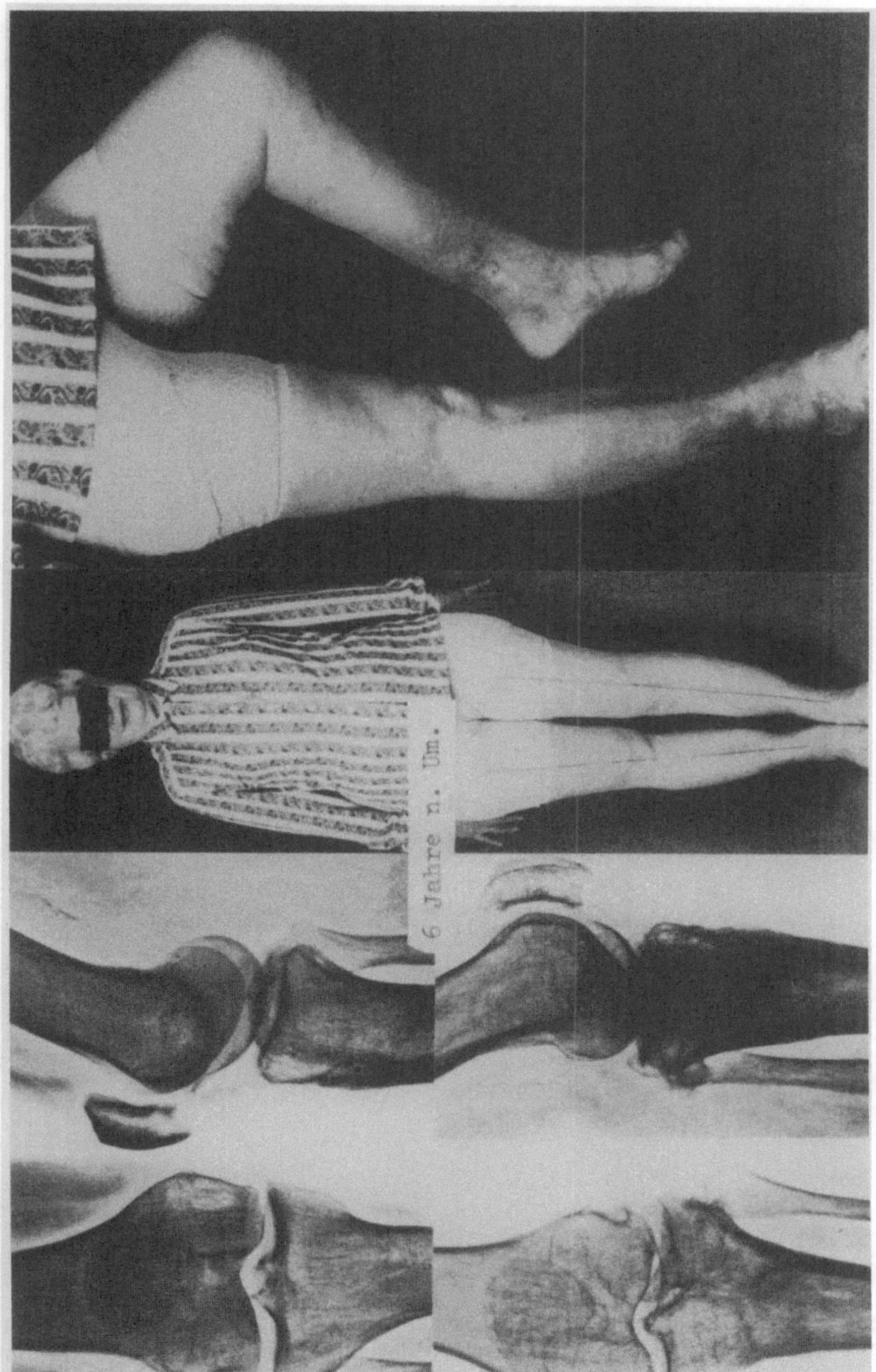

Fig. 2d

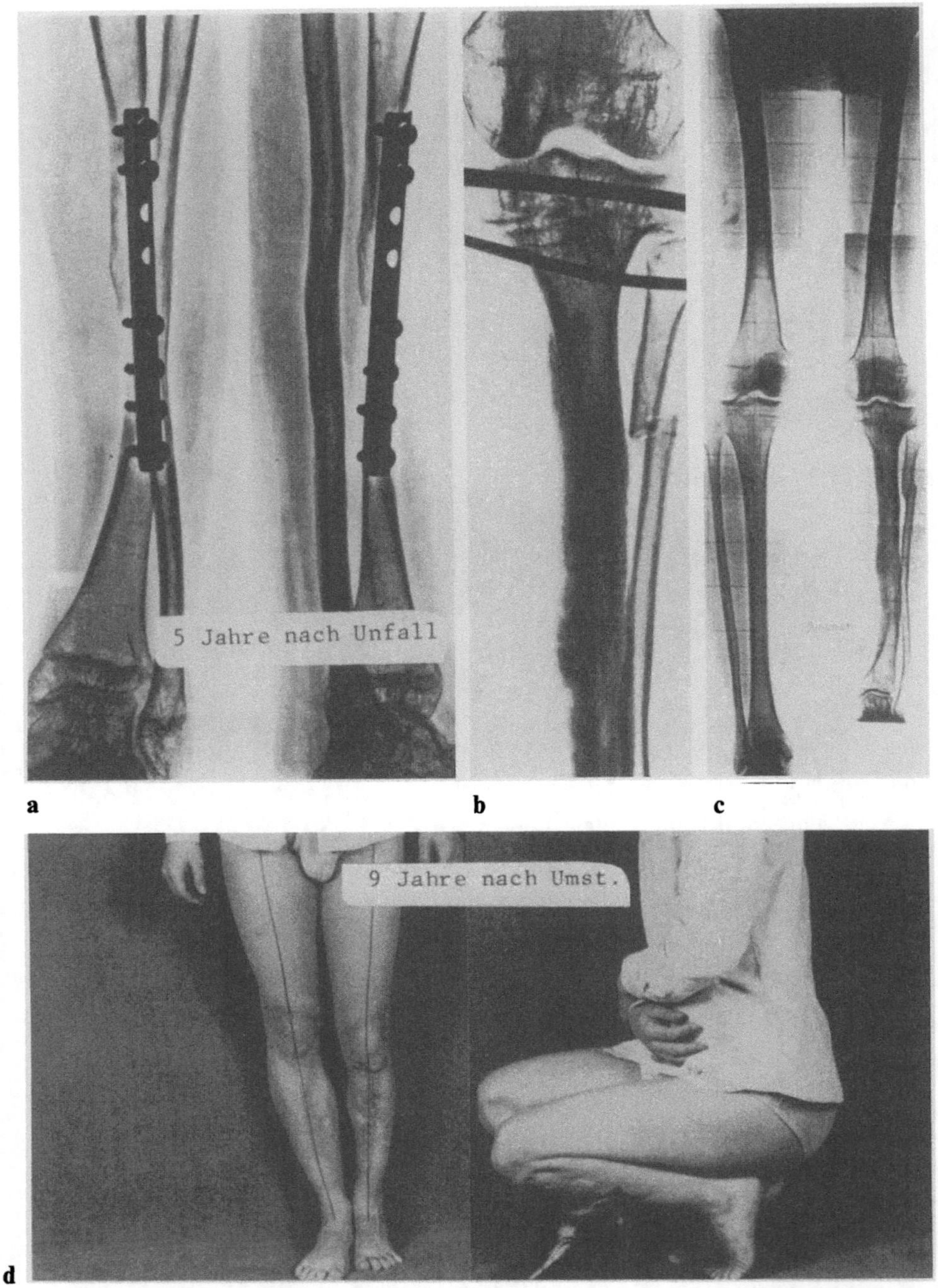

Fig. 3 a – d. H. F., male, medical student, sustained left tibial fracture with bone loss at age 7 in traffic accident. Osteomyelitis developed after multiple operations (threatening amputation), and a nonunion ensued. **a** 5 years postinjury the bone was refractured, causing 10 cm of limb shortening and significant varus angulation. The bone healed after 7 years of therapy. **b** At 10 years postinjury a valgus osteotomy (15°) was performed and healed uneventfully. **c** Roentgenographic and **d** clinical findings 9 years after corrective surgery: excellent knee motion, restricted ankle flexion. There is muscular atrophy and 10 cm of limb shortening, which is corrected with an elevated shoe. The patient is active recreationally (sailing, dancing)

References

1. Debrunner AM (1970) Die operative Behandlung von Gonarthrosen. In: L. Nicod (Hrsg) Die Gonarthrose. Huber, Bern Stuttgart Wien
2. Dolanc B (1973) Die Behandlung des instabilen Kniegelenks mit Achsenfehlstellung durch intraligamentäre Anhebe-Tibiaosteotomie. Arch Orthop Unfallchir 76:280
3. Hierholzer G, Voorhoeve A, Kleining R, Kehr H (1975) Reintervention nach Schienbeinkopfbrüchen. Chirurg 46:352
4. Hohmann D, Legal H, Seidel K (1975) Hohe Tibiakopfosteotomien in der Behandlung der Gonarthrose des alten Menschen. Orthopäde 4:172
5. Müller KH, Biebrach M (1977) Korrekturosteotomien und ihre Ergebnisse bei kniegelenknahen posttraumatischen Fehlstellungen. Unfallheilkunde 80:359
6. Müller KH, Biebrach M (1977) Korrekturosteotomien und ihre Ergebnisse bei idiopathischen kniegelenknahen Achsenfehlstellungen. Unfallheilkunde 80:464
7. Müller KH, Thelen E (1976) Ergebnisse und posttraumatische Arthrose nach operativ versorgten Tibiakopffrakturen. Aktuel Traumatol 6:55
8. Müller ME (1967) Posttraumatische Achsenfehlstellungen an den unteren Extremitäten. Huber, Bern Stuttgart Wien
9. Nicod L (1970) Die Gonarthrose. Huber, Bern Stuttgart Wien
10. Wagner H (1976) Indikation und Technik der Korrekturosteotomien bei der posttraumatischen Kniegelenkarthrose. Hefte Unfallheilkd 128:155

Summary: Corretive Osteotomies after Trauma about the Knee

L. Gotzen

Malunited fractures involving the knee joint, distal femur and proximal tibia are a cause of joint incongruity, instability, and angulation. They are regarded as preosteoarthritic deformities.

Pain and disability often are a primary result of altered joint mechanics, but they tend to be most severe when they develop secondarily as a result of progressive joint wear. The pathogenic mechanism of osteoarthritis is the local overloading of cartilage, menisci and bone by excessive pressure.

Deformities of the articular surfaces create a highly unfavorable biomechanical situation in which degenerative changes tend to be rapid. Motion of the joint is permanently impaired through incongruity and subluxation, and damaging compressive and shear forces are exerted on the articular surfaces.

With simple limb angulation, the progression of osteoarthritis is more gradual because the abnormal load on the joint is less severe and can be further alleviated by muscular compensation. The abnormal distribution of stresses leads to a usually circumscribed joint destruction in which mechanical wear and enzymatic breakdown of the cartilage incite a reactive synovitis, characterized by pain and swelling of the capsule and effusion.

The end result is the complete picture of osteoarthritis of the knee with painful limitation of motion from localized destruction of the joint surfaces, synovitis, insertion tenopathies, and muscular atrophy and contractures. Elimination of the mechanical disturbance by corrective surgery is the prime requisite for preventing or interrupting the vicious cycle. Even advanced osteoarthritis and advanced age are not necessarily contraindications to corrective osteotomy if there is a chance of achieving a reasonably normal joint position. Surgery that restores a normal weight-bearing alignment often produces remarkable recoveries with a regression of complaints and improvement of function, as the results of follow-up examinations clearly demonstrate.

A detailed analysis of the abnormal mechanics of the knee joint in the presence of posttraumatic deformity and its functional and morphologic consequences provides the rationale for operative therapy. It is essential that every corrective operation be preceded by a comprehensive clinical and roentgenographic evaluation to determine the precise nature and extent of the deformity. Preoperative reontgenograms are used to make scale drawings indicating the site and amount of the correction, the sequence of operative steps, the result of the correction, and the technique of stabilization.

Simple angulations usually pose no serious problems of diagnosis, case selection, planning, or operative technique. The correction is planned in such a way that the mechanical axis of the limb is returned to the center of the knee

Corrective Osteotomies of the Lower Extremity
Edited by G. Hierholzer, K. H. Müller

joint, and the knee baseline is horizontal. This will ensure that symmetrical, purely axial compressive loads are imposed on the joint surfaces.

Only in advanced osteoarthritis with varus deformity should one consider overcorrecting the limb into about 2–4° of valgus in order to unload the medial compartment. This is paricularly beneficial in elderly patients who may have little potential for muscular compensation. Open wedge osteotomies offer the advantage of preserving limb length. They are particularly useful in younger patients as a means of restoring anatomic and functional integrity.

Joint instabilities that result from stretching of the ligaments by deformities do not require special treatment and can usually be dynamically compensated following joint realignment and muscle strengthening. Corrective osteotomy must be combined with ligament reconstruction in cases where a decompensated instability exists secondary to trauma.

Far more troublesome are malunited intraarticular fractures, especially those involving the femoral condyles. Usually an intraarticular correction is possible only in the early stage, at which time the original fracture site may be osteotomized and the fragments anatomically reduced. But often the procedure must be limited to an extraarticular correction whose aim is simply to improve mechanical alignment.

Malunited tibial condylar fractures with depression of the articular surfaces are more common. Joint incongruity and angular deformity are complicated by the presence of joint instability. An intraligamentous elevating osteotomy in these cases will align the limb and restore ligamentous tension. The tibia must be osteotomized close to the articular surface, especially on the lateral side, to achieve this ligament–tightening effect.

The anterior intraligamentous elevating osteotomy has also proved useful in the treatment of posttraumatic genu recurvatum. If the corticocancellous wedge graft is solidly interposed between the osteotomy surfaces, additional fixation is unnecessary.

Corrective osteotomies about the knee for posttraumatic deformity are among the most rewarding procedures in reconstructive surgery. Proper case selection requires a detailed knowledge of the functional anatomy and biomechanics not only of the knee joint but ot the entire lower extremity. The surgeon must know the material properties of the various components of the extremity as well as their mechanical and biological behavior under normal and abnormal conditions. Operative success also requires a mastery of the entire spectrum of bone and joint surgery. The knowledge, skills and experience of the surgeon are critical in determining the fate of the affected knee joint and the extent to which the anatomy and function of the limb can be restored.

V. The Ankle and Foot

Indications and Technique of Corrective Osteotomies of the Distal Tibia and Ankle Mortise

S. Weller

The successful treatment of injuries about the distal tibia and ankle joint, like all intraarticular and periarticular fractures, requires an anatomic restoration of all damaged structures [4]. Specifically, it is necessary to repair lesions of the osseous, cartilaginous and ligamentous structures which act in concert to maintain the integrity of the ankle mortise and ensure the normal function, stability and loading of the extremity.

Numerous experimental and clinical studies have shown that the fibula and tibiofibular syndesmosis play a pre-eminent role in the complicated biomechanics of the ankle joint [8,9,10,12].

Given the frequency of injuries about the ankle joint, physicians will continue to be confronted with poor therapeutic results despite appropriate case selection and the competent administration of operative or nonoperative treatment. It then becomes necessary to decide whether corrective surgery is needed to prevent late or permanent damage or improve secondary reactions and disability that have already occurred [5,6,11,14].

When we examine this question, we find that the early and late sequelae, i.e. the causes of deformity after previous conservative and operative treatment of fractures in or about the ankle, can be subdivided into five groups (Figs. 1–3):

1. Elongated fibula with varus tilting of the talus.
2. Shortened fibula with valgus tilting of the talus.
3. Supramalleolar distal tibial fractures with angular deformities (including compression fractures of the distal tibia).

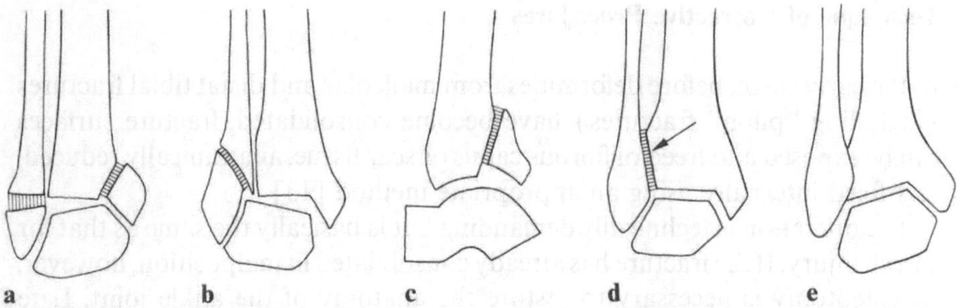

Fig. 1 a–e. Classification of characteristic deformities and posttraumatic changes about the ankle. **a** Elongated fibula with varus tilting of the talus. **b** Shortened fibula with valgus tilting of the talus. **c** Step in the joint surface. **d** Ossification of the tibiofibular syndesmosis. **e** Supramalleolar deformity of the ankle joint

Corrective Osteotomies of the Lower Extremity
Edited by G. Hierholzer, K. H. Müller

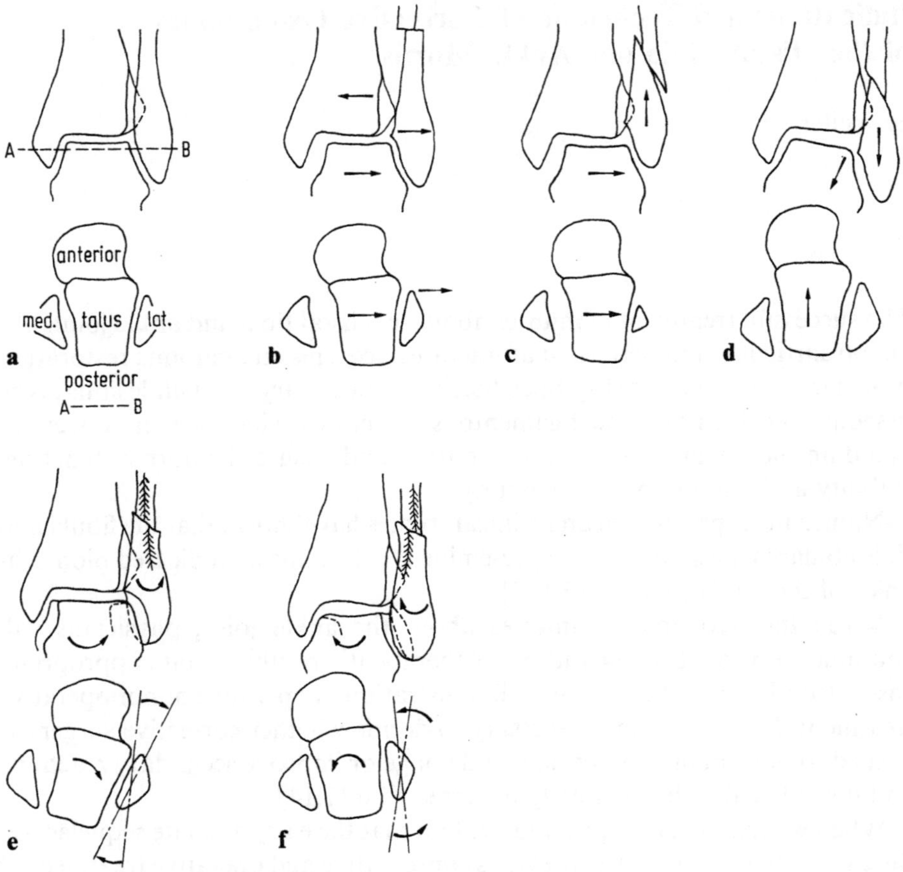

Fig. 2 a–f. Possible causes of subluxation of the talus

4. A step in the joint surface and inadequate reduction of anterior and posterior edge fragments.
5. Ossification of the tibiofibular syndesmosis and periarticular ossification of capsular and ligamentous tissues.

Technique of Corrective Procedures

In the early stage, before deformities from malleolar and distal tibial fractures (including "pilon" fractures) have become consolidated, fracture surfaces can be exposed and freed of fibrous callus or scar tissue, anatomically reduced, and fixed internally using an appropriate method [13].

The operation is technically demanding but is basically the same as that for a fresh injury. If the fracture has already consolidated in malposition, however, an osteotomy is necessary to restore the anatomy of the ankle joint. Late corrections of this type are very challenging technically, and their outcome is difficult to predict. They are a rational option only if the ankle joint is free of significant secondary osteoarthritis [2,5,6,8,14].

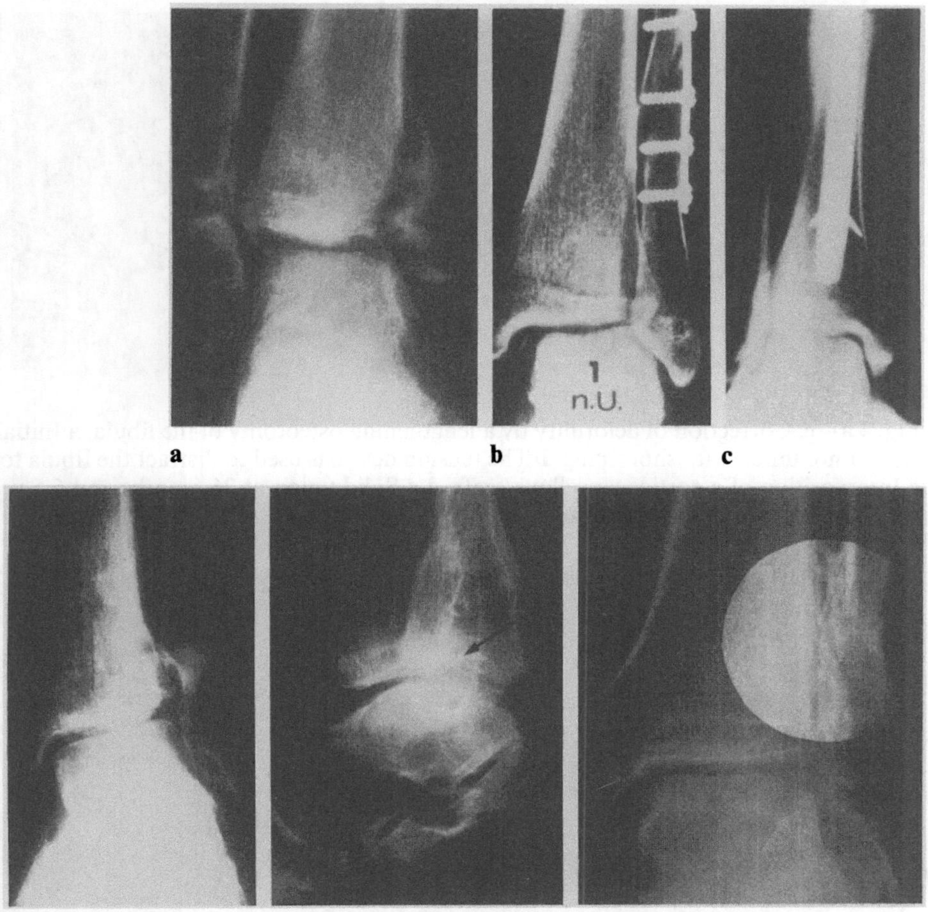

a b c

d e f

Fig. 3 a–f. Roentgenograms illustrating typical sequelae of trauma about the ankle. **a** Nonunion of the fibula with elongation (and nonunion of the medial malleolus) with varus tilting of the talus. **b** Internal fixation of the fibula with shortening, causing valgus tilting of the talus. **c** Malunited distal tibial fracture with secondary osteoarthritis from compensatory varus of the talus. **d** Fibular fracture that united with shortening, joint opening, and valgus deviation of the hindfoot with secondary osteoarthritis. **e** Formation of a step by a large posterior tibial fragment (Volkmann's triangle) that healed in a displaced position; secondary osteoarthritis. **f** Ossification of the tibiofibular syndesmosis

Experience has shown that certain fractures of the fibula have a tendency to unite with shortening and external rotation of the distal fragment [3]. This necessarily leads to deficiency of the ankle mortise, usually with some degree of subluxation of the talus. Not infrequently, a ruptured and incarcerated deltoid ligament or nonunion of the medial malleolus is encountered on the medial side (Figs. 4 and 5).

In these cases the first step is to clear the medial joint space or correct the deformity of the medial malleolus [2,14]. This is followed by reduction of the talus, which usually is "rotationally" subluxated. The next step is to restore the anatomic length and rotational alignment of the fibula by means of a

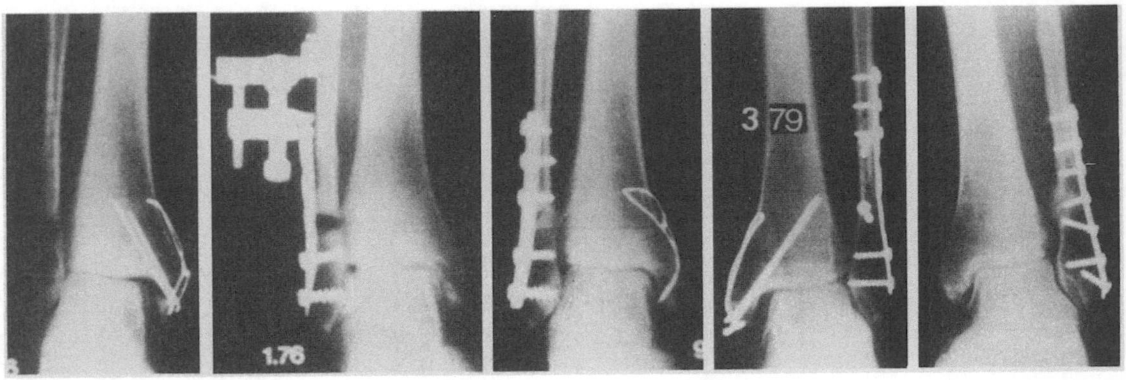

a b c d e

Fig. 4 a–e. Correction of deformity by a lengthening osteotomy of the fibula. **a** Initial roentgenogram of fibular nonunion with shortening. **b** The tension devise is used to distract the fibula to its original length. **c** Interposition of a corticocancellous graft. **d,e** Solid union at 26 months and 6.5 years after operation with no evidence of osteoarthritis

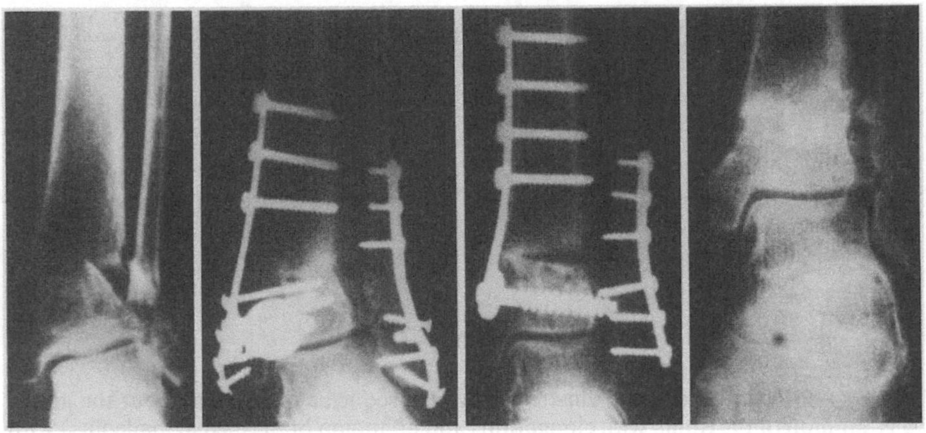

Fig. 5. Corrective osteotomy of a distal tibial deformity and the result at 3 years

suprasyndesmotic osteotomy. This is most easily and accurately accomplished by using the tension device in the distraction mode. It is impressive to observe how neatly the talus is returned to the ankle mortise, and the subluxation reduced, as the fibula is lengthened and internally rotated. The resultant defect in the fibula is bridged with a segment of autologous corticocancellous bone. The lateral malleolus is fixed with a semitubular or one-third tubular plate.

If the original deformity involves a supramalleolar valgus or varus angulation (greater than 10°!), it can be corrected by conventional osteotomy and plate osteosynthesis (Fig. 6). The open wedge type of osteotomy is recommended and often does not require additional buttressing.

At this point it must be stressed that every corrective or secondary operation on bone is more difficult than the primary treatment of a fresh injury, because the surgeon lacks many important landmarks provided by fracture surfaces and ligament stumps. For this reason, corrective procedures should be

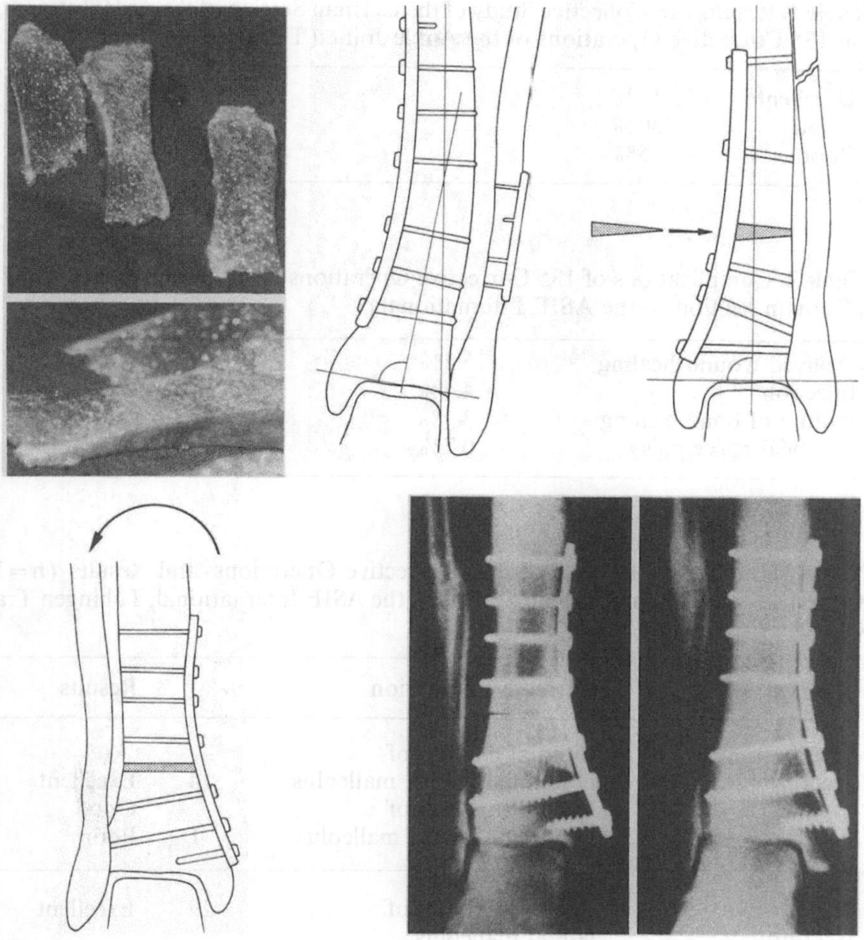

Fig. 6 a,b. Corrective osteotomy of a distal tibial fracture that united with angulation and malrotation. **a** Preoperative planning of an open wedge osteotomy with insertion of a corticocancellous wedge graft. **b** Correction of a malrotated distal tibial fracture; preoperative drawing, roentgenograms after surgery and after union of the osteotomy

performed by the most experienced surgeon available. They should not serve as a learning experience for beginners in the belief that the limb is already damaged and the corrective procedure has the status of a "patch-up" job.

If, after carefully weighing the factor of technical cost and tissue traumatization against the best result that can reasonably be expected, the surgeon elects to undertake a corrective procedure, he should make every effort to translate into reality that which is technically feasible.

Clinical Material

The capabilities and limitations of the corrective procedures are illustrated by two series of our own patients with follow-ups. The first series is from a 1977

Table 1. Results of a Collective Study of the German Section of the ASIF International on 135 Corrective Operations of the Ankle Joint (Tübingen Trauma Clinic)

Excellent	15%
Good	30%
Poor	55%

Table 2. Complications of 135 Corrective Operations of the Ankle Joint (German Section of the ASIF International)

Delayed wound healing	5.2%
Infection	4.4%
Failure of bone healing	3 %
Peroneal nerve palsy	0.7%

Table 3. Injuries of the Ankle Joint, Corrective Operations, and Results (n=135), Collective Study of the German Section of the ASIF International, Tübingen Trauma Clinic)

Injury	Corrective operation		Results	
Dislocation-fracture type A (n=15)	Internal fixation of nonunited medial malleolus	14	Excellent	6
			Good	5
	Internal fixation of nonunited lateral malleolus	1	Poor	4
Dislocation-fracture type B (n=44)	Internal fixation of lateral malleolus	29	Excellent	11
	Internal fixation of nonunited medial malleolus	20	Good	12
	Lengthening osteotomy of the fibula	5		
	Shortening of the fibula	1		
	Ligament plasty or repair	9	Poor	21
Dislocation-fracture type C (n=56)	Lengthening osteotomy of the fibula	35	Excellent	3
	Internal fixation of nonunited medial malleolus	31	Good	21
	Internal fixation of fibular nonunion	13		
	Ligament plasty or repair	23	Poor	32
Distal tibial compression fracture (tibial pilon) (n=20)	Supramalleolar corrections	15	Excellent	1
	Internal fixation of tibial nonunion	3	Good	3
	Internal fixation of fibular nonunion	2	Poor	16

retrospective study of the German Section of the ASIF International covering 135 corrective operations of the ankle performed between 1962 and 1974 [10,11] (Tables 1 and 2). Patients included in the study had had reconstructive surgery a minimum of 2 months after their injury and had presented for follow-up a minimum of 12 months after the operation. The results of this series are shown in Table 3.

A second series of 44 patients who had undergone supramalleolar corrective osteotomies at our Tübingen clinic between 1974 and 1980 for angular deformities secondary to fractures of the middle and distal (supramalleolar) thirds of the tibia were studied retrospectively between 4 months and 29 years after the traumatizing event [11].

Discussion

In both populations that were followed, very strict criteria were applied to the evaluation of late results. If preosteoarthritic changes or signs of early osteoarthritis were noted, the operation was classified as a failure even if improvement of subjective complaints, gait and ankle motion was apparent at follow-up. This stringent approach to evaluation was prompted by the experimental studies of Riede et al. [7], who found a high association between even very minor joint incongruities and secondary osteoarthritis.

In evaluating the late results of corrective operations of the ankle, we regard preosteoarthritic changes as a poor prognostic sign even if they are causing little or no interference with the patient's work or recreational activities at the time of the examination. We are more tolerant of small anatomic irregularities of the medial malleolus, because weight-bearing stresses and shock loads associated with walking and running are always directed onto the lateral malleolus, and the intact syndesmosis provides a highly effective shock-absorbing structure [12,13]. Thus, when treating bimalleolar fractures it is possible to dispense with an anatomic fixation of the medial malleolus if necessary, although a perfect reduction is required for the lateral malleolus [6]. Even if the medial malleolus is lost, the ankle joint will still have adequate function and stability if the distal fibula and syndesmosis are intact. This is not to say, of course, that lesions of the medial malleolus never require treatment. The incongruity caused by a deformity or nonunion of the medial malleolus can easily incite a locally painful degenerative arthritis. Moreover, normal tension and position of the deltoid ligament are desirable on mechanical grounds, because tension on this ligament during the first half of the stance phase is important in counteracting the valgus tendency of the ankle joint in that phase.

The special significance of the lateral malleolus in joint mechanics underscores the necessity of operative intervention to correct deformities or nonunions of that structure [2,5,6,11,14]. The good late results (52%!) after the operative stabilization of a nonunion of the lateral malleolus, which may coexist with nonunion of the medial malleolus, fully justify a reconstructive operation [11].

As one might expect, late corrections of malunited fibular fractures have less favorable outcomes. Shortening of the malunited fibula is a common occurrence and is often followed by valgus deviation of the talus, especially if there is a coexisting nonunion of the medial malleolus. Considering the severity of the preosteoarthritic deformity of the ankle joint, the good late results obtained in 43% of our cases after distal advancement of the lateral malleolus are particularly noteworthy.

Greater restraint is advised in operations on the syndesmosis. If the posterior syndesmosis is intact, simple distal advancement (lengthening) of the lateral malleolus is sufficient to correct mortise laxity. Only in the rare cases where the syndesmosis and interosseous membrane are completely deficient should the syndesmosis be reconstructed using a piece of peroneus tendon, skin or other tissue, at which time a temporary suprasyndesmotic retention screw is placed to aid healing of the graft. This operation is very often followed by ossification of the reconstructed syndesmosis with subsequent stiffness and degeneration, although the resulting complaints are fairly mild and are a relatively late occurrence.

It is not surprising that corrective procedures after tibial "pilon" fractures have by far the poorest late results, considering the unfavorable presenting situation of joint comminution and associated cartilage damage. Usually it is in the best interests of the patient to perform an early arthrodesis of the irreversibly damaged joint rather than attempt a reconstruction.

In patients with posttraumatic deformities (valgus, varus or torsion) of the distal supramalleolar region that are unaccompanied by significant disruption of the ankle joint (i.e., the distal articular surface of the tibia), it is usually possible to obtain good late and long-term results through early corrective osteotomy.

Summary

Based on a critical assessment of the results of follow-up examinations after corrective operations of the distal tibia and ankle, the following statements may be made with regard to the selection of patients for surgery:

1. Generally speaking, the prospect of a sucessful corrective operation declines with passage of time, patient age, and the complexity of the deformity. Hence, very strict criteria should be applied to the selection of patients for corrective surgery of the ankle joint.
2. The corrective procedure should be performed as early as possible; i.e., early corrections should be undertaken before the onset of osteodystrophy, and late corrections before secondary osteoarthritis appears. We feel that the ordeal and expense of a corrective operation should reward the patient with at least a decade of pain-free or essentially pain-free function.
   If no secondary osteoarthritic changes are visible in roentgenograms, a corrective operation should be attempted if at all possible, especially in younger individuals.

3. Many corrective procedures are technically challenging and should be reserved for centers that have the necessary experience and equipment. The corrective procedure is more than just a surgical task; it requires specialized supportive facilities with regard to physical therapy and the temporary or definitive fitting of orthopedic footwear and other orthopedic care measures.
4. Corrective surgery requires cooperation and understanding on the part of the patient. Without them, the best efforts of the physician may be in vain. A detailed talk with the patient prior to treatment can contribute greatly to a successful outcome.
5. The extent to which total arthroplasty of the ankle joint will provide a rational option for severe, irreversible joint damage remains unclear, because so far this treatment has not been used on a widespread basis [1]. Unfortunately we have no experience of our own to relate, and no long-term follow-ups of ankle arthroplasties are yet available in the literature.
   A sound arthrodesis of the ankle joint can provide a painless and reasonably normal gait, particularly when there is good compensatory motion in the subtalar joint. This fact is reassuring on the one hand, but on the other it can make the decision to attempt corrective surgery difficult, especially if the success of the surgery is in doubt.

References

1. Buchholz HW, Engelbrecht E, Siegel A (1973) Totale Sprunggelenksendoprothese, Modell "St. Georg". Chirurg 44:241
2. Lauge Hansen N (1948) Fractures of the ankle. Analytic-historic survey as the basis of new experimental, roentgenologic and clinical investigations. Arch Surg 56:259
3. Lauge Hansen N (1963) Knöchelbrüche und Bandverletzungen des Fußgelenks und des Fußes. Zentralbl Chir 15:545
4. Leitz G (1967) Korrekturoperationen bei in Fehlstellung verheilten Knöchelfrakturen. Hefte Unfallheilkd 92:137
5. Leitz G (1971) Die operative Korrektur veralteter Knöchelgabelsprengungen. Arch Orthop Unfallchir 70:36
6. Meeder PJ, Keller E, Weller S (im Druck) Die supramalleoläre Korrekturosteotomie – Indikation, Technik und Ergebnisse. Springer, Berlin Heidelberg New York Tokyo
7. Riede U, Willenegger H, Schenk R (1969) Experimenteller Beitrag zur Erklärung der sekundären Arthrose bei Frakturen des oberen Sprunggelenks. Helv Chir Acta 36:343
8. Weber BG (1966) Die operative Behandlung der Knöchelbrüche. Hefte Unfallheilkd 92:25
9. Weber BG (1966) Die Verletzungen des oberen Sprunggelenks. Huber, Bern Stuttgart Wien
10. Weller S, Lenapp U, Eck T (1977) Ergebnisse nach Korrektureingriffen am oberen Sprunggelenk (Sammelstudie der Deutschen Sektion der AO-International). Unfallheilkunde 80:213–219
11. Weller S, Knapp U (1981) Korrigierende Eingriffe am OSG. In: Arthrose und Instabilität am oberen Sprunggelenk. Hefte Unfallheilkd 133:57–63. Springer, Berlin Heidelberg New York

12. Willenegger H (1961) Die Behandlung der Luxationsfrakturen des oberen Sprunggelenks nach biomechanischen Gesichtspunkten. Helv Chir Acta 28:225
13. Willenegger H, Weber BG (1963) Malleolarfrakturen. Technik der operativen Frakturenbehandlung. Springer, Berlin Göttingen Heidelberg
14. Ziller R, Seyfarth H (1970) Erfahrungen bei der operativen Behandlung veralteter Verletzungen im Bereich des oberen Sprunggelenks. Zentralbl Chir 95:772

Statics and Dynamics of the Foot

E. H. Kuner and W. Schlickewei

The statics and dynamics of the foot have long been integral components of orthopedics, especially with regard to the diagnosis and treatment of congenital and acquired foot deformities. In trauma surgery, these issues must be considered when sequelae of trauma directly involve the foot. Similar issues are raised by posttraumatic changes occuring elsewhere in the lower extremity, such as alterations of the mechanical limb axis that produce an abnormal weight-bearing alignment. At this point we leave the field of biomechanics and enter the realm of pathomechanics, which, through an equally complex set of laws and mechanisms, disrupts the normal sequence of events that occur during stance and gait. Pathomechanics causes abnormal loads to be placed on one or more parts of the foot, leading to sometimes severe subjective complaints, abnormalities of gait, and disability. Objectively, the motion of certain joints of the foot is limited or abolished, and changes are apparent in the external shape of the foot and in the footprint. A change in the distribution of weight-bearing stresses leads to hyperkeratosis. During evaluation, attention should be given not so much to the thickness of the callosities, which is influenced by autonomic innervation, blood flow, metabolism and age, as to the pattern of their distribution. Sustained or chronic abnormal loads also produce obvious roentgenologic changes that permit areas of abnormal stress concentration to be identified.

For better understanding of trauma-related disturbances of foot statics and dynamics, we shall review some essential aspects of the biomechanics of the foot. The skeleton of the foot consists of many separate parts that are assembled into a functional unit. The general architecture of the foot is often compared to a vault, although it does not possess all the characteristics of a true architectural vault [6]. While certain bones of the foot do exhibit a wedge-like shape, the intrinsic weight of the bones and even the pressure of weight bearing does not wedge the bones together in a manner that causes them to bear loads more efficiently [5]. The strength of the plantar vault depends entirely on the individual tension-resistant connections that hold the pedal skeleton together. These connections, consisting of various tissues with different properties, form the basis of the static and dynamic loading of the foot. They ensure a smooth heel-to-toe rolling of the foot during evolution of the step and are capable of absorbing large peak stresses that accompany strenuous exertion.

Corrective Osteotomies of the Lower Extremity
Edited by G. Hierholzer, K. H. Müller

The footprint normally shows three main points of support [2]. These are:
- the heel,
- the head of the first metatarsal,
- the head of the fifth metatarsal.

These points of support are interconnected by three arches. The first in the *lateral arch*, extending from the base of the calcaneus to the head of the fifth metatarsal. The second is the *medial arch*, extending from the base of the calcaneus to the head of the first metatarsal. The third is the *transverse* or *anterior arch*, which extends from the head of the first metatarsal to the head of the fifth metatarsal. During weight bearing, the transverse arch is completely flattened so that all the metatarsal heads rest on the ground. The lateral arch also flattens completely during weight bearing. Even so, both of these arches are important functionally. This is demonstrated by quantitative measurements of the footprint, which show that the points of support listed above bear much greater loads than the other parts of the foot [9].

Functionally the foot may be divided into three parts:
- the subtalar plate (lamina pedis),
- the toes,
- the talus.

The subtalar plate contains all pedal bones except for the talus and phalanges [2]. It consists of a lateral and a medial part. The lateral part is formed by the fourth and fifth metatarsals anteriorly and the calcaneus posteriorly, with the cuboid interposed as a keystone. This lateral arch is made tense by the plantar aponeurosis and abductor digiti minimi muscle. The medial part of the subtalar plate is formed by the first through third metatarsals, the first through third cuneiforms, and the navicular. This bony bridge is held against the calcaneus by the powerful plantar calcaneonavicular ligament.

The height of the medial arch is determined mainly by the position of the calcaneus. When the calcaneus is in a position of valgus, the sustentaculum tali and thus the posterior buttress of the medial arch are lowered. In the extreme case the sole of the foot below the navicular touches the ground. Conversely, the sustentaculum tali and the navicular are raised farther from the ground when the calcaneus is rotated into varus; this is accompanied by an elevation of the medial arch. The bones of the foot are united by tight ligaments in a way that enables them to resist strong bending moments with a minimum expenditure of material and effort [6]. This comprehensive system of tension-resistant connections spans the plantar vault and prevents excessive splaying of its supports when weight is placed on the foot. Thus, short fibers span neighboring bones, more superficial fibers span a greater length, and the plantarmost fibers unite the more widely spaced supporting surfaces of the pedal skeleton.

The different elements of this osteofibrous chain have varying degrees of mobility. For example, the first metatarsal has a fairly large range of motion relative to the first cuneiform. Its range of plantar flexion/dorsal extension reaches 22°, compared with a range of only about 10° for the rest of the metatarsals [3]. The transverse connections between the metatarsals allow the anterior part of the subtalar plate to rotate about a longitudinal axis. This movement, known as supination or pronation of the forefoot, occurs mainly at Chopart's joint line. During pronation the fifth metatarsal is raised while the first metatarsal is simultaneously plantar flexed. The opposite movement, supination, produces dorsal extension of the first metatarsal and plantar flexion of the fifth metatarsal. On passive manipulation the average range of supination of the forefoot is 35°, and its range of pronation is 15°. The active range of motion is usually much less. The intrinsic mobility of the subtalar plate allows for an economical utilization of muscular activity. The ligaments are arranged in such a way that when the forefoot is supinated they are taut and thus hold the entire osseous system together. Pronation of the foot decreases tension on the ligaments, allowing the individual elements of the subtalar plate to move relative to one another to some degree. This means that supination is the only position in which the subtalar plate can form a rigid support for the body weight without the need for strong muscular intervention. When weight is placed on the pronated foot, muscular activity is necessary for stability [6].

The bony trabeculae, moreover, exhibit a pronounced trajectorial alignment as they traverse the bones of the foot [6].

Bipedal stance is an active process. An erect posture is controlled by the labyrinthine system and maintained through a process of continual adjustments involving a varying, alternating innervation of the muscles of posture and stance [2]. The position of the foot and leg are constantly regulated in such a way that a perpendicular dropped from the center of gravity passes approximately through the navicular bone [5] and thus slightly anterior to the axis of rotation of the ankle joint. Balance is maintained by the pull of the triceps surae acting on the tuber calcanei through the Achilles tendon, while the deep muscle layer at the calf provides for fine control. Interaction with the dorsal extensors of the foot is important in this process. The reflex control of muscular activity is accomplished through feedback from proprioceptors occurring in the muscles, tendons, joint capsules, and fasciae. These receptors respond to mechanical stimuli associated with the position and movements of the foot and lower extremity [2].

Debrunner [2] divides the weight-bearing phase of normal gait into four stages: contact of the heel with the ground, full contact of the sole with the ground, raising of the heel, and raising of the balls of the toes. These stages are accompanied by movements at the ankle joint, subtalar joint, and movements within the subtalar plate. Due to the association of inversion/eversion and pronation/supination, the subtalar plate is lax and compliant at the stage of heel contact, while during pushoff the subtalar plate and talus become immobile as a result of combined dorsal extension and inversion. This mechanism facilitates adaptation of the foot to uneven ground features when the heel is put down, and it aids in the transmission of propulsive forces during pushoff.

Debrunner [2] has measured the dynamic forces exerted on the Achilles tendon during strenuous activities such as jumping and skiing. Jumping on both feet exerts forces on each foot equal to about 1.3 times the body weight.

During running, pushoff exerts a force of approximately 170 kp on the ground, which corresponds to a tensile force of 230 kp on the Achilles tendon. Wittmann [10] measured the loads on the balls of the feet during skiing and found that this force seldom exceeds 130 kp during skiing on bumpy terrain. A pressure of 130 kp on the ball of the foot is equivalent to a tensile force of 176 kp on the Achilles tendon and a load of 360 kp on the ankle joint. During ordinary athletic activities, central nervous mechanisms operate to ensure that the Achilles tendon is not stressed to the point of rupture. However, in competitive athletics the loads may closely approach the tolerance limit, and the extra forces caused by a fall forward with the heel stationary may be sufficient to rupture the tendon [10].

Pedal statics and dynamics can be disturbed by direct or indirect trauma to the foot, tibia, or femur. For example, a tibial fracture that has united with rotational deformity can upset the fine balance of pressure and tension in the foot in such a way that irreversible changes develop over time. Generally speaking, internal malrotation of the tibia or excessive anteversion of the femoral neck decreases the curvature of the medial arch, resulting in pes planus. It would be pointless to treat the flatfoot in this case without also correcting the causative deformity [8].

With regard to direct pedal trauma, the most critical injuries are those involving the talus, calcaneus, and the first and fifth metatarsals, for these are the elements that receive and transmit forces. The multiple articular surfaces and vulnerable blood supply of the talus make that bone a central problem in the foot-injured patient. In the calcaneus, Vidal type II and III fractures can greatly restrict the motion of the subtalar plate and thus alter a key component of pedal statics and dynamics. Traumatic shortening of the first ray, as in a malunited fracture of the first metatarsal, causes a recession of the anterior buttress of the medial arch and thus places greater loads on the heads of the second and third metatarsals. Also, plantar displacements and angulations of the metatarsal heads lead to flattening of the transverse arch, usually accompanied by severe pain and the formation of callosities at unphysiologic sites. This example demonstrates the fundamental importance of normal anatomy to function, and that an alteration of even one component disturb the entire system. Besides bony injuries, pedal function is also subject to disturbance by lesions of soft structures (unstable ligament sprains, tendon injuries) and Sudeck's dystrophy.

Amputations also change the statics of the foot [7]. This effect is not so pronounced with amputations at the forefoot (e.g., toe amputations) as at the metatarsus. For example, an amputation at the line of Lisfranc interrupts the medial arch at its summit.This leads to a predominance of the action of the triceps muscles, producing an equinovarus deformity [1]. This is even more pronounced with an amputation at Chopart's line. For these reasons it is recommended that an arthrodesis of the ankle joint also be performed in the same operation.

Given the peculiar biomechanics of the foot, every attempt should be made during primary treatment to restore anatomic integrity, especially of the talus and the first and fifth metatarsals, so that loads can be received and distributed to the normal points of support. With the calcaneus fracture no method is yet available for effecting a complete anatomic restoration, and so the main goal is to preserve the posterior point of support and the central site where the force of the body weight is applied.

All treatments aimed at alleviating posttraumatic conditions should be guided by biomechanical and pathomechanical principles. The main concern is to protect the area of injury from excessive loads by conservative or operative means (corrective osteotomy, arthrodesis, etc.) and create compensatory capabilities for a reasonably normal pattern of movement.

References

1. Baumgartner R (1972) Die orthopädietechnische Versorgung des Fußes. Thieme, Stuttgart
2. Debrunner HU (1974) Biomechanik und Orthopädie. Orthopäde 3:102
3. Fick R (1904) Handbuch der Anatomie und Mechanik der Gelenke, Bd3, Fischer, Jena
4. Helfet A, Lee D (1980) Disorders of the foot. Lippincott, Philadelphia
5. Kummer G (1961) Torsionsprobleme der unteren Extremität. 49. Kongreß. Verh Dtsch Orthop Ges S.115
6. Lanz T v, Wachsmuth W (1972) Praktische Anatomie, Bd I/4. Springer, Berlin Heidelberg New York
7. Matthiaß HH, Berndt S (1965) Fußbefunde bei Beinamputierten. Arch Orthop Unfallchir 58:341
8. Nicod L (1972) Zur Ätiologie des Knickplattfußes. In: Baumgartner R (Hrsg) Die orthopädietechnische Versorgung des Fußes. Thieme, Stuttgart
9. Scholder P (1972) Funktionelle Anatomie und Biomechnik des Fußes. In: Baumgartner R (Hrsg) Die orthopädietechnische Versorgung des Fußes. Thieme, Stuttgart
10. Wittmann G (1973) Biomechanische Untersuchung zum Verletzungsschutz im alpinen Skisport. Inaugural – Diss., Techn. Universität München

Corrective Osteotomies of the Foot

J. Probst

Of the 50,322 compensatable first injuries treated at clinics serving the German commercial trade associations between 1976 and 1979, 6128 were injuries of the foot, and 405 of these involved the ankle joint. The calcaneus was involved in 2012 cases. Injuries of the trasus, metatarsus and phalanges were present in 2750 cases (5.46%, or 9.46% including calcaneal injuries). Injuries of the tibial shaft (2135=4.24%) and distal tibia including the malleolar region (3514=6.98%), which totaled 5649 cases in this series (11.22%), invariably have effects on the foot as a result of shortening, angulation, malrotation, atrophy, dystrophy, dysfunction or infection, but these effects cannot be dealt with in statistical terms. It is noteworthy that direct (6168) and possible indirect (5649) sequelae of foot injuries together (11,817=23.48%) total less than the number of direct hand injuries. The hand, including the distal, articular ends of the radius and ulna, was involved in 12,975 injuries. The tremendous number of corrective operations performed on the hand contrasts with the very few performed on the foot. At our Murnau Clinic we performed only 9 corrective osteotomies of the foot after trauma during the 5-year period from 1978 to 1982. By comparison, 1571 patients were treated with orthopedic (nonprosthetic) footwear for a variety of indications during the period from 1977 to 1981 (1982 not yet evaluated).

The number of possible osteotomies of the foot between the tarsus and phalanges is very great. We owe their development to classical orthopedics [3,5]. Most corrective osteotomies of the foot were conceived and tested for congenital foot deformities or deformities acquired during the growth period.

N=50,322	N	%	
Talus	138	0.27	
Calcaneus	2012	4.00	5.04
Tarsus	386	0.77	
Metatarsus	1417	2.81	
Phalanges	385	0.77	4.42
Other	425	0.84	
	4763	9.46	

Fig. 1. Statistical overview of the injuries about the foot and ankle which were compensated for the first time by the German mutualities, 1976–1979, average per annum

Corrective Osteotomies of the Lower Extremity
Edited by G. Hierholzer, K. H. Müller

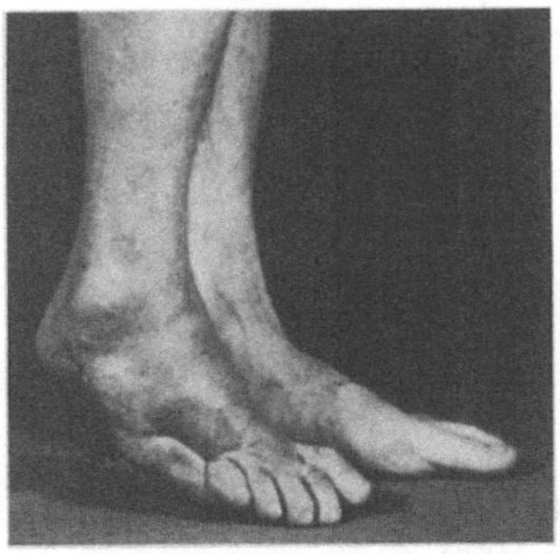

Fig. 2. Rigid equinus deformity of the right foot accompanied by scar contractures of the forefoot and metatarsal region. Typical result of tarsal and metatarsal injury with secondary healing, dystrophy, and dysfunction. Orthopedic footwear restored a useful gait

The chief purpose of these osteotomies is to correct disturbances of gait secondary to deformities of the foot or more proximal parts of the extremity as well as dysfunctions, especially when referrable to paralysis [7].

Orthopedic deformities tend to have certain features in common: As a rule, the foot has not been previously operated; there is no significant abnormality of the skin, the epi- and subfascial spaces and layers, or of the structural connections between the soft tissues, joints and bones; there is good function of the vascular and neurotrophic systems; and the extremity, while disabled to some degree, is still being used by the patient.

A quite different situation exists in cases of posttraumatic deformity, for which the corrective osteotomy is designed (Fig. 3):

Key morphologic and functional elements are damaged or destroyed. Generally there is considerable dystrophy or atrophy of skeletal tissues, and the joint motion necessary for a complete functional recovery is irrevocably lost. The gliding surfaces and sheaths for muscles and tendons, annular ligaments and fulcra are obliterated, and their mobility is hampered by cicatrization and contraction of surrounding soft structures. The quantity and quality of blood flow are diminished, and the capacity for functional adaptation is compromised or lost. In contrast to foot deformities that are congenital or acquired in the growth period, the posttraumatically deformed foot probably has been in a state of disuse for weeks or months. As a result, the

Orthopedic deformity	**Posttraumatic deformity**
Undamaged, accustomed to function	Damaged, disaccustomed to function
Skin, subcutaneous tissue	Skin, subcutaneous tissue = scarred
Fascia, structures	Fascia, structures = scarred
Tendon sheaths	Tendon sheaths = obliterated
Muscles	Muscles = dystrophic
Joints, ligaments	Joints, ligaments = obliterated
Bone	Bone = dystrophic, atrophic
Blood vessels, nerves	Blood vessels = obliterated
	Nerves = ?
Good healing potential	Poor healing potential

Fig. 3. Contrast between the presenting characteristics of orthopedic and posttraumatic deformities

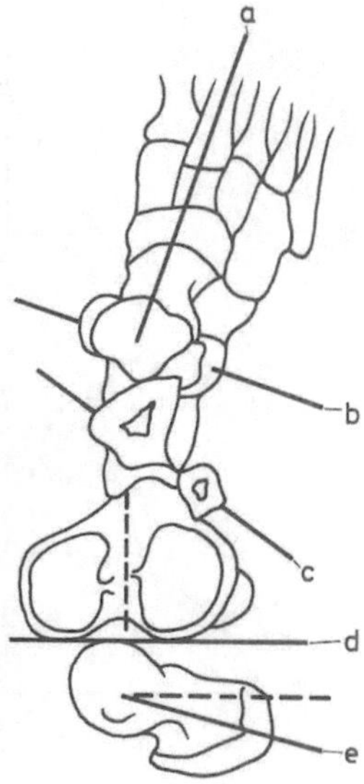

Fig. 4. Torsional diagram of the leg and foot: metatarsus and tarsus (a), plane of ankle joint (b), tibia and fibula (c), femur (d), femoral neck (e)

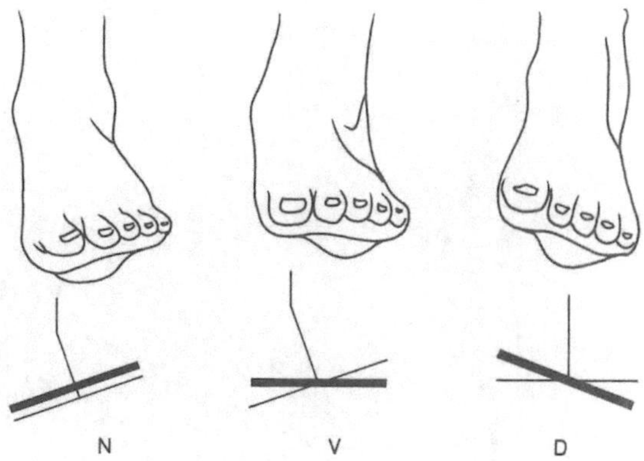

Fig. 5. Loads applied to the foot are balanced by the interaction of the metatarsus and forefoot with the hindfoot: N = Normal foot in pronated position. V = With valgus deformity loads are balanced by pronation of the hindfoot. D = Derotation of the metatarsus and forefoot with compensated valgus (after G. Brandt)

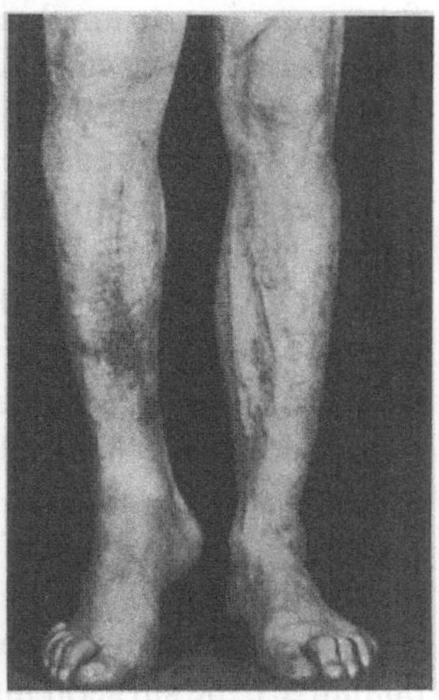

Fig. 6. Functionally uncompensated equinus deformity of the right foot. Note the elevation of the right knee and clawing of the toes. Operative treatment or a corrective shoe is indicated

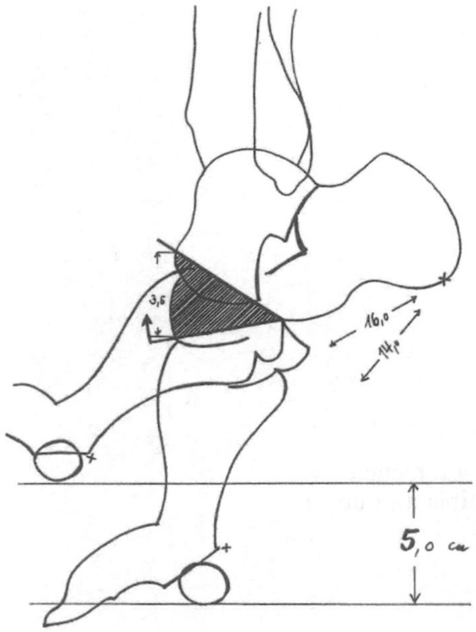

Fig. 7. Compensation of equinus-related limb lengthening by an osteotomy of the tarsal region, e.g., at the talo-calcaneo-naviculo-cuboid articulation. A wedge resection in this region is very effective in equalizing limb lengths and is also favorable functionally because it spares the ankle joint and the joints of the forefoot (original drawing)

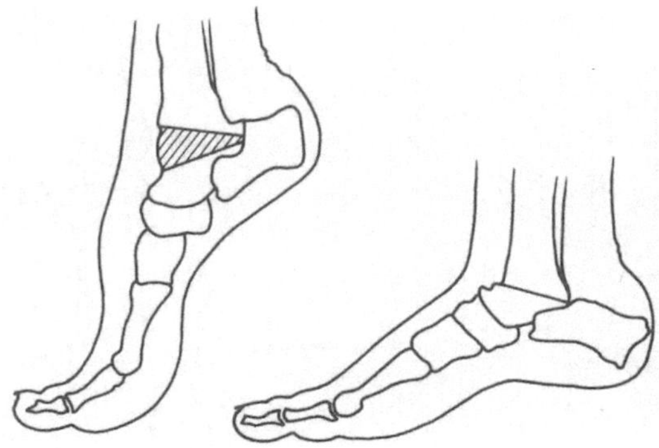

Fig. 8. Elimination of equinus deformity by resection arthrodesis of the ankle joint. Owing to the shortness of the lever arm there is relatively little motion on the posterior side of the joint, and so an Achilles tenotomy is usually unnecessary

foot loses important load-bearing elements in the skin, connecting layers, articular cartilage (if present) and skeleton and is no longer able to bear the body weight [4].

Given these fundamentally contrasting situations, we find that many orthopedic osteotomies designed to improve the function of foot are no longer appropriate because of tissue deficiencies or an excessive risk of healing difficulties. Procedures that are widely used in orthopedics because of their proven efficacy are not always applicable to traumatology. In some cases they will appear questionable from the outset or even futile and thus will be contraindicated. While classical orthopedics emphasizes the primacy of form as the basis of function, traumatology must adopt a somewhat different approach, for the goal of functional recovery often must rely on "abnormal" forms that can be modified only to a limited degree.

Thus, in selecting patients for corrective osteotomy between the tarsus and phalanges, the surgeon must look beyond the proposed alteration of form and

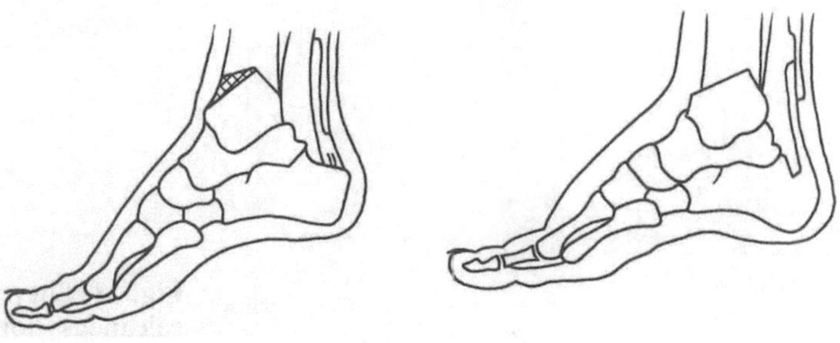

Fig. 9. Repositioning osteotomy of Max Lange. Advantage: The osteotomy is done above the malleoli and therefore spares the ankle joint. Disadvantage: The long lever arm places considerable tension on the Achilles tendon and may necessitate a tenotomy

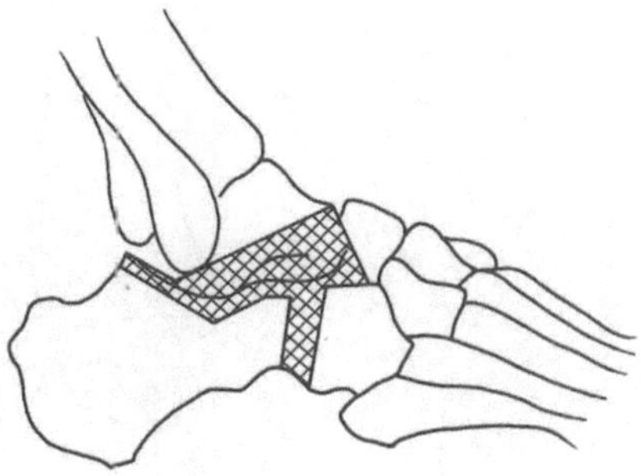

Fig. 10. Arthrodetic resection of Lambrinudi. The wedge-shaped resection is open anteriorly to allow for correction of equinus deformity

determine whether the operation will create the morphologic and functional conditions necessary to restore or significantly improve the usefulness of the foot, or whether morphologic conditions can be directly or indirectly created that will contribute to the enhancement of function [1].

An important consideration is the anticipated functional capacity of the involved limb. That is, the indication for surgery is not localized to the area between the talus and phalanges, but must include the entire leg or even both legs and the pelvis. Thus, besides an evaluation of conditions intrinsic to the foot, the corrective osteotomy requires a functional analysis of the extremity as a whole [2]. At this point it will be helpful to review briefly the static, mechanical, and functional relationships of the foot and leg:

The application of the body weight to the foot is mediated by the muscular tension of the limb and by the anatomic torsion of the limb segments. A stable stance on the pronated foot is made possible by supination at the hindfoot, supplemented medially by support on the ball of the great toe as an extension of the medial ray. Just as acquired foot deformities have effects on the remainder of the extremity, causing damage to the proximal joints and muscles, traumatic lesions of the femur, tibia, hip and knee produce static changes in the foot in the form of angulation and torsion. Deformities of the foot that are associated with changes in the relative positions of the forefoot and hindfoot lead to abnormalities of position and movement. Supination deformity of the foot causes external rotation of the talus and ankle joint, while pronation deformity has the opposite effect, i.e., internal rotation of the talus and ankle [1].

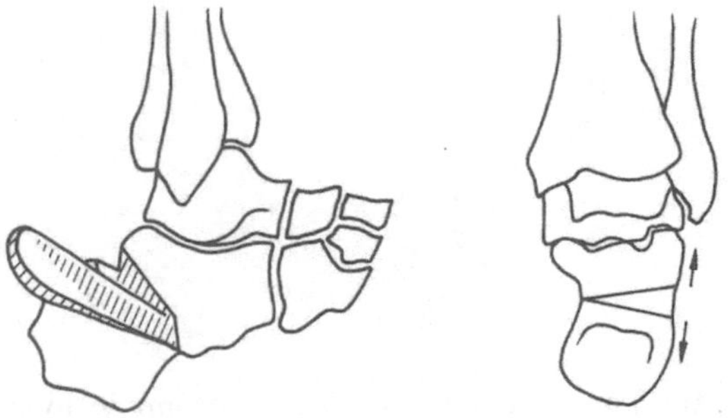

Fig. 11. Dwyer osteotomy of the calcaneus for varus deformity (after Morscher)

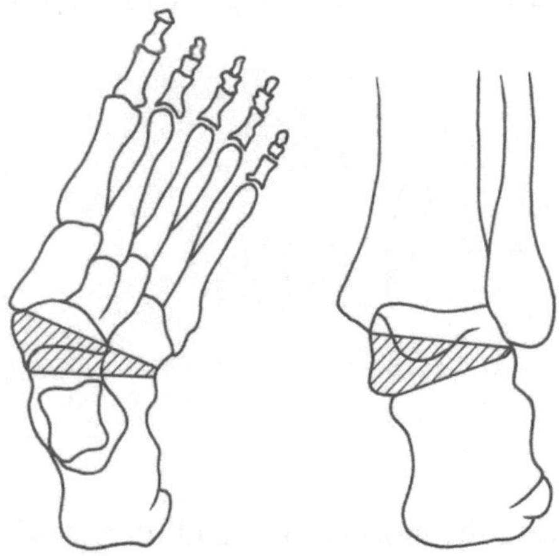

Fig. 12. Osteotomy for valgus deformity. A spherical resection is made to correct both abduction and valgus angulation

These associations, which are relatively easy to appreciate in classical orthopedics, are more difficult to demonstrate in traumatology on account of the underlying injury, even in cases where tibial trauma gives rise to a very conspicuous foot deformity [2]. It would be too simplistic to regard indirect foot deformities purely as local phenomena. Conversely, primary traumatic deformities of the foot cannot be considered in isolation from the tibia and the knee.

These relationships underlie the frequent secondary involvement of the foot in more proximal injuries.

But if the number of corrective operations on the foot (excluding arthrodeses, which usually are done for direct trauma) is relatively small, this is mainly because secondary posttraumatic foot deformities occur in the presence of severe primary tibial and femoral injuries, and they fail to satisfy the above-mentioned requirements for surgical correction or else pose an unacceptable surgical risk. At the same time, a great many of these deformities can be managed conservatively with external orthopedic aids.

A typical example of a purely functional, secondary deformity of the foot is the equinus deformity. Prolonged immobilization, inadequate physical therapy, and patient errors can lead to the development of a fixed equinus deformity (in contrast to the mobile, paralytic form). Because the onset of this deformity is often insidious, tarsal and metatarsal joints may already be

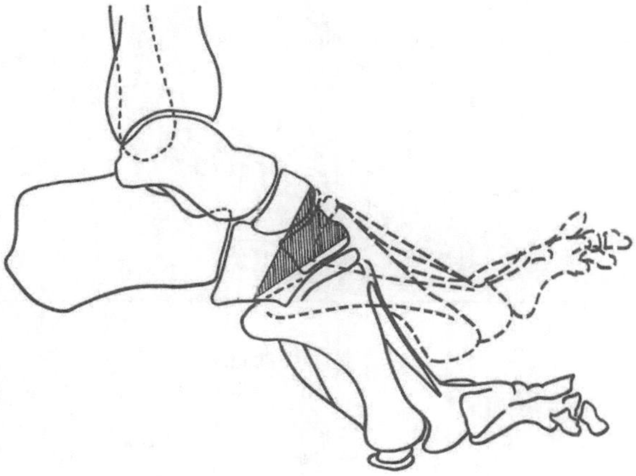

Fig. 13. Resection osteotomy at Lisfranc's joint line, a frequent site of involvement in comminuted fractures (original preoperative drawing)

obliterated when corrective osteotomy is elected, so that the foot presents as a more or less rigid structure. If residual motion exists in the ankle joint, it is usually painful and necessitates an arthrodesis of that joint, which can be utilized to correct the equinus deformity.

The most important step in patient selection is to determine whether the deformity is accompanied by limb shortening – for the equinus deformity is an excellent biological means of compensating for a short limb. In making this determination, it is necessary to test the behavior of the Achilles tendon. If this tendon is contracted or otherwise shortened, it must be lengthened and the foot deformity corrected by a sustained program of physical therapy, possibly combined with supportive orthopedic footwear.

If the limb is too long, as in paralytic equinus deformity, a wedge resection is indicated. The site of the osteotomy should be that which is most favorable from the standpoint of the soft-tissue envelope, i.e., the site where the surgery will pose the smallest risk. Always, care is taken to avoid any lateral tilting of the foot that would have to be corrected by a high-risk secondary operation. Care also is taken to avoid excessive positive or negative torsion, as this will probably also require a second operation, being difficult to correct with a shoe.

In suitable cases the osteotomy is performed not in the foot but in the supramalleolar region of the tibia, as suggested by Lange [5]. This option is always preferred when the tarsal joints are still mobile and functional.

The procedure of Lambrinudi, which involves a resection arthrodesis of the calcaneocuboid joint, is especially appropriate for cases where there is pronounced angulation of the metatarsus and forefoot. One difference between resection arthrodesis and corrective osteotomy is that the former often can create more favorable spatial relationships through the removal of bone. In this respect resection arthrodeses are usually more advantageous and are suitable for a wider range of indications.

Fractures of the proximal tarsus require corrective surgery either primarily as a result of joint comminution or secondarily as a result of abnormal statics with associated changes in the components of the ankle joint. Usually this surgery takes the form of an arthrodesis.

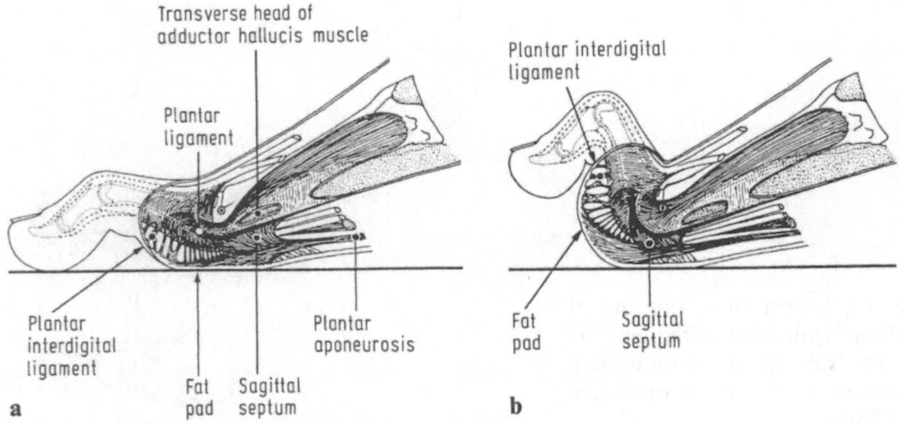

Fig. 14 a, b. The submetatarsal pad and its behavior in hammertoe deformity: **a** Transverse, longitudinal and vertical ligamentous fibers form a resilient pad below and proximal to the metatarsal head. The tendons of the interossei insert on the plantar side anterior to the axis of the metatarsophalangeal joint (circled black dots). **b** In hammertoe deformity the pad is displaced over the metatarsal head while the sagittal septa are drawn beneath it. The tendons of the interossei are displaced dorsally and cross the axis of the metatarsophalangeal joints (0), thereby losing their function as plantar flexors. (From F. Bojsen-Møller, "Normal and pathologic anatomy of the forefoot," *Orthopäde 11* (1982(, 148–153)

The Dwyer valgus osteotomy of the calcaneus is excellent for correcting lateral ligament laxity caused by varus deformity. A simple tightening operation would allow recurrent stretching of the ligaments with each step. Preservation of the ligaments requires correction of the causative deformity. The calcanean osteotomy also improves steadiness of gait and eliminates "wobbling." This elegant procedure, which originally was designed for the treatment of pes cavus, is rational only if satisfactory long-term function of the posterior talocalcanean joint is anticipated. Besides steadying the gait, the osteotomy also removes abnormal stresses from the talocalcanean joint.

Operations on the distal tarsus are limited to resections, most commonly in the form of arthrodeses involving the navicular bone. In some cases a posttraumatic adduction or abduction deformity of the foot may require a corrective wedge resection of the lateral or medial side. Because the plantar vault generally is already destroyed, its integrity need not be considered. The usual intent of this operation is to improve heel-to-toe rolling of the foot during gait while an orthopedic shoe is worn.

Quite common and severe foot deformities are associated with comminuted fracture-dislocations at the Lisfranc joint line [9]. A true reconstruction is possible only in fresh injuries, and some deformity or disability usually remains. In most cases osteotomy is unable to provide dramatic improvement of function, and so its main purpose is to facilitate treatment with an orthopedic shoe.

Abnormal stresses secondary to deformities of the middle tarsal heads can be relieved by the operation of enclavement [8].

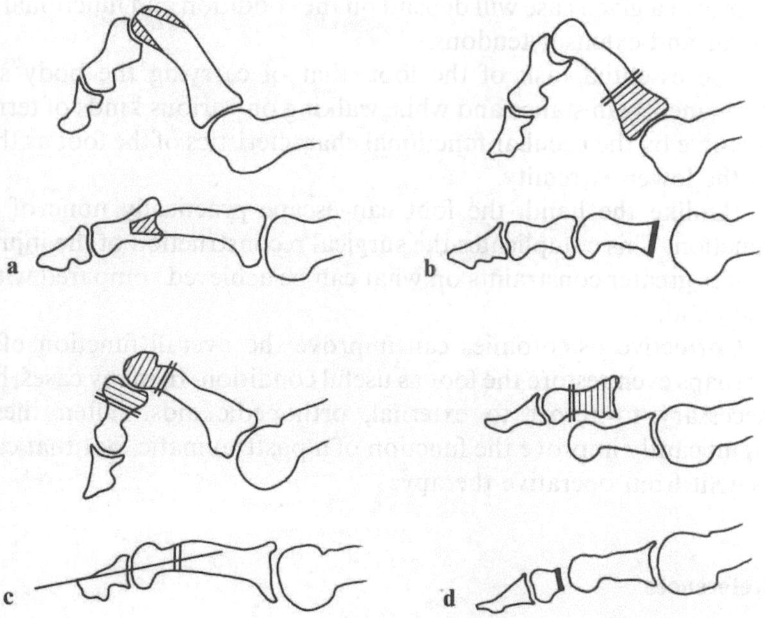

Fig. 15 a–d. Resection osteotomies of the phalanges: **a** Young arthrodesis of the proximal interphalangeal joint. **b** Gocht resection of the metatarsophalangeal joint. **c** Campbell resection of the proximal interphalangeal joint. **d** Hohmann resection of the base of the middle phalanx for dislocation of the proximal interphalangeal joint

Often too little attention is given to the significance of the toes and their deformities. The preservation of their form and function is a major concern during the treatment of other injuries of the leg and foot. If deformities occur, such as hammertoes and claw toes, it must be understood that they not only hamper the evolution and pushoff of the step but also weaken the important point of pedal support at the junction of the metatarsals and phalanges.

In hammertoe deformity the tissue pad below the metatarsal head, consisting of a functionally adapted fibrous structure, becomes displaced dorsally as the proximal phalanx slides over the dorsal aspect of the metatarsal head. As a result, the sagittal septum, which is not competent to withstand loads, is moved below the metatarsal head, which now closely underlies the skin on the plantar surface of the foot. In this condition the forefoot is unable to bear weight.

This situation justifies a phalangeal osteotomy, particularly when one considers the rapid obliteration and stiffening of the involved joints that occur once the lateral extensor fibers become permanently active as flexors. The resulting contracture of the forefoot and metatarsus, the disturbance of gait and weight bearing, and the alteration of the soft-tissue envelope complete the picture.

The resection osteotomies of Gocht, Hohmann, Campbell, and Young [3,5] are available for the treatment of hammertoe deformity. Hammertoe with dislocation is corrected by the procedure of Imhäuser [3,5]. The procedure of choice in a given case will depend on the condition and functional status of the flexor and extensor tendons.

The essential task of the foot, that of carrying the body securely and permanently in stance and while walking on various kinds of terrain, is made possible by the peculiar functional characteristics of the foot as the end organ of the lower extremity.

Unlike the hand, the foot can escape practically none of its intended function. This complicates the surgical reconstruction of the injured foot and places greater constraints on what can be achieved compared with surgery of the hand.

Corrective osteotomies can improve the overall function of the foot or perhaps even restore the foot as useful condition. In many cases, however, it is necessary to resort to external, orthopedic aids. Often these aids will significantly improve the function of a posttraumatic foot that can no longer benefit from operative therapy.

References

1. Bojsen-Møller F (1982) Normale und pathologische Anatomie des Vorfußes. Orthopäde 11:148–153
2. Brandt G (1959) Eingriffe an den Extremitäten. In: Breitner B, Zukschwerdt L, Kraus H (Hrsg) Chirurgische Operationslehre. Bd IV/2. Urban & Schwarzenberg, München
3. Hackenbroch M, Witt AN (1973) Orthopädisch-chirurgischer Operationsatlas Bd V. Thieme, Stuttgart
4. Hüsing U (1978) Der posttraumatische Knicksenkfuß. Orthop Prax 14:926–929
5. Lange M (1962) Orthopädisch-Chirurgische Operationslehre 2. Aufl. Bergmann, München
6. Morscher E, Baumann JU, Hefti F (1981) Die Kalkaneus-Osteotomie nach Dwyer, kombiniert mit lateraler Bandplastik bei rezidivierender Distorsio pedis. Z Unfallmed Berufskr 74:85–90
7. Rabl CRH, Nyga W (1982) Orthopädie des Fußes, 6. Aufl. Enke, Stuttgart
8. Regnauld B (1982) Das diaphyso-epiphysäre Enclavement der Metatarsalia. Orthopäde 11:191–199
9. Steinhäuser J (1975) Luxationsfrakturen im Lisfranc-Gelenk und ihre Behandlung. Z Orthop 113:720–722

Results of Corrective Osteotomies of Posttraumatic Deformities about the Ankle Joint

H. Conradi and U. Gras

Introduction

Posttraumatic deformity of the ankle is the product of failed conservative or operative efforts to restore normal axial and articular relationships after osseous and ligamentous injuries in the region of the ankle joint [2,3].

The result of the deformity is an abnormal biomechanical situation which, depending on severity, can lead to osteoarthritis and painful limitation of motion.

The goal of corrective surgery in such cases is to restore function and weight-bearing ability by accurate reconstruction of axial and articular relationships before symptoms of posttraumatic osteoarthritis become manifest [2,3,7,8,11]. Compared with the treatment of fresh injuries, corrective procedures are more demanding in their planning and conduct and less certain in their outcomes [4,5]. Success depends on such factors as age, severity of primary joint damage, duration of residual preosteoarthritic deformity, and the accuracy of the reconstruction [6,13,14,15].

In our follow-up of 65 corrective operations about the ankle joint, we sought to determine whether a close correlation exists between the foregoing criteria and the result of the operation, or whether the result is significantly influenced by additional, uncontrollable subjective and biological factors [2,14]. Three approaches were used in evaluating the results:

1. An "objective" approach (using the Weber point system) in which results are scored according to complaints, walking ability, function, and level of occupational and recreational activity, with special allowance for roentgenologic findings [12].
2. Clinical function and complaints [2,3].
3. Subjective evaluation.

A point system was used to rate the results as "excellent," "good" or "poor." A fourth rating, "fair" was added to the subjective evaluation to obtain a better differentiation [2,3].

A late result was rated as excellent (score of 0) if the patient was free of complaints, had a normal gait, could engage in usual occupational and recreational activities, had free motion in the ankle and subtalar joints, and had an anatomically reconstructed ankle that showed no roentgenographic signs of osteoarthritis.

A "good" result was one in which follow-up showed an improvement of complaints and function after corrective surgery, and roentgenograms showed no evidence of osteoarthritis. The scores for these cases ranged between 1 and

Corrective Osteotomies of the Lower Extremity
Edited by G. Hierholzer, K. H. Müller

5. If the score exceeded 5 points, the result was rated as poor. These cases were characterized by severe complaints with impairment of gait and significant losses of function at the ankle. Degenerative changes were apparent in roentgenograms.

Technique and Tactics of the Corrective Procedures

The surgical correction of deformities of the lateral and medial malleoli relied on proven, standarized procedures. The indication for a supramalleolar osteotomy was more than 10 degrees' angular deformity of the limb axis relative to the plane of the ankle joint. The deformity, which resulted from the inadequate treatment of a distal-third or pilon tibial fracture, was corrected either by a simple wedge resection or by an open wedge osteotomy with insertion of a corticocancellous graft. The osteotomy was fixed by plate of osteosynthesis or with an external frame if soft-tissue conditions or a previous infection prohibited internal fixation. Generally the tibia was osteotomized at the level of the vertex of the correction angle. Some deformities necessitated simultaneous corrections in multiple planes. The procedure followed in reconstructing the distal articular surface of the tibia was guided by the presenting situation. The object was to obtain a congruent joint with normal axial relationships [11].

Clinical Material

Our clinical population consists of 65 patients (42 men and 23 women) who presented for follow-up examinations after corrective surgery about the ankle. Sixty-six patients were treated at the Bergmannsheil Bochum Clinics between 1974 and 1981. Fifty-one patients from this series were followed, in addition to 14 others treated at the Duisburg-Buchholz Clinic between 1977 and 1981. Sixty of these patients had been referred from abroad. Primary treatment had been conservative in 30 cases and operative in 35. We limited our review to reconstructive procedures that were done 2 months or more (maximum of 24 years) after the original injury. The interval between corrective surgery and follow-up was at least 1 year (maximum of 9 years).

The original injuries were distributed by type as follows:
32 Fracture-dislocations (11 type B, 21 type C)
11 Compression fractures
22 Distal tibial fractures.

Type B and C fracture-dislocations: The most frequent operation was a lengthening osteotomy of the fibula, combined in four cases with the internal fixation of a nonunited medial malleolus (Tables 1 and 2).

In almost all cases the medial malleolar region had to be explored and scar tissue removed from the joint before the dislocated talus could be reduced. Then the fibula was osteotomized at the level of the malunited fracture and distracted until a normal articulation of the ankle joint was obtained. The

Table 1. Results of the Primary Treatment of 32 Fracture-Dislocations

Nonunion of lateral malleolus	5
Shortening of lateral malleolus	18
Valgus deformity of lateral malleolus	3
Varus deformity of lateral malleolus	4
Nonunion of medial malleolus	9
Disruption of ankle mortise	11
Tibial edge fragment with step in joint surface	5

Table 2. Corrective Operations of the Ankle Joint Performed in 32 Patients

Internal fixation of a nonunion of the medial malleolus	9
Internal fixation of a nonunion of the lateral malleolus	5
Lengthening osteotomy of the fibula	26
Shortening osteotomy of the fibula	–
Supramalleolar corrective osteotomy	2
Ligament reconstruction or repair	11

Table 3. Site of Corrective Operation for 32 Type B and C Fracture-Dislocations

Correction of a nonunion	5
Osteotomy at the fracture site	19
Osteotomy above the fracture site	2
Osteotomy below the fracture site	1
Supramalleolar corrective osteotomy	2
Osteotomy not required	3

defect in the fibula was bridged with a corticocancellous graft and fixed with a one-third tubular plate or, rarely, a semitubular plate. With a coexisting rupture of the anterior syndesmosis and deficiency of the interosseous membrane, we inserted a temporary suprasyndesmotic retention screw (Table 3).

In 9 cases there was also a posterolateral or posteromedial tibial edge fragment that involved more than 1/3 of the articular surface and created a step-like incongruity.

The joint incongruity was not corrected in any of these cases. A supramalleolar correction was necessary in two adolescents.

The average age of the surgical patients was 37 years, with a range from 12 to 75 years. The mean interval from injury to corrective surgery was 12 months (2 months to 7 years). The mean interval between surgery and follow-up was 3 years (1 year to 9 years) (Fig. 1).

Of the 32 corrective osteotomies performed after fracturedislocations of the ankle, only 1 was given an excellent objective rating. Ten were rated as good, and 21 were rated as poor. Based solely on function and severity of complaints, 17 cases were rated as good and "only" 14 as poor.

When subjective evaluations were elicited, 21 patients rated the result as good, 8 as fair, and only 3 as poor.

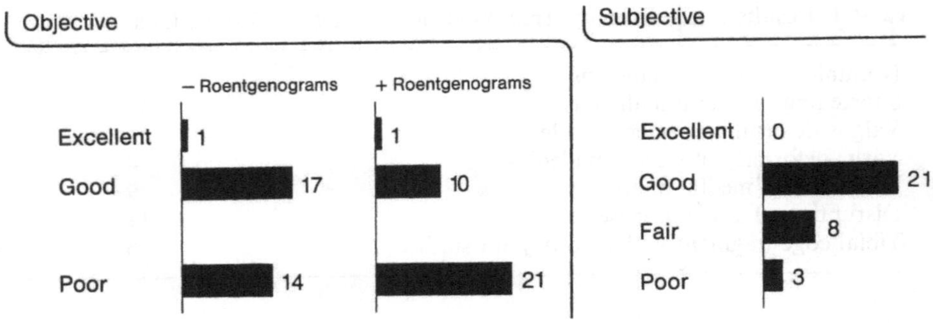

Fig. 1. Result of corrective surgery in 32 fracture-dislocations

Analysis of the results indicates the following: The average patient age in cases rated good or excellent was 33.9 years, as opposed to 39 years in cases rated poor. The average interval between primary treatment and corrective surgery was 15.3 months in the "good" and "excellent" cases, versus 10 months in the "poor" cases. The relatively large number of poor late results was due mainly to the severity of the original trauma. Fifteen of the patients with "poor" results had sustained a bimalleolar fracture-dislocation of the ankle joint (7 type B and 8 type C). A tibial edge fragment was present in seven. Five patients had an isolated fracture of the lateral malleolus (3 type B and 2 type C, 1 with an associated tibial edge fragment).

In 8 of the 21 cases given a poor objective rating, osteoarthritis increased after corrective surgery [9,15]. Examples are shown in Figs. 2 and 3.

Distal tibial compression fractures (Table 4 and 5): Eight patients in this group had corrections in one plane for valgus or varus deformity, and two had simultaneous corrections in two planes for a combined deformity (valgus with forward displacement and valgus with external rotation). Four patients underwent wedge resections of the tibia, and six underwent open wedge osteotomies with insertion of a corticocancellous graft. In one case it was still possible to reconstruct the tibial articular surface by cancellous bone grafting of the fracture zone (Table 5).

The mean patient age at reoperation was 36 years (range of 15 to 59). The mean interval from primary treatment to corrective surgery was 3 years (2 months to 5 years). The average interval from corrective surgery to follow-up was 3.5 years (1 year to 7 years) (Fig. 4).

Based on the strict Weber scoring system, a good result was obtained in only two cases while the remaining nine had to be classified as poor. Roentgenographic findings did not significantly effect the scores. It is possible that corrective surgery was excessively delayed in this group.

Surprisingly, the patients gave the result of their surgery a substantially higher subjective rating. One patient rated the result as excellent, five as good, three as fair, and only two as poor. The average patient age in the good case was 16.5 years, as opposed to 40.1 in the poor cases. Surgery was performed an average of 3.4 years after the original trauma in the good cases, and 1.5 years in the poor cases. The severity of osteoarthritis increased postoperatively in six of the poorly rated cases. Figs. 5 and 6 show examples.

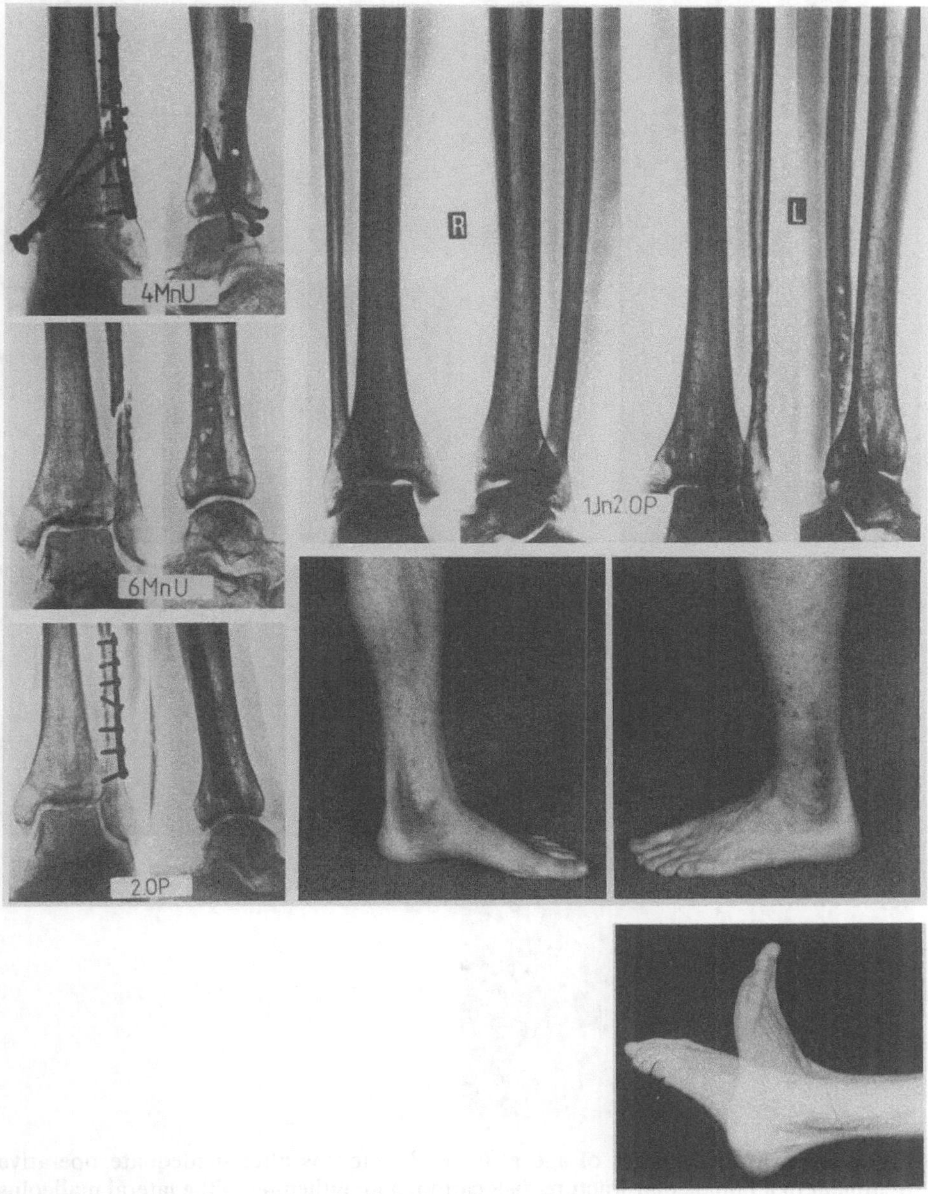

Fig. 2 a – e. Man 28 years of age **a** 4 and 6 months after operatively treated bimalleolar fracture-dislocation. **b** Second operation fixing the nonunited fibula and lengthening it by 5 mm. **c** Roentgenograms at 12 months after operation show complete healing. **d, e** Clinical appearance at 12 months: Gait is normal with 10° loss of ankle flexion. The result is rated as good

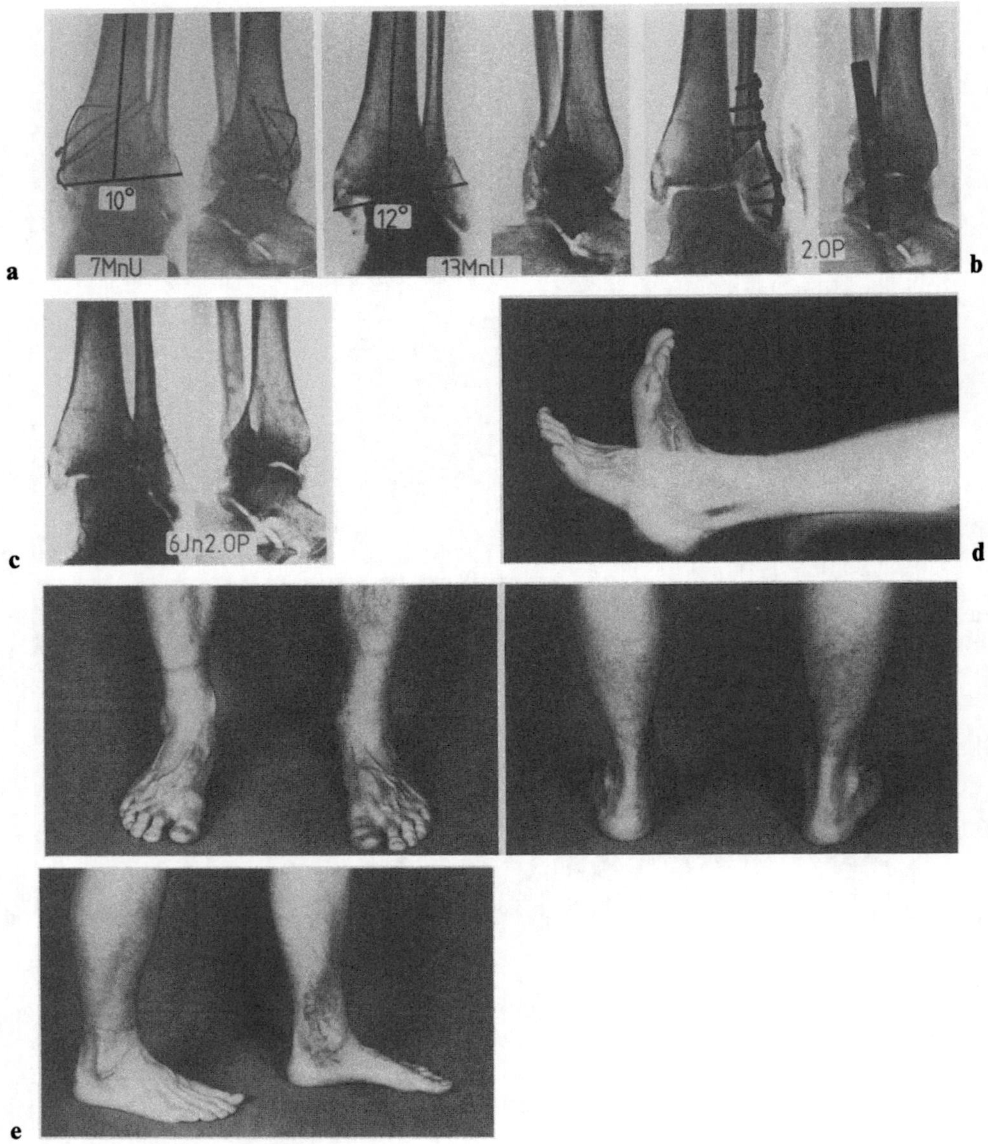

Fig. 3 a–e. Man 27 years of age **a** 7 and 13 months after inadequate operative treatment of a bimalleolar fracture-dislocation. **b** Lengthening of the lateral malleolus by 10 mm. **c** Roentgenograms at 6 years after correction show evidence of posttraumatic osteoarthritis; result is rated as poor. **d** Clinical appearance: Gait is normal, function is fair with 10° loss of ankle flexion and 50% limitation of subtalar motion. **e** Appearance at follow-up 6 years after correction: subjective pain on weight bearing

Table 4. Results of the Primary Treatment of 11 Compression Fractures

Valgus	10–15°	6
Varus	10–30°	2
Combined deformity:		
Valgus and forward displacement	20 and 15°	1
Valgus and external rotation	15 and 10°	1
No deformity		1
Joint incongruity		4

Table 5. Supramalleolar Corrective Operations Performed for 11 Compression Fractures

Varus osteotomy	6
Valgus osteotomy	2
Combined osteotomies:	
Varus and backward displacement	1
Valgus and joint reconstruction	1
Arthrodesis of the ankle joint	1

Table 6. Site of Corrective Surgery in 11 Compression Fractures (Tibial Pilon Fractures)

Osteotomy at the fracture site	7
Osteotomy above the fracture site	3
(Osteotomy of the fibula	6)
Arthrodesis	1

Distal tibial fractures (Tables 7 and 8): Sixteen tibial fractures that had united with more than 10° of angulation required correction in one plane only. Six required simultaneous corrections in two planes. In most cases the site of the deformity coincided with the level of the original fracture. Nine cases were treated by wedge insertion, five by wedge resection, and the remaining eight by cancellous bone grafting. In two cases axial realignment was followed by the internal fixation of a nonunion. External skeletal fixation was used in 6 cases, internal plating in 15 cases, and simple screw fixation in 1 case (Table 9).

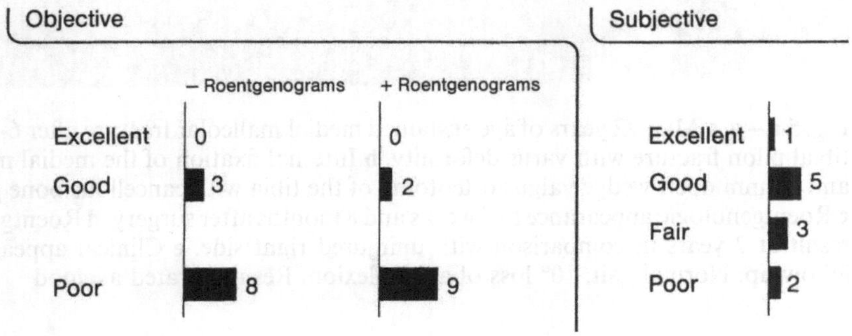

Fig. 4. Result of corrective surgery in 11 pilon fractures

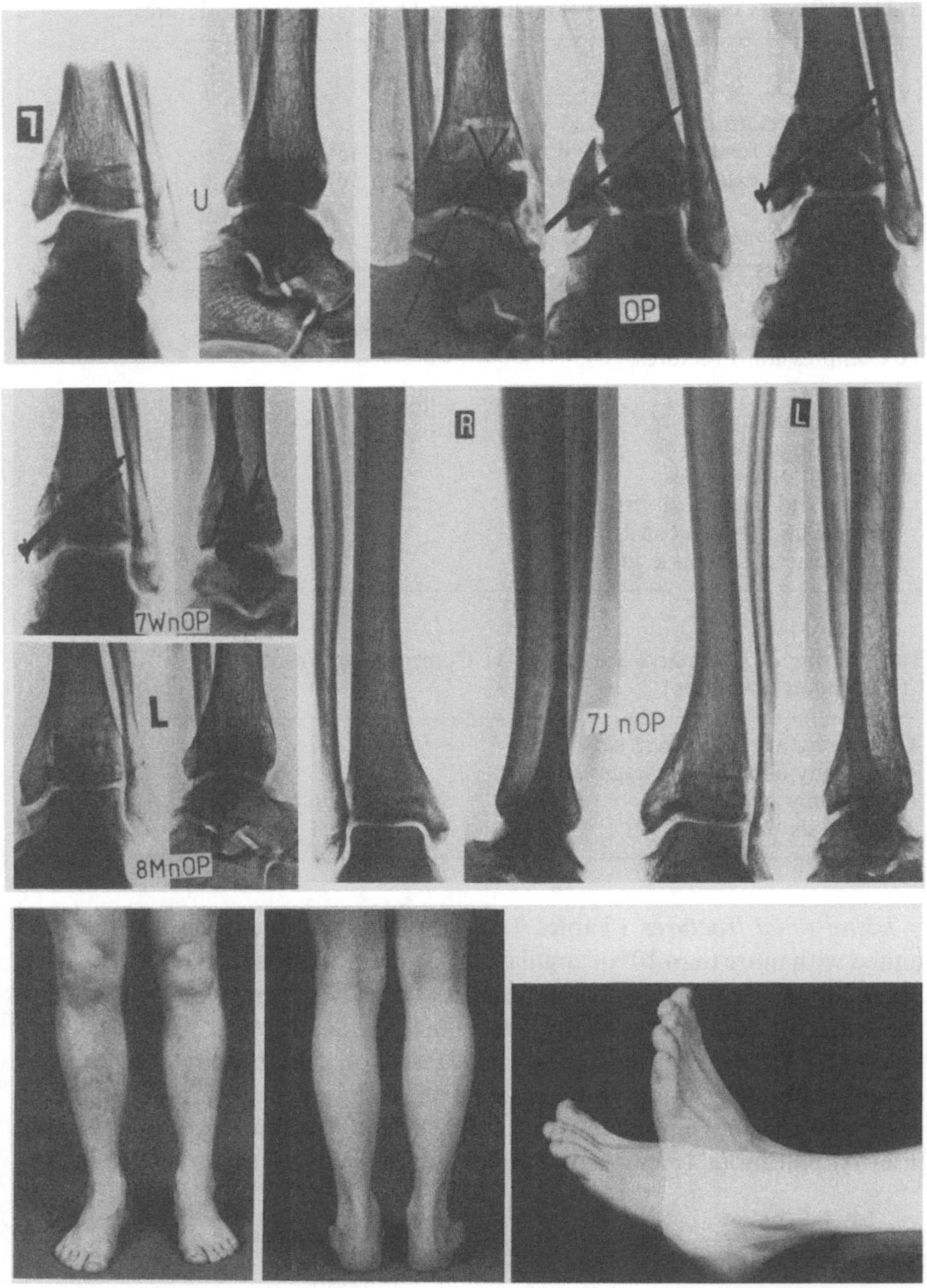

Fig. 5 a – e. a Man 22 years of age sustained medial malleolar fracture after 6-year-old tibial pilon fracture with varus deformity. **b** Internal fixation of the medial malleolus and 10-mm open-wedge valgus osteotomy of the tibia with cancellous bone grafting. **c** Roentgenologic appearance at 7 weeks and 8 months after surgery. **d** Roentgenologic result at 7 years in comparison with uninjured right side. **e** Clinical appearance at follow-up: Normal gait, 10° loss of ankle flexion. Result is rated as good

a b c d

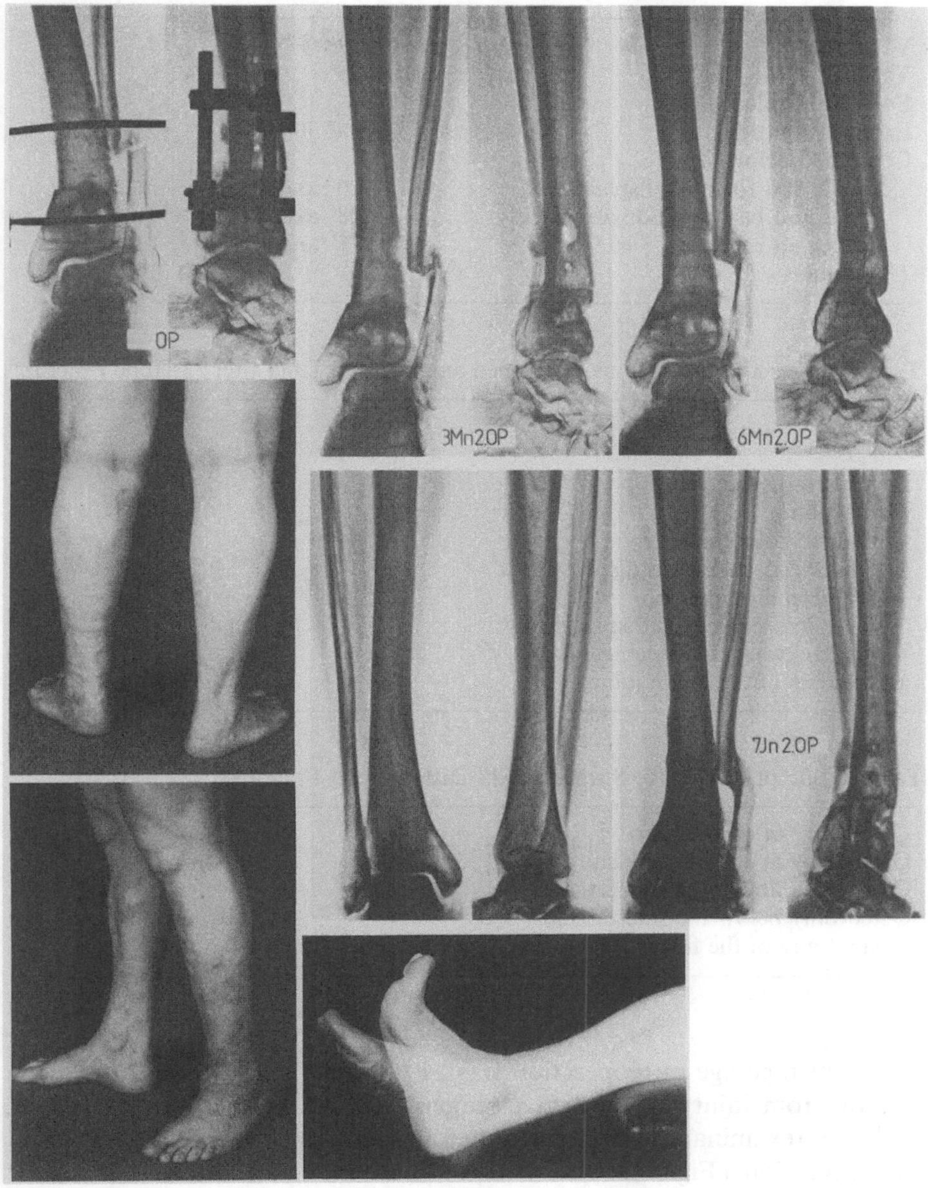

Fig. 6 a–d. Man 58 years of age 1 year after an operatively treated compression fracture. **a** Supramalleolar varus (15°) and derotation (10°) osteotomy stabilized with an external frame. **b** Roentgenograms at 3 and 6 months after operation. **c** Roentgenologic status at 7 years. **d** Ckinical appearance at follow-up: Mobile 10° equinus deformity, 10° of external malrotation, 1 cm of limb shortening, posttraumatic osteoarthritis with pain at rest and impaired gait. Result is rated as poor

Table 7. Results of the Primary Treatment of 22 Distal Tibial Fractures

Valgus	10–20°	7
Varus	10–15°	6
Forward displacement	15°	1
External rotation	10 and 30°	2
Combined deformity:		
Valgus and forward displacement	10–20° and 10–20°	3
Varus and backward displacement	18° and 25°	1
Varus and rotation	8–15° and 10–20°	2
(Nonunion		2)

Table 8. Corrective Operations Performed on the Distal Tibia after 22 Tibial Fractures

Valgus	6
Varus	7
Backward displacement	1
Derotation	2
Combined osteotomies:	
Valgus and backward displacement	1
Valgus and derotation	2
Varus and backward displacement	2
Varus backward displacement with arthrodesis of the ankle joint	1

Table 9. Site of Corrective Surgery in 22 Distal Tibial Fractures

Correction of a nonunion	3
Osteotomy at the fracture site	10
Osteotomy above the fracture site	2
Osteotomy below the fracture site	7
(Osteotomy of the fibula	8)

The average age at reoperation was 31.5 years (9 to 73), and the mean interval from injury to corrective surgery was 3.5 years (1 to 24 years). Follow-up examinations were performed an average of 3 years (1 to 8.5 years) after operation (Fig. 7).

Of the 22 patients in this group who were followed, only one late result merited an excellent objective rating, and 8 were rated as good. Thirteen were rated as poor. Similar ratings were made on the basis of function and severity of complaints. As in the two previous groups, the subjective evaluation was more favorable. Fifteen patients rated their present condition as good compared with their previous status, one patient rated the result as fair, and three rated it as poor. Three patients were unable to give a definitive rating.

The average patient age in the 9 good and excellent cases was 21.5 years. The mean interval form trauma to corrective surgery was 3 years. In the poor cases, the mean patient age at corrective surgery was 35 years, and the mean interval from primary treatment to correction was 2.4 years. The severity of

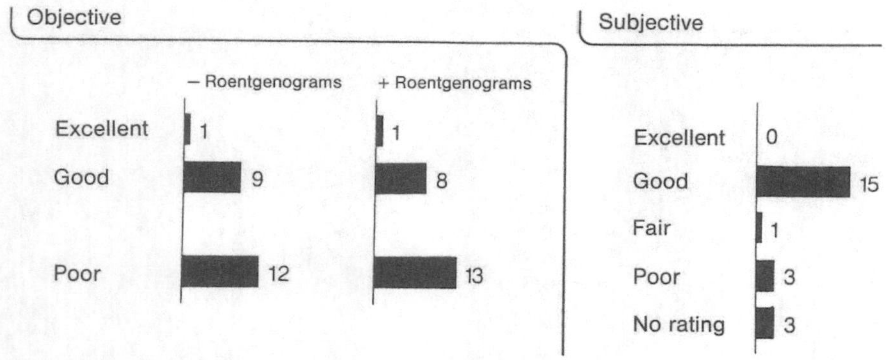

Fig. 7. Result of corrective surgery in 22 distal tibial fractures

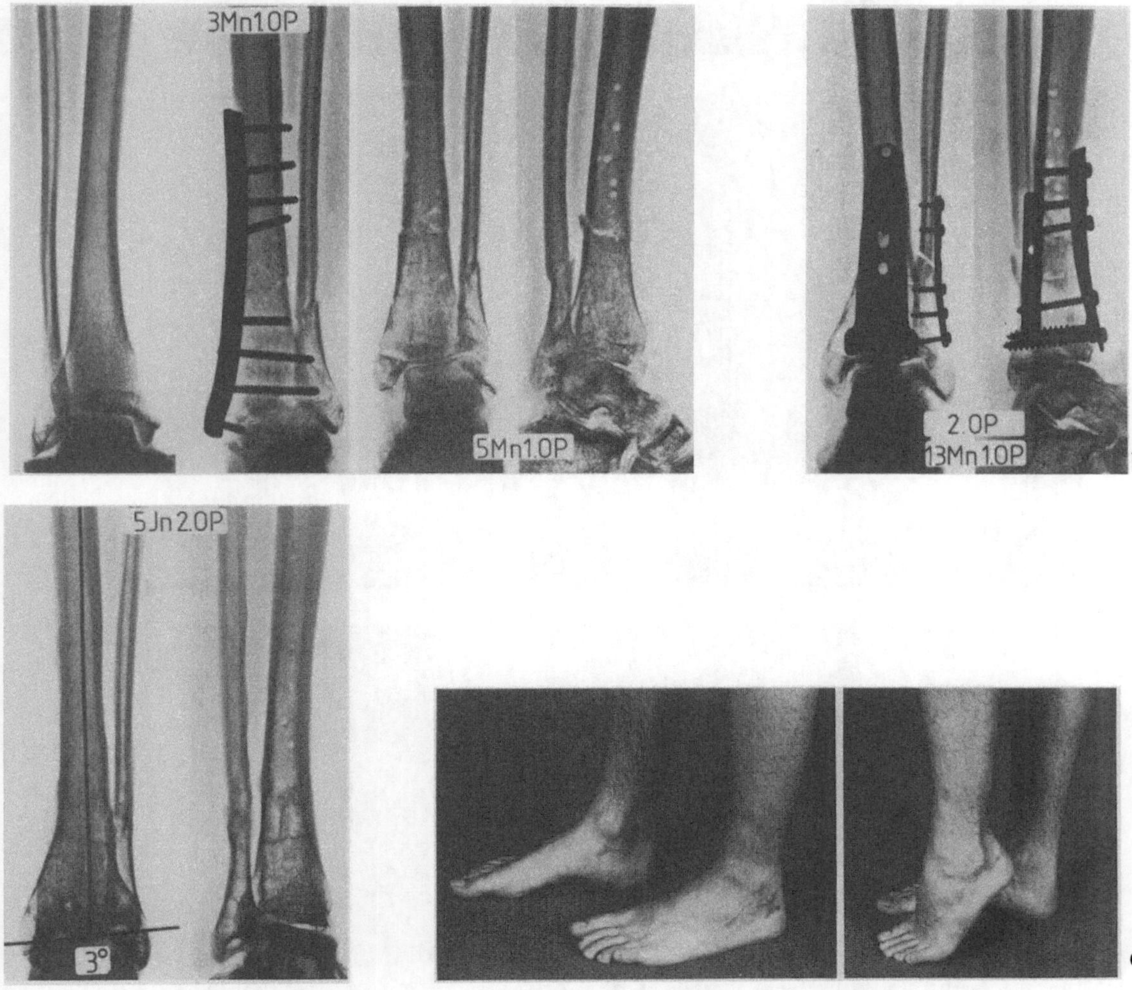

Fig. 8 a–d. Man 23 years of age. **a** 3 and 5 months after an operatively treated distal tibial fracture. **b** Closed-wedge varus osteotomy of the tibia (12°) with lengthening of the fibula. **c** Roentgenologic status at 5 years after surgery. **d** Clinical appearance at follow-up: Unimpaired gait, 10° of ankle flexion. Result is rated as good

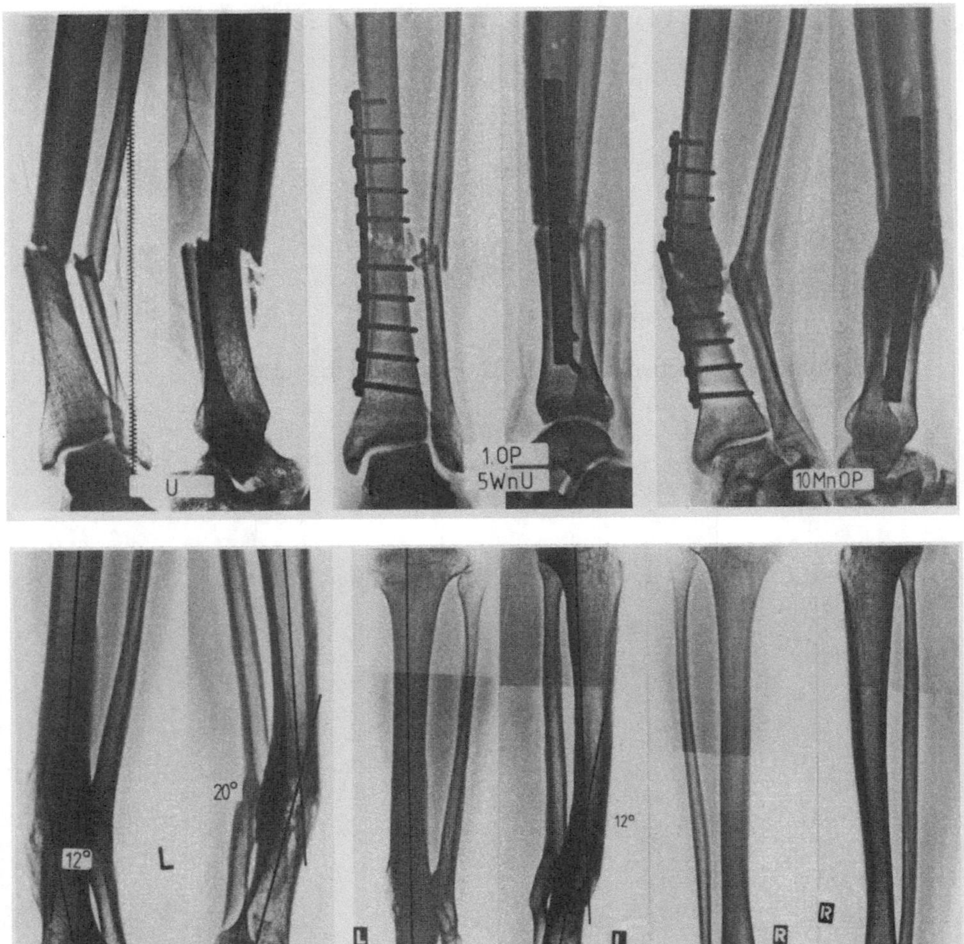

a b c d

osteoarthritis increased in seven cases, four of which among those rated poorly. Five patients already had mild preexisting osteoarthritis before surgery [10]. Examples are shown in Figs. 8 and 9.

Complications

The principal complications were infection and impaired wound healing (Table 10), which were present in a total of 11 operations.

Table 10. Postoperative Complications of the Corrective Surgery

	Disturbances of wound healing		Nonunion	Peroneal palsy
	Aseptic	Septic		
Fracture-dislocations 32	1	3	0	0
Compression fractures 11	0	2	1	2
Distal tibial fractures 22	2	3	0	0
Total	3 (4.6%)	8 (12.3%)	1 (1.5%)	2 (3.1%)

Summary

Evaluation of the late results of 65 corrective osteotomies about the ankle according to an objective point scale yielded 2 excellent, 20 good and 43 poor results (Fig. 10). Thus, 33.8% of the results were rated as good or excellent, and 66.2% were rated as poor. Taking function and severity of complaints as criteria, we find that the good and excellent results increase to 31 (47.7%) while the poor results decrease to 34 (52.3%).

The average age of patients with good objective late results was 27.7 years; the average age in the poor cases was 39. The mean interval between primary treatment and corrective surgery was 2.1 years in the good cases and 1.9 years in the poor cases. In 25 cases roentgenograms showed a progression of osteoarthritis by one grade of severity according to the classification of Bargon [1]. Eighteen of these cases had poor objective ratings.

Fig. 9 a–d. Man 33 years of age sustained an open supramalleolar tibial fracture that progressed to osteomyelitis and malunion after plate osteosynthesis. **b** Seven years after infected nonunion of the tibia. **c** The limb was corrected with 12° of varus and 20° of anterior angulation by wedge resection, and an external frame was applied; bone was solid at 8 months. **d** Roentgenologic status at 4 years after operation: 12° backward displacement, 10° loss of ankle flexion. There is gait impairment and pain on weight bearing. The result is rated as poor

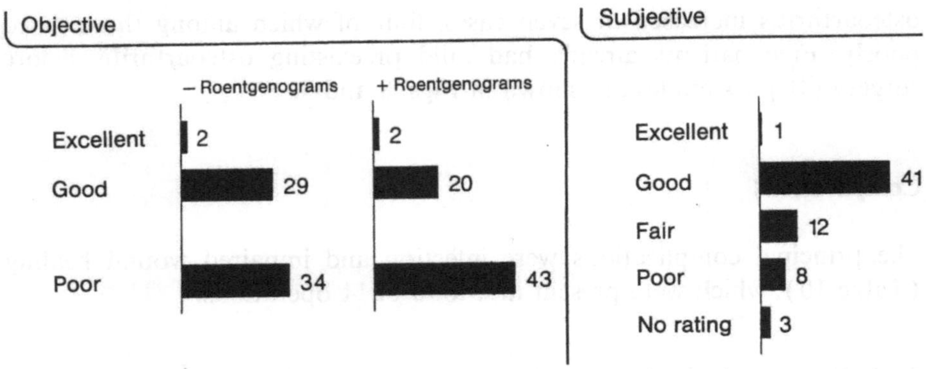

Fig. 10. Overall results of the corrective operations (65 patients)

Analysis of the data does not allow precise statistical conclusions to be drawn on account of the small case numbers involved. Nevertheless, the following observations may be made:

1. Cases should be selected for corrective osteotomy as early as possible and in accordance with strict criteria.
2. The more complex the original injury and the older the patient, the lower the success rate of corrective surgery.
3. In cases where posttraumatic osteoarthritis is already advanced, it must be decided whether reconstructive measures have a reasonable prospect of improving function, or whether arthrodesis would be a more rational means of obtaining a stable, pain-free ankle.
4. Within the limits stated, the surgical correction of preosteoarthritic deformity about the ankle apparently is rewarding even if a perfect reconstruction is no longer possible. This is demonstrated by the large percentage of patients who were subjectively pleased with their operation and by the better results of rating based on clinical criteria alone.
5. This observation does not mitigate the importance of creating normal axial and articular relationships during reconstructive surgery.

References

1. Bargon G (1978) Röntgenmorphologische Gradeinteilung der posttraumatischen Arthrose im oberen Sprunggelenk. Hefte Unfallheilkd 133:28–34
2. Friedebold G (1978) Spätversorgung nach Malleolarfrakturen. Technik – Ergebnisse. Hefte Unfallheilkd 133:45–63
3. Friedebold G (1978) Ergebnisse der Spätversorgung von Luxationsfrakturen des oberen Sprunggelenks. Hefte Unfallheilk 131:76–88
4. Kehr H (1977) Knöchelfrakturen, Sekundäreingriffe. Bericht über die Unfallmed. Tagung des Landesverbandes Rheinland-Westfalen der gewerbl. Berufsgenossenschaft. Heft 30
5. Knapp U (1978) Ergebnisse nach Korrektureingriffen am oberen Sprunggelenk. Therapiewoche 28:1541–1542
6. Lehrberger K (1979) Korrektureingriffe bei fehlverheilten Knöchelbrüchen. 22. Unfallseminar, 20.10.1979, Hannover, S 127–131

7. Leitz G (1967) Korrekturoperationen bei in Fehlstellung verheilten Knöchelfrakturen. Hefte Unfallheilkd 92:137
8. Leitz G (1971) Die operative Korrektur veralteter Knöchelgabelsprengungen. Arch Orthop Unfallchir 70:36–50
9. Platzgummer H (1964) Spätergebnisse und Erfahrungen mit der operativen Wiederherstellung der Knöchelgabel (tibiofibulare Arthrose) nach deform verheilten Knöchelbrüchen und Syndesmosen-Sprengungen. Arch Orthop Unfallchir 56:639
10. Ruedi T, Allgöwer m (1978) Spätresultate nach operativer Behandlung der Gelenkbrüche am distalen Tibiaende (sogen. Pilon-Frakturen). Unfallheilkunde 81:319–323
11. Wagner H (1977) Prinzipien der Korrekturosteotomie am Bein. Orthopäde 6:145–177
12. Weber BG (1972) Die Verletzung des oberen Sprunggelenks. Huber, Bern Stuttgart Wien
13. Weller S, Knapp U (1979) Ergebnisse nach operativer Behandlung von frischen und veralteten Verrenkungsbrüchen im oberen Sprunggelenk. Unfallmed. Tagung des Landesverbandes der gewerbl. Berufsgenossenschaften, 36:63
14. Weller S, Knapp U, Eck T (1977) Ergebnisse nach Korrektureingriffen am oberen Sprunggelenk. Sammelstudie der Deutschen Sektion der AO-international. Unfallheilkunde 80:213
15. Ziller R, Seyferth H (1970) Erfahrungen bei der operativen Behandlung veralteter Verletzungen im Bereich des oberen Sprunggelenks. Zentralbl Chir 95:772

Results of Corrective Osteotomies for Posttraumatic Deformities of the Foot

A. Skuginna, E. Peternek

The growing prevalence of incapacitating foot injuries among out patients – most resulting from vehicular accidents involving cyclists [3] and crushing injuries sustained at work – prompted us to conduct a thorough critical review of corrective operations performed on the foot. Arthrodeses were reviewed only if an open or closed wedge osteotomy was concurrently performed for treatment of an angular deformity. In corrective operations of the forefoot, only the operative procedure for deformities of the great toe are discussed.

The results reviewed in the present article represent a compilation of cases treated at the Bergmannsheil Bochum and Duisburg-Buchholz trauma clinics.

Evaluation of the functional outcomes of corrective foot operations is difficult because of the great variation in operative sites, and because the procedure is specifically tailored to the individual case. In most cases the presenting condition is one of conspicuous foot deformity [2]. Because the construction of a normal-appearing foot is not a realistic goal, we regard the improvement of foot statics as the main evaluation criterion.

In follow-up examinations we performed comparative range-of-motion measurements in the lower extremity, evaluated the soft-tissue and circulatory status of the feet, and also evaluated the statics of the feet by using a podometer to measure loads on the plantar surface. Roentgenograms of the feet in three planes also were obtained.

The key points of the evaluation scale are shown in Table 1.

The wearing of orthopedic shoes was disregarded in our evaluation because of the diversity of presenting deformities and because an anatomic restoration was not a reasonable goal in the majority of cases.

Table 1. Scale Used to Evaluate the Results of Corrective Operations for Posttraumatic Foot Deformities

Good:	Marked improvement of foot statics, unrestricted walking ability, absence of pain
Fair:	Improvement of foot statics, gait impairment and pain on heavy exertion Roentgenograms: Desired correction nearly achieved
Poor:	Marked residual foot deformity, no improvement of gait, constant pain on weight bearing Roentgenograms: Desired correction not achieved

Corrective Osteotomies of the Lower Extremity
Edited by G. Hierholzer, K. H. Müller

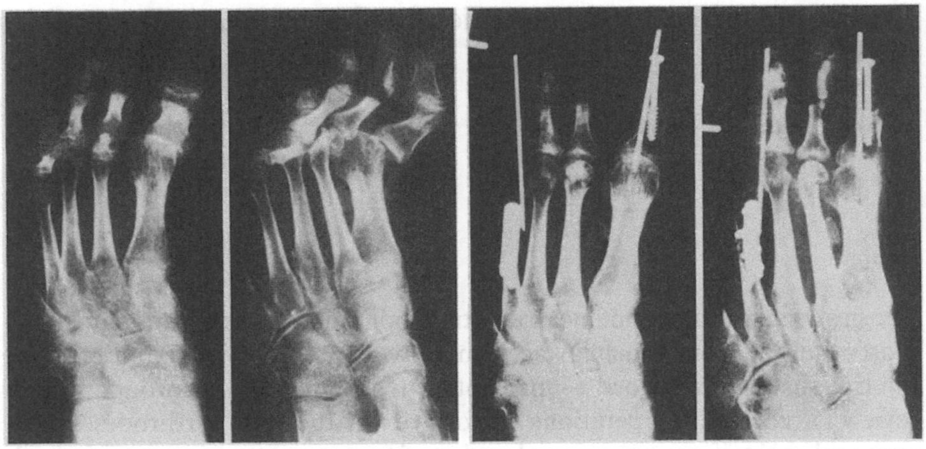

a b

Fig. 1 a,b. Operative treatment of phalangeal deformities. The deformity was corrected and the distal joint of the great toe fused with a small-fragment cancellous screw (inserted as a lag screw). **a** Before surgery; **b** after surgery

Most of the operations were closed wedge osteotomies; open wedge procedures were exceptional. Fixation was accomplished with the ASIF small-fragment set, Blount staples, and in some cases with external fixation, large cancellous screws and Kirschner wires. In deformities involving the distal phalanx of the great toe, we realign the phalanx and arthrodese the distal joint with a small-fragment cancellous screw (Fig. 1).

Results

During the period from 1972 to 1981, 31 corrective osteotomies were performed at the Duisburg-Buchholz and Bergmannsheil Bochum trauma clinics for the treatment of posttraumatic foot deformities. The etiologies of the deformities are shown in Table 2. The patients consisted of 25 men and 6 women, the high prevalence of injuries sustained at work according for the preponderance of males. The patients ranged in age from 22 to 53 years. Most of the deformities involved the region of the hindfoot (Table 3), but on the whole the range of deformities was extremely wide and diverse. In the operations for equinus deformity, the degree and rigidity of the deformity

Table 2. Corrective Osteotomies of Posttraumatic Foot Deformities (Duisburg-Buchholz and Bergmannsheil Bochum Trauma Clinics, n=31)

Trauma etiologies:	
Work	16
Traffic	10
Home	2
Recreation	3

Table 3. Sites of Posttraumatic Foot Deformities (Excluding Phalangeal Deformity, n=31)

Hindfoot	12	25 men, 6 women
Tarsus	7	*Age*: 22 to 53 years
Metatarsus	8	
Combined deformity	4	

Table 4. Types of Foot Deformity Corrected (n=31)

Equinus	8
Posttraumatic clubfoot	6
Varus or valgus deformity of the hindfoot	7
Posttraumatic splayfoot	3
Pes cavus	2
Other foot deformity[a]	5

[a] Isolated deformity of a metatarsal bone, adduction or abduction deformity

proved so severe that Achilles tenoplasty and arthrolysis were no longer sufficient to relieve the deformity. In all the cases selected for corrective surgery, there was marked concomitant involvement of the pedal joints adjacent to the deformity [1]. This was confirmed by roentgenography. The deformities are listed by type and distribution in Table 4 (see example in Fig. 2).

In 29 cases the correction was effected by a wedge resection osteotomy, combined in 11 cases with cancellous bone grafting. The bone was osteotomized such that the base of the resected wedge was on the convex side of the deformity. Only two cases were treated by open wedge osteotomy with insertion of a corticocancellous graft.

Most osteotomies were stabilized with Blount staples. Some were fixed with small-fragment cancellous screws placed in the tension-band mode and with

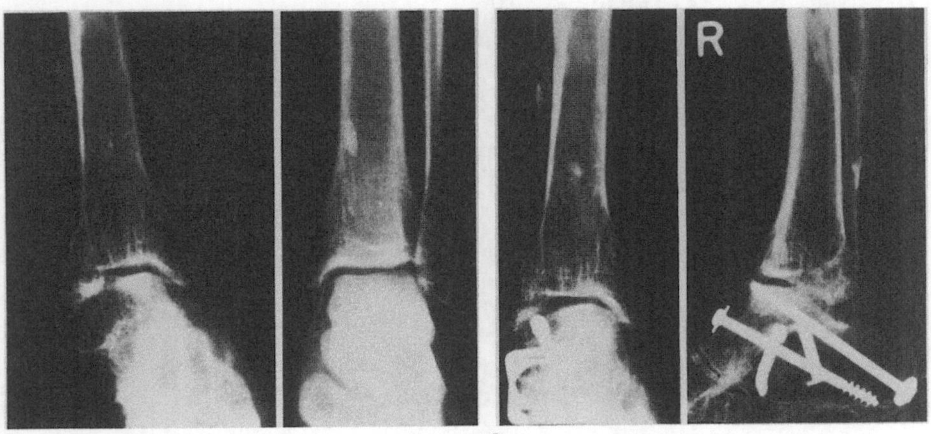

a b

Fig. 2 a,b. Operative correction of a varus deformity of the hindfoot. **a** Before surgery; **b** after bony consolidation with metal implants still in place

ASIF neutralizing plates. In three cases an external frame was used because of soft-tissue problems. Three osteotomies were fixed with large cancellous screws, which gave good compression across the osteotomy site (Table 5).

Table 5. Types of Metallic Fixation (n=31)

Blount staple	13
Small-fragment set → Cancellous screw	2
Small-fragment set → Plate and screws	3
Combination of Blount staple and small cancellous screw	2
Wire fixation (Kirschner wire, Steinmann pin)	4
Combination of drill wire and screws	1
Large cancellous screws	3
External frame	3

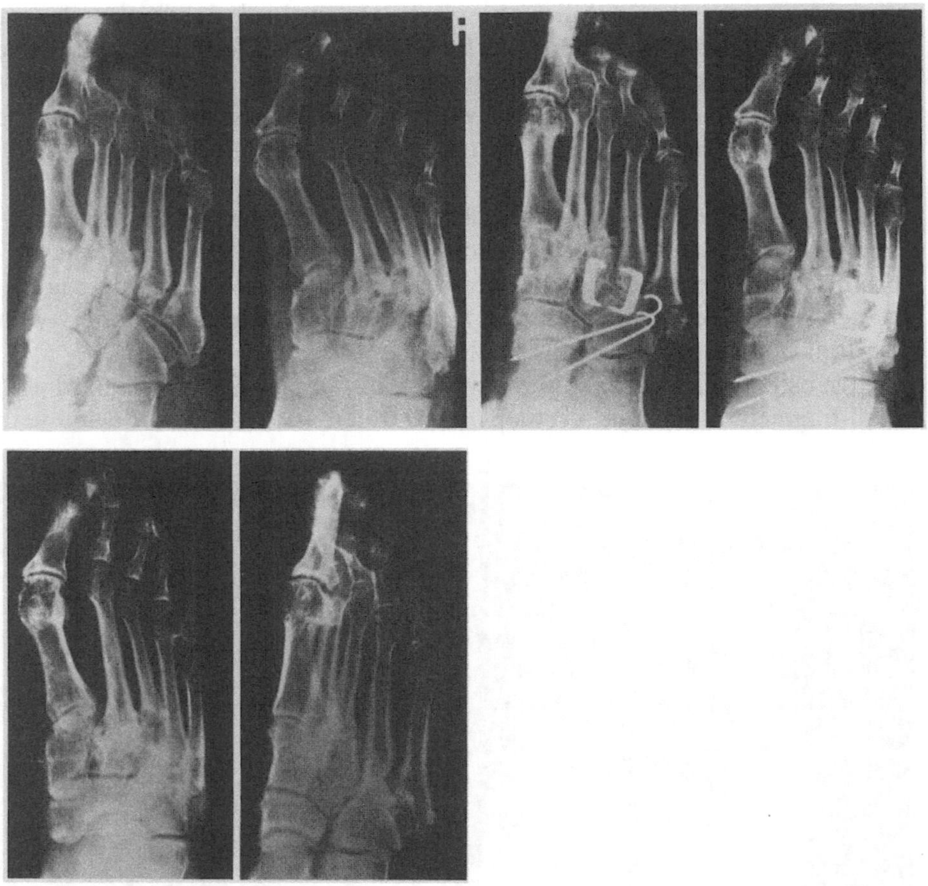

a b c

Fig. 3 a–c. Operative correction of a posttraumatic varus deformity of the trasus. **a** Before surgery. **b** Correction by wedge resection, fixation with Kirschner wires and Blount staples. **c** Status after removal of fixation material

Generally the implants were removed 8 months after surgery. This varied from a minimum of 5 weeks to a maximum of 4 years (Fig. 3).

An average of two months passed before full weight was placed on the operated foot. The shortest time to full weight bearing was one month, and the longest was four months. The foot was kept in plaster for about five weeks postoperatively except in cases where an external frame was used. Early, active exercises were initiated at 14 days if the osteotomy was sufficiently stable.

Four patients developed postoperative infections. However, these were clearly related to the presenting condition of the foot. Two of the patients had had previous soft-tissue infections.

The average interval from foot injury to corrective surgery was 3.5 years, with a range from 4 months to 18 years.

Of the 31 patients who underwent corrective foot surgery, 23 presented for follow-up. Using the evaluation criteria listed above, we rated the results of 19 operations as good or fair. The correction was judged to be inadequate in the remaining four (Table 6).

On reviewing the results of our follow-up examinations, we find that the operative method and fixation material cannot be standardized due to the diversity of presenting conditions. Given the complex morphology and statics of the foot, there is a need to adapt the operating technique and material to each individual case. Thus, screw fixation is not appropriate in every case, and a few cases even require the use of an external frame. On evaluating the planes of correction, especially in the tarsal and metatarsal regions, we observed that individual revisions of the tarsal joints are unnecessary, and that it is preferable to utilize a single plane of correction across the tarsal region, taking care that the base of the corrective wedge is at the vertex of the convex side of the deformity. Generally this will provide a satisfactory improvement of tarsal statics, which can be documented by the improved pressure load on the plantar surface of the foot. All the surgical patients had to wear orthopedic shoes postoperatively. Even if the surgery did not normalize the pedal skeleton, it still contributed significantly to the improvement of pedal statics (Fig. 4).

Bone healing was generally uneventful following the corrective surgery. Cancellous grafting was necessary when bony atrophy was severe.

Given the relatively poor soft-tissue conditions that accompany post-traumatic foot deformity, it is not surprising that corrective operations in that region carry an increased risk of infection. We feel that plaster immobilization and elevation of the operated foot are essential for the prevention or treatment of postoperative swelling, and that the use of large plate implants should be avoided.

Table 6. Clinical Results of Corrective Foot Surgery (n=23)

Good	9
Fair	10
Poor	4

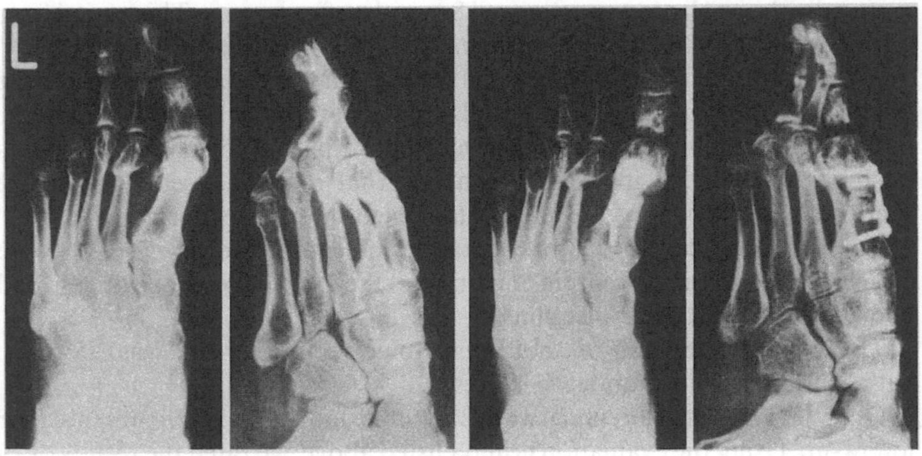

a b

Fig. 4. a Posttraumatic deformity of the first metatarsal. **b** Correction by dorsal wedge resection and fixation with a small-fragment plate

The results of our follow-ups indicate that the corrective operations significantly improved the statics and appearance of the foot in the great majority of cases treated. For this reason, we feel that the traditional attitude of restraint toward the use of surgery to correct posttraumatic foot deformities is no longer justified.

References

1. Hierholzer G (1974) Indikation und Technik der Arthrodese des unteren Sprunggelenks. Hefte Unfallheilkd 133:110–118
2. Hierholzer G, Hörster G, Gretenkord K (1981) Spätzustände nach Luxationen und Frakturen der Knöchelgabel des Fußes (Kongreßbericht). Langenbecks Arch Chir 355:443–448
3. Kuner EH, Müller T, Lindenmaier HL (1978) Einteilung und Behandlung der Talusfrakturen. Hefte Unfallheilkd 131:197–211

Summary: Corrective Osteotomies after Trauma about the Ankle and Foot

U. Pfister

Little attention is given in the literature to postraumatic deformities of the ankle and foot. The increasing reliance on corrective surgery in the treatment of angular deformities about the hip and knee apparently has bypassed the foot. This is remarkable when one considers that, unlike other deformities of the lower extremity, the pain and disability of the deformed foot often are perceived with every step.

Althoug Probst points out that pure foot injuries account for only about 4.2% of compensatable injuries sustained at work, there can be no question that the foot is secondarily involved by many injuries to more proximal structures. Postraumatic deformities that are secondary to malunited tibial and ankle fractures, nerve lesions, circulatory disturbances and dystrophy; equinus deformities; supination-adduction deformities; valgus deformities in hindfoot injuries; deformities of the longitudinal and transverse arches in tarsal and metatarsal injuries; and toe deformities secondary to fractures or disturbances of neurovascular function after complete or incomplete compartment syndrome are such frequent sources of complaints that a detailed study of their sequelae is both necessary and rewarding.

In principle, classical orthopedics offers many corrective operations that are suitable for deformities of the foot and ankle. However, the prerequisites for these operations are fundamentally different in the posttraumatic foot. While most nontraumatic deformities feature an intact foot with healthy soft tissues, a normal blood supply and stable articular connections, posttraumatic deformities are associated with cicatricial and dystrophic changes in the soft tissues, bones, and joints.

Probst speaks of a fundamental derangement of function and morphology. A disturbance of adaptive capacity is also charcteristic, especially in late cases.

These postraumatic changes increase the risks of a corrective operation. Weller states that operations for deformity of the ankle joint, which are relatively favorable in terms of primary healing, are associated with a 10% rate of postoperative infection and disturbed wound healing. Presumably this rate is somewhat higher in osteotomies of the dystrophic pedal skeleton. In many cases the increased risk is acceptable only if all options for conservative, orthopedic management have been exhausted. Expectations must be realistic with regard to the outcome of surgery. Usually the patient must be satisfied with an improvement over his preoperative status; he should not expect a perfect reconstruction.

Despite the risks involved, the decision to undertake corrective surgery of the ankle is fairly straightforward. The trauma surgeon finds himself on

Corrective Osteotomies of the Lower Extremity
Edited by G. Hierholzer, K. H. Müller

familiar ground, and the goal of the procedure will be dictated by the extent to which normal anatomic relations can be restored. The classification of Weller recognizes five major types of deformity about the ankle:

1. Elongation of the fibula with varus tilting of the talus
2. Shortening of the fibula with valgus tilting of the talus
3. Supramalleolar angulation
4. A step in the joint surface
5. Rigidity of the ankle mortise from damage to the syndesmosis.

Deformities of categories 1–3 are readily managed by restoring the original length of the fibula or by correcting the supramalleolar angulation. If these procedures are done early enough, their results are almost always good. On the other hand, the technically demanding operations to treat deformities of categories 4 and 5 often produce unsatisfactory end results. Taking all 5 categories together, we find that the results of corrective surgery for all ankle deformities are good or satisfactory in only about 50% of cases according to the collective statistics to the ASIF. Many of these cases eventually necessitate an arthrodesis of the ankle, which when correctly performed offers a valuable recourse and should be presented to the patient before surgery as a workable alternative in the event the first operation is a failure.

The categorization of posttraumatic foot deformities is more difficult than in the ankle. Probably the most frequently diagnosed deformities are talipes planovalgus after calcanean fracture; equinus deformity caused by a contracture at the ankle joint, which is often accompanied by supination of the foot; and equinus deformity of the forefoot secondary to metatarsal lesions. No specific data are available on the prevalence of these conditions, and no guidelines have been established with regard to the corrective procedures of choice. However, individual reports and personal experience indicate that wedge-resection osteotomy of the metatarsal region is a good and useful treatment for equinus of the forefoot and for abduction and abduction deformities. In the absence of painful ankyloses or partial ankyloses in an abnormal position, arthrodesis of the ankle or subtalar joint can correct the position of the foot and alleviate pain. Probst and Witt point out that a supramalleolar osteotomy can also correct equinus deformity if there is normal motion in the ankle joint.

Osteotomies of the calcaneus for posttraumatic planovalgus deformity have been widely performed only in acutely injured patients, are variable in their result, and have a high association with problems of wound healing. In late conditions, arthrodesis of the subtalar joint with correction of the valgus deformity by the closed or open wedge method often gives an excellent result.

So far there have been no systematic follow-up studies of posttraumatic corrective operations on the first and fifth rays, which, as buttresses of the plantar vault, are critically important to the anatomy and function of the foot. With all arthrodeses and osteotomies of the foot, it may be assumed that results will be satisfactory only if neighboring joints are able to adapt to the altered situation, i.e., are free of significant degenerative disease.

For the patient, the late sequelae of fractures of the phalanges or posttraumatic deformities of the toes represent a constant source of pain. In this area classical orthopedics offers a number of surgical options for various kinds of deformity.

In most posttraumatic affections of the foot, the dystropic changes and compromised blood flow make it necessary to perform corrective operations in stages. Thus, it is recommended that deformities of the tarsus and metatarsus and deformities of the phalanges be corrected in successive operations rather than concurrently.

Proper orthopedic care during rehabilitation is equal in importance to the operation itself in contributing to a successful outcome.

It remains to be added that posttraumatic deformities of the ankle, foot and toes are frequently underestimated despite their great functional significance. Their effects are often trivialized, and their responsiveness to surgical intervention has not been adequately explored. Even so, it is clear that the prognosis of these deformities is favorable with early intervention, and that even in late operations patients have a tendency to rate any degree of improvement very positively.

VI. Posttraumatic Deformity of the Growing Skeleton

Growth Disturbance after Epiphyseal Plate Injuries

A. Betz and L. Schweiberer

Processes of endochondral ossification are of special relevance to longitudinal growth in the epiphyses. They underlie the formation of the epiphysis and are responsible for its regeneration and remodeling.

Schenk (Fig. 1) subdivides the ephihyseal plate anatomically and functionally into two regions:

1. the epiphyseal part with the proliferating zone and cartilaginous columns, and
2. the metaphyseal part with its hypertrophic cartilage cells and zone of provisional calcification.

The *epiphyseal part of the plate* contains a pool of proliferation chondroblasts extending from the resting cartilage to the border of the hypertrophic zone. Functional loading of the plate by tension and compression aligns the chondroblasts and stimulates them to mature. Here we observe the cell proliferation that is essential for longitudinal bone growth, which is why this

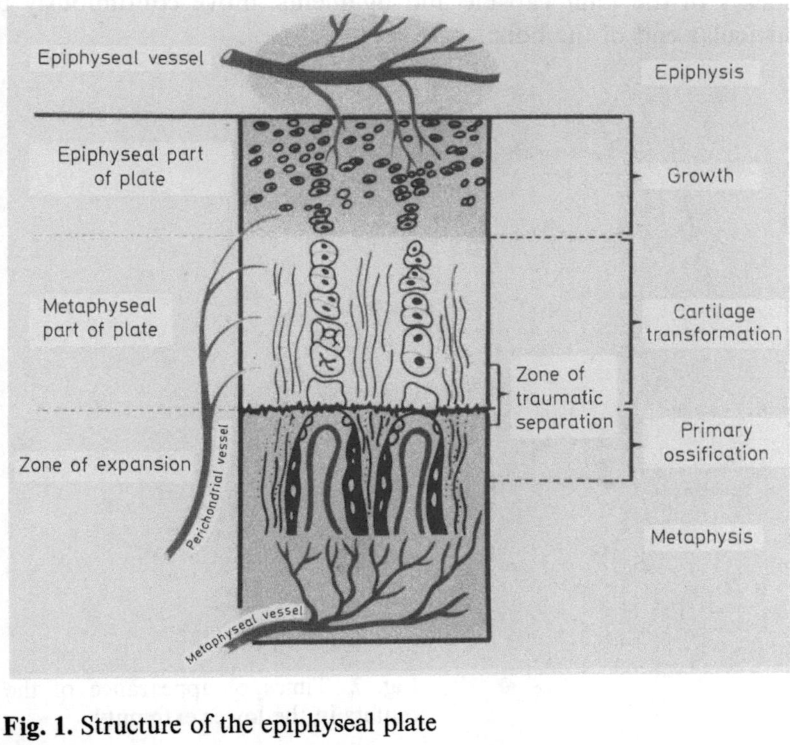

Fig. 1. Structure of the epiphyseal plate

Corrective Osteotomies of the Lower Extremity
Edited by G. Hierholzer, K. H. Müller

region is so susceptible to traumatization and why the effects of trauma can be so severe.

In the *metaphyseal part of the plate* the chondrocytes mature, enlarge through fluid absorption, and lose their ability to proliferate. The cellular hypertrophy contributes purely to longitudinal growth as the cells increase in length by about a factor of three.

At the *junction of the epiphyseal plate with the metaphysis* the zone of expansion begins, marked by processes of chondrolysis, followed by the zone of ossification with the deposition of fiber bone. Mineralization in this region takes place on the longitudinal, intracolumnar cartilaginous septa. This pattern of mineralization gives the advancing capillaries access to the base of the individual cell columns and opens the way for invasion by chondroblasts and osteoblasts leading to resorption of the calcified cartilage. As in the columnar region, the structure of the metaphyseal cancellous bone becomes aligned in response to functional loads.

Originally the *epiphysis* (Fig. 1) is entirely cartilaginous. With the appearance of the ossification centers (Fig. 2), the growth cartilage becomes separated from the joint cartilage. These centers enlarge as endochondral ossification progresses. The connection between the epiphyseal plate and joint cartilage remains cartilaginous during growth.

The *perichondrium* (Fig. 3) is a zone of appositional growth which increases the diameter of the epiphyseal plate and thus provides for its latitudinal growth. It overlies the growth cartilage on its external surface and blends with the periosteum on the metaphyseal side. During growth, the border between the perichondrium and periosteum, and with it the attachments of the joint capsule and ligaments, move continuously toward the articular end of the bone.

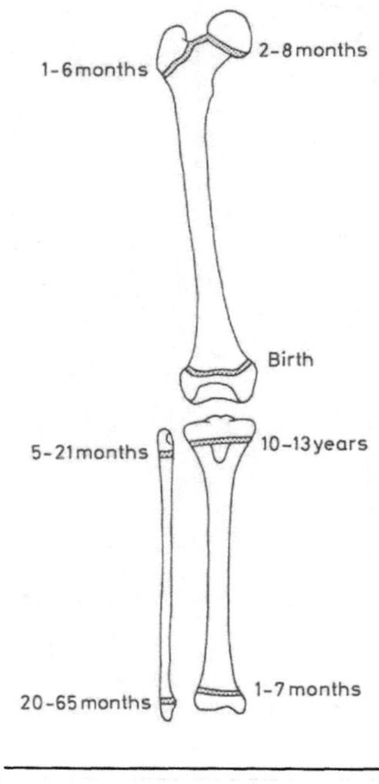

Fig. 2. Times of appearance of the epiphyseal centers in the lower extremity

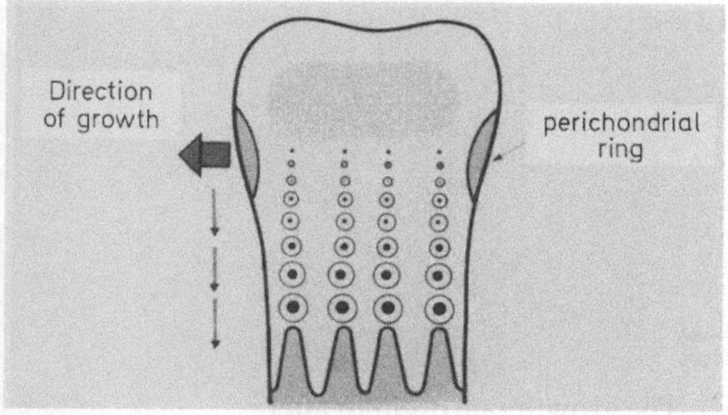

Fig. 3

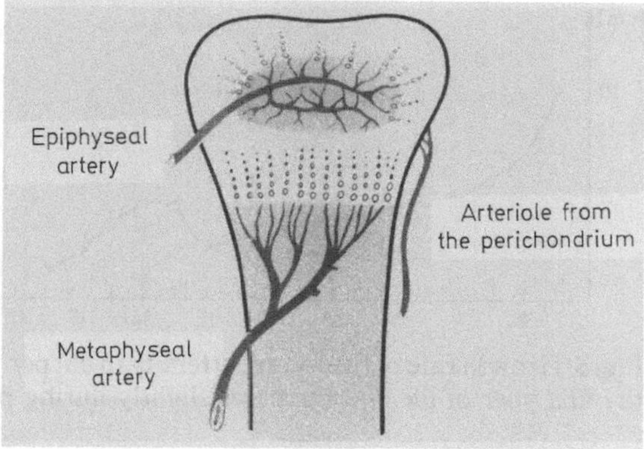

Fig. 4

Fig. 3. Scheme of latitudinal and longitudinal growth in the epiphyseal plate. Perichondrium: Increase in diameter (latitudinal growth) of the plate
Fig. 4. Schematic diagram of the blood supply of the epiphyseal plate

Because of this arrangement, a unilateral arrest of growth can result if trauma at the level of ligamentous attachment causes the formation of an osseous bridge between the epiphysis and metaphysis.

The blood supply of the epiphyseal plate is of particular significance (Fig. 4). The epiphysis, metaphysis and perichondrium each have their own vascular systems. There is still disagreement as to whether the epiphyseal vessels anastomose with the periosteal and metaphyseal vessels via the perichondrial ring; in this way the epiphyseal plate would be affected by hyperemia at a fracture site that is distant from the plate.

The blood vessels do not penetrate the epiphyseal plate itself. Thus, changes in the status of vascular perfusion can result in disturbances of plate function.

There are only *two ways* in which the epiphyseal plate can respond to pathogenic influences: through *stimulation* or *inhibition* of its function.

Stimulation of the function of the growth cartilage causes an acceleration of longitudinal growth. This occurs whenever perfusion of the epiphyseal vessels is increased by processes affecting the plate itself or adjacent tissues, such as diaphyseal fractures. Similar reactions are observed in inflammatory diseases such as hematogenous osteomyelitis. Another example is Klippel-Trénaunay-Weller syndrome with hypervascularity of the epiphyses, which may cause excessive longitudinal growth.

Complete stimulation is the most common type of growth disturbance. Its clinical significance is greatest in the lower extremity due to the alteration of hip and spinal statics that accompanies a discrepancy of leg lengths.

The degree to which the epiphyseal plate can respond to trauma with increased longitudinal growth depends basically on the patient's growth potential and age: the younger the child, the greater the growth potential (Fig. 5). Thus, the significance of hyperemia and its duration is in direct proportion to the age of the patient at the time of injury.

Various authors have shown that the duration of increased blood flow and thus the amount of lengthening depends directly on the duration and intensity of the remodeling processes that occur during fracture repair.

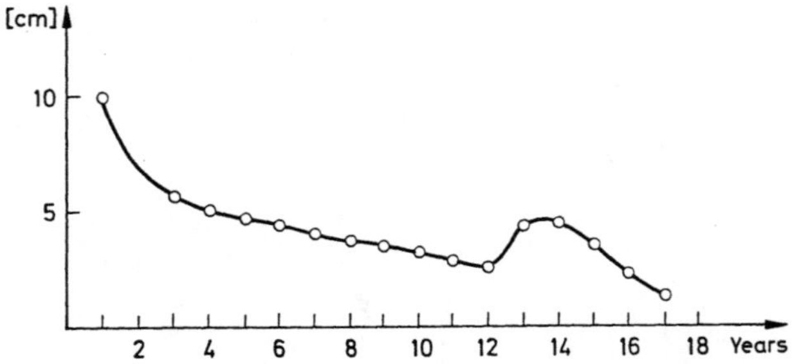

Fig. 5. Growth rate of the lower extremity in cm per year. The growth rate declines after the first year of life and increases slightly during puberty

Flach et al. and von Laer state that complete stimulative growth disturbances can be treated only by indirect means – specifically, by reducing the duration of bone remodeling. With this in mind, they advise the primary correction of deformities by the simplest means possible. Delayed reduction maneuvers and operations should be avoided.

However, there is no primary treatment that can influence leg length discrepancy during posttraumatic growth.

Partial stimulation results from injuries near or across growth plates that involve a localized delay of consolidation. Von Laer states that prolonged remodeling on one side of the metaphysis leads to a localized increase in blood flow, causing a partial stimulation that increases growth in one portion of the adjacent epiphyseal plate. This growth disturbance can greatly exacerbate the deformity produced by the trauma. After the fracture consolidates, the stimulation ceases and the epiphysis can again align itself at right angles to the prevailing load, assuming sufficient growth potential remains (this will depend on the age and sex of the patient and the condition of the affected plate).

Partial stimulation is the only growth disturbance that can be influenced by primary treatment.

With *primary compression* it is possible to shorten the duration of anticipated partial remodeling processes and thus shorten the period of partial growth stimulation.

The early *inhibition* of epiphyseal plate function by trauma leads to retardation or arrest of longitudinal growth and is equivalent to unphysiologic closure of the growth plate. The balance between proliferation and chondrolysis is shifted in favor of lysis, leading to vascular invasion of the plate region and increased ossification.

If the injury involves only the *metaphyseal part of the plate* where chondrolysis prevails, there may be a temporary depression of lytic processes resulting in a *widening of the plate*. The good vascularity of the metaphysis ensures a rapid regeneration.

The *epiphyseal part of the plate* with the germinal layer reacts much more sensitively to trauma. Besides disrupting the functional equilibrium of the plate, trauma to this region causes destruction of true growth cartilage and promotes the spread of mineralization processes to the plate itself until a

Table 1. Prognostic Factors (Epiphysis and Metaphysis)

1. Age and sex
2. Location
3. Primary displacement

partial or complete osseous connection is established with the epiphyseal ossification center.

In the literature the formation of a bony bridge between the epiphysis and metaphysis is variously attributed to:
1. necrosis of the growth cartilage from direct damage in a crushing injury,
2. necrosis of the growth cartilage from damage to the blood supply, and
3. the vascular invasion of a longitudinal discontinuity in the growth plate with subsequent ossification.

Complete plate closure with total degeneration of the growth cartilage is very *rare* and leads to a *complete* arrest of growth.

The severity of the growth disturbance depends on the growth activity of the plate and the age of the patient, i.e., the expectation of future growth. Even more significant because of its frequency and presentation is *partial* closure of the plate like that often caused by fractures across the growth plate with osseous bridging between the epiphysis and metaphysis.

The prognosis of a partial growth arrest (Table 1) also depends largely on the *age* and *sex* of the patient – sex being a factor only to the extent that bone growth and maturation begin at a somewhat earlier age in girls than in boys. The closer the patient is to skeletal maturity, the less conspicuous will be the effect of a localized inhibition of growth. Because the epiphyseal plates in different locations close at different times, and because their growth potentials vary, the location of the injury represents another important evaluation criterion (Fig. 6).

The greater the amount of primary displacement, the greater the danger of a growth disturbance. The process of longitudinal growth on the injured side is analogous to the operation of a feedback control system (Fig. 7) which gradually recovers from an initial, excessive oscillation to an undisturbed state by means of a damped counteroscillation.

In a system of this type, a disturbance acting on the controlled process (Fig. 8) affects the measured quantity M, which is used by the internal program as an input for correction of the process by means of the control quantity S.

In the literature we find varying and seemingly contradictory hypotheses on posttraumatic growth changes. According to the law of functional adaptation (Fig. 9) as elucidated by Pauwels (1957), unequal longitudinal bone growth is a compensatory mechanism whereby a deviated growth plate is realigned so that it is again perpendicular to the prevailing pressure load. Supposedly a change in the direction of this resultant or a change in the position of the epiphyseal plate leads to correction and adaptation through increased longitudinal growth on the side of greater pressure.

Hueter and Volkmann, on the other hand, favor the theory that increased longitudinal epiphyseal growth is a result of unloading. This is consistent with

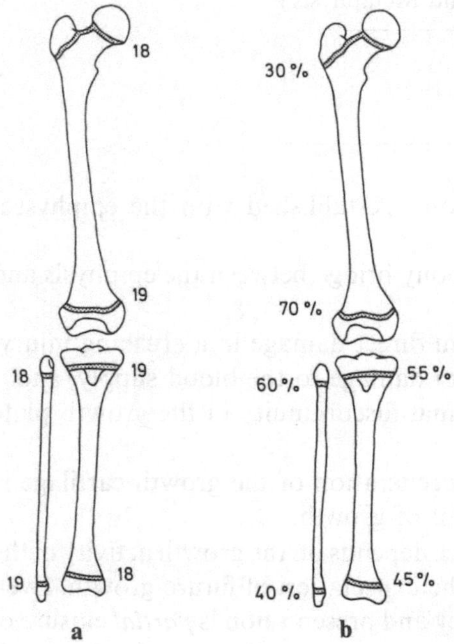

Fig. 6. a Age at epiphyseal plate closure and **b** contributions of the individual epiphyseal plates to longitudinal growth

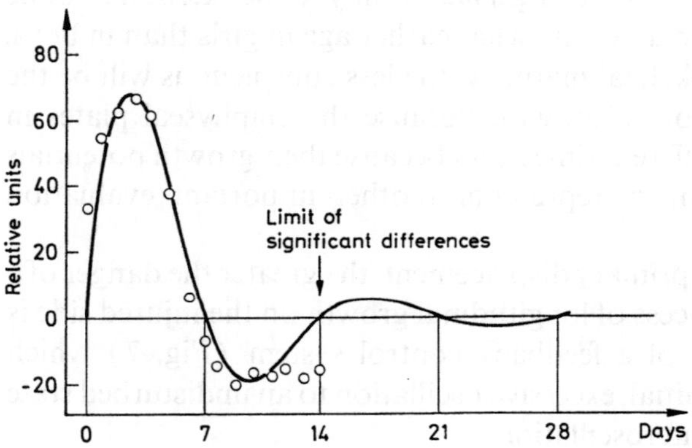

Fig. 7. Fluctuation of the daily growth rate in an injured limb (after Cotta). The curve has the shape of a damped oscillation

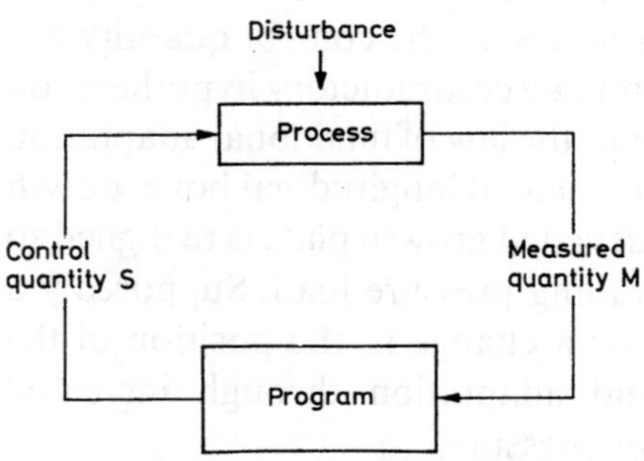

Fig. 8. Diagram of the feedback mechanism that regulates daily longitudinal growth in an injured limb (after Cotta)

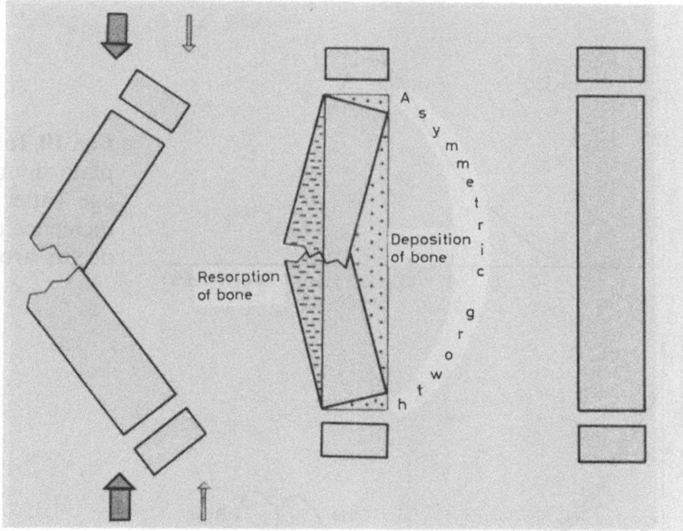

Fig. 9. Functional mechanism for the spontaneous correction of osseous deformity. A deviated growth plate is realigned through asymmetric longitudinal growth

the results of Klapp et al. indicating that growth disturbance occurs only in the absence of local control by the periosteum and muscle tone, i.e., only if the restraining structures (periosteum, soft-tissue envelope) are divided or at least deficient.

Thus, it is suggested that an inequality of pressure or a failure of restraint stimulates growth on the side where loads are deficient and inhibits growth on the side where loads are excessive, and that this mechanism allows for the spontaneous correction of deformities in and around the epiphysis.

According to these views, the epiphyseal reaction also aids in the compensation of angular deformities affecting the diaphysis and metaphysis.

An asymmetric acceleration of growth in the epiphyseal plate makes the most important contribution to the restoration of normal axial relationships in the limb.

In contrast to these *specific* corrective mechanisms, the response to a *posttraumatic increase or decrease of limb length* seems to be essentially *nonspecific*.

Thus, a primary shortening deformity can be corrected only by an increase of epiphyseal plate function during growth, while the equally nonspecific correction of a *lengthening deformity* is possible only by somewhat premature closure of the growth plate, i.e., early cessation of growth on the formerly injured side during prepubescence.

Clinically, the biological characteristics of skeletal growth are a two-edged sword: On the one hand, they can assist therapy by allowing for the spontaneous correction of deformities. On the other hand, the same mechanisms can make treatment more difficult by aiding the progression of angulations and other deformities (e.g., hypoplasia of the lateral malleolus after trauma to the distal fibular epiphysis).

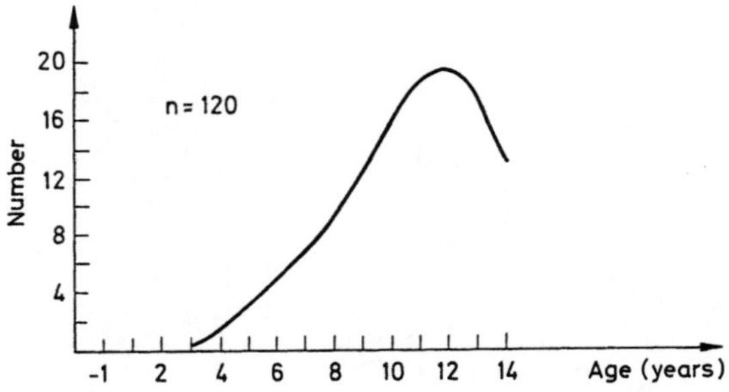

Fig. 10. Incidence of epiphyseal plate injuries as a function of age (after Steinert). The peak incidence of epiphyseal injuries occurs around puberty

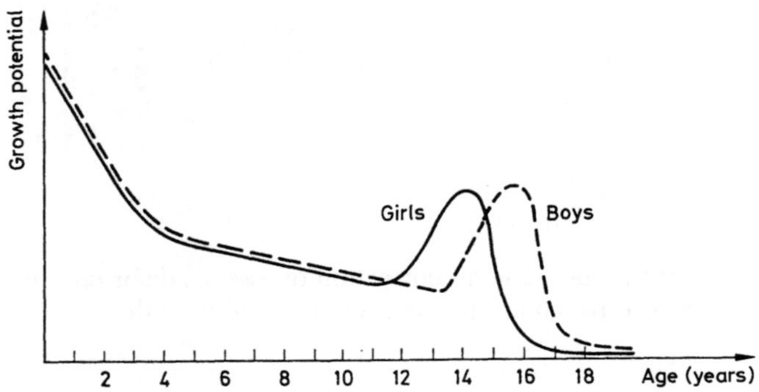

Fig. 11. Longitudinal growth as a function of age (after Fankoni)

Fortunately, the peak incidence of epiphyseal plate injuries (Fig. 10) is in the vulnerable pubertal period, at which time growth disturbances usually have minimal impact because little growth potential remains (Fig. 11). However, the same circumstance precludes the possibility of significant spontaneous correction.

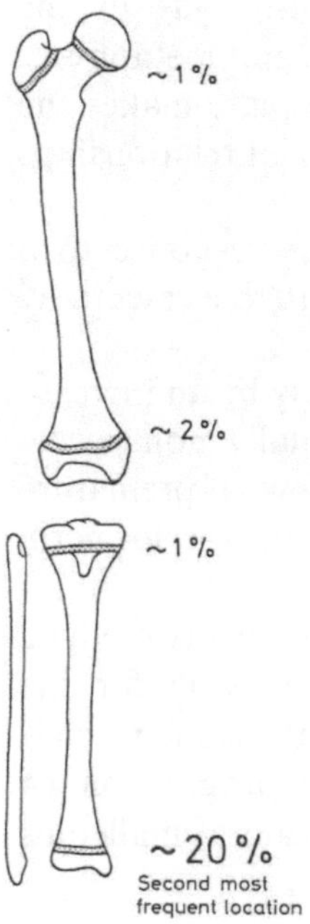

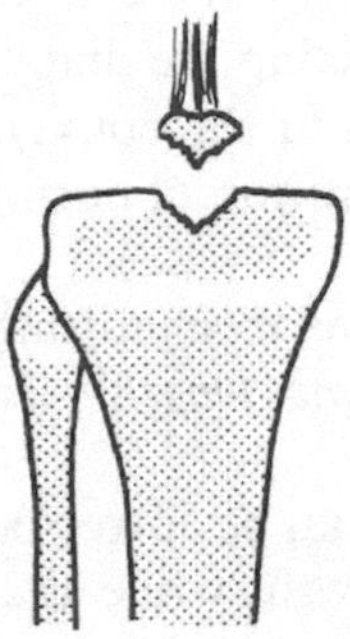

Fig. 13. Epiphyseal avulsion fracture of the intercondylar eminence

Fig. 12. Frequency distribution of epiphyseal plate injuries in the lower extremely

Thus, the earlier in growth an epiphyseal plate injury is sustained, the greater the tendency for the deformity to worsen as growth progresses.

Approximately 10% of pediatric fractures involve injuries of the epiphyseal region, and growth disturbances may be expected to occur in 10% of the injured epiphyses.

Statistically, the distal tibia ranks second only to the distal radius in its susceptibility to epiphyseal injury (Fig. 12).

The various classifications based on mechanism of injury or anticipated posttraumtic growth disturbance are well known.

Metaphyseal and epiphyseal avulsion fractures vary in their prognoses:

Epiphyseal avulsion fractures (Fig. 13) cause no problems other than instability. With proper treatment (Fig. 14) that leaves the epiphyseal plate intact, iatrogenic growth arrest is not a danger since the actual growth area is not violated.

Metaphyseal avulsion fractures, such as avulsions of the lateral collateral ligament from the epicondyle, may lead to *valgus deformity* due to the formation of a callus bridge between the epiphysis and metaphysis (Fig. 15).

Besides deformities in the *frontal plane*, growth disturbance is also possible in the *sagittal plane*. An example is genu recurvatum caused by an anteroposterior growth discrepancy from premature apophyseodesis of the tibial tuberosity (Fig. 16).

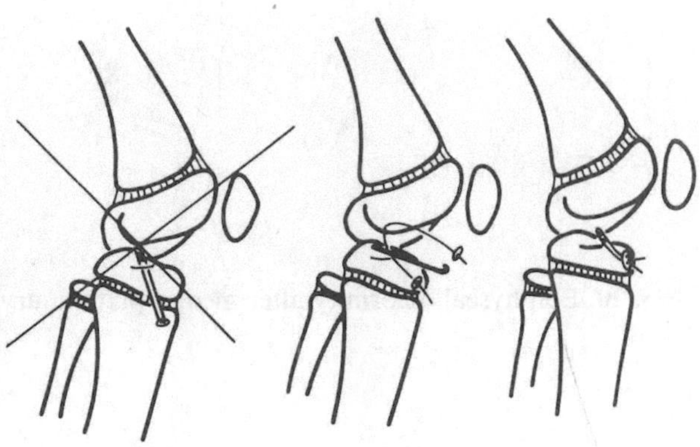

Fig. 14. Principle of the treatment of epiphyseal avulsion fractures: Screws should not violate the tibial tuberosity or the epiphyseal plate

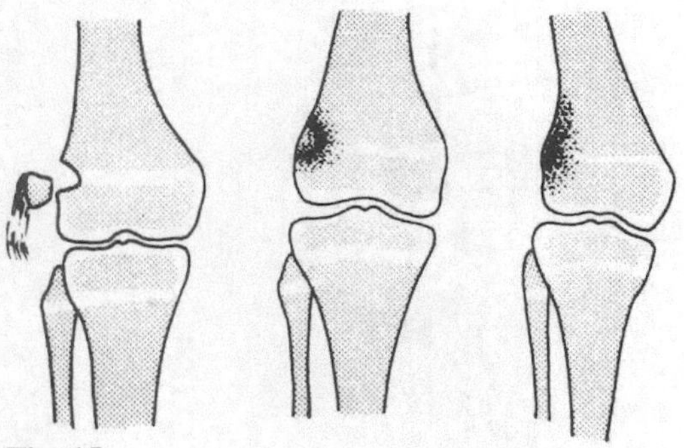

Fig. 15

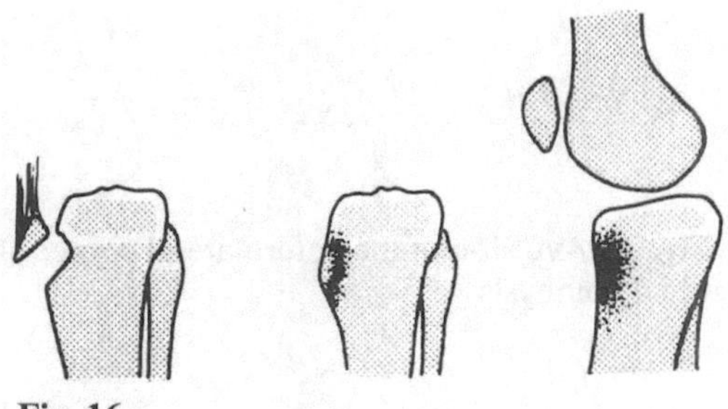

Fig. 16

Fig. 15. Metaphyseal avulsion fracture. Here: Avulsion of the lateral collateral ligament from the femoral epicondyle → valgus deformity

Fig. 16. Apophyseodesis of the tibial tuberosity leads to genu recurvatum

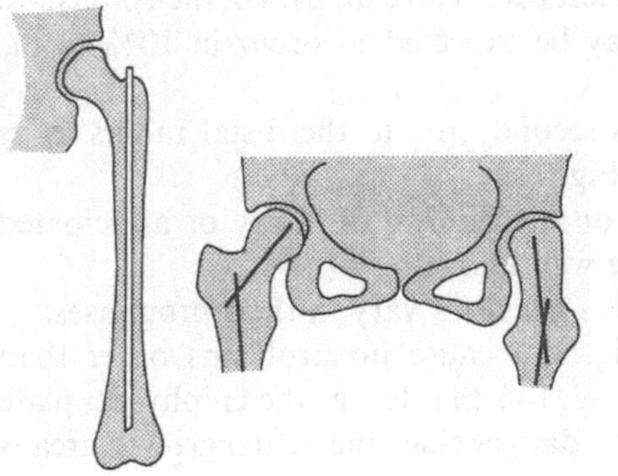

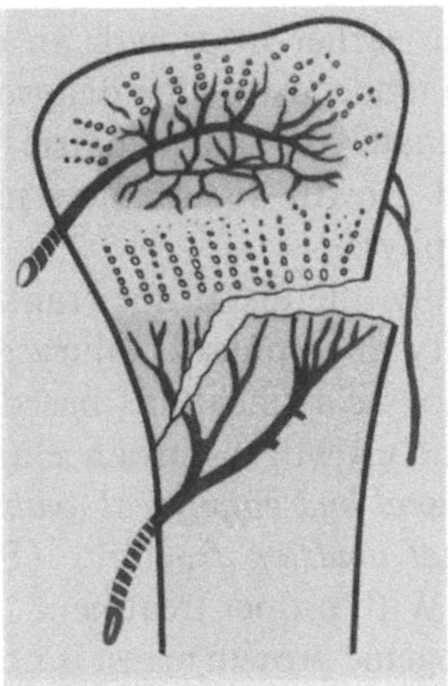

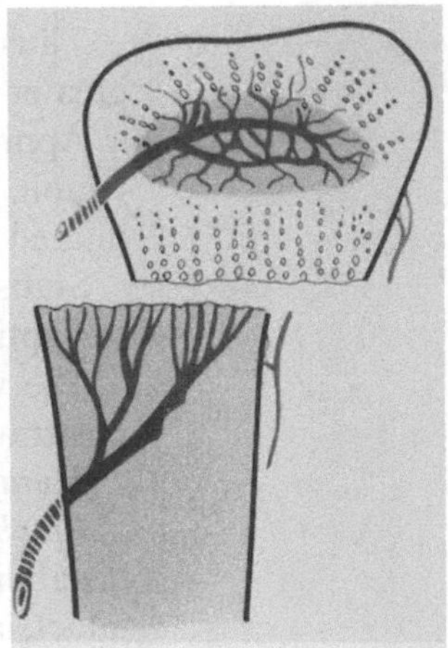

Fig. 17 **Fig. 18** **Fig. 19**

Fig. 17. Apophyseodesis of the greater trochanter (e.g., from improper medullary nailing) leads to coxa valga
Fig. 18. Fracture-separation of the epiphysis with a metaphyseal fragment
Fig. 19. Simple separation of the epiphysis without metaphyseal involvement

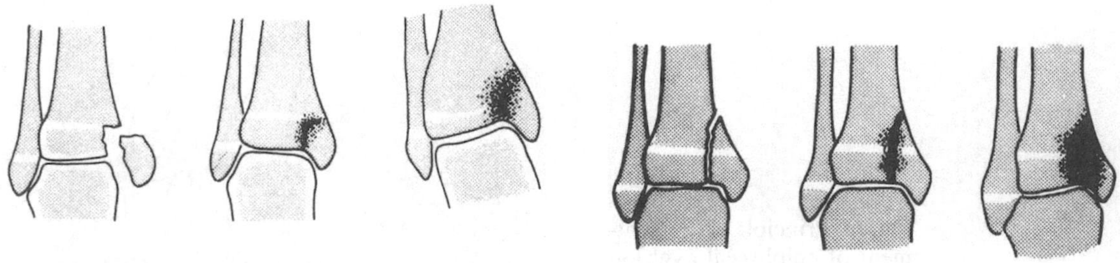

Fig. 20. Epiphyseal deformity after medial plate injury in the distal tibia → varus deformity

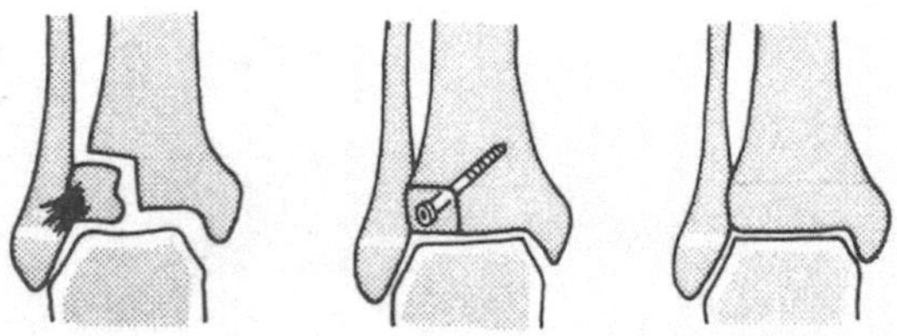

Fig. 21. Avulsion of the anterolateral corner of the tibial epiphysis

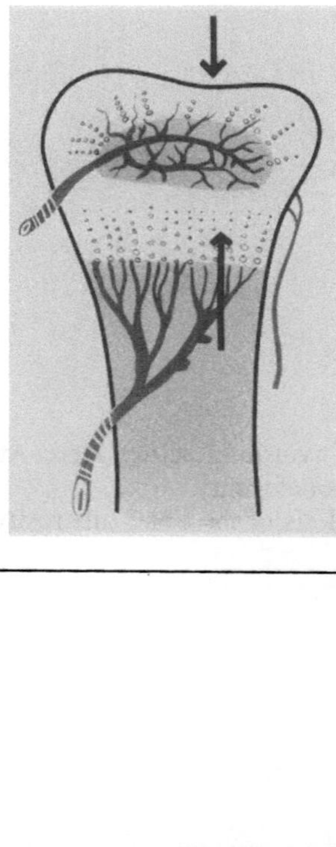

Fig. 22. Axial compression as the mechanism of crushing injury to the epiphyseal plate

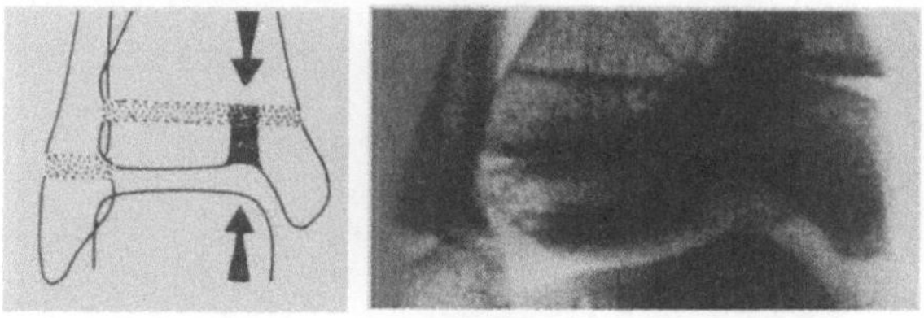

Fig. 23. Right: Roentgenogram of a crushing injury with osseous bridging. Left: The mechanism of the injury by axial compression

Apophyseodesis of the greater trochanter, like that caused by improper intra-medullary nailing, produces a *coxa valga* deformity (Fig. 17).

Separations of the epiphysis with (Gig. 18) and without (Fig. 19) a metaphyseal fragment do not involve the germinal layer of the plate and generally do not cause growth disturbance.

The *majority* of epiphyseal deformities are located in the distal tibia. Most plate injuries occur on the *medial* side and result in *varus deformity* (Fig. 20).

The *valgus deformity* that would be expected after avulsion fractures of the anterolateral corner of the tibial epiphysis (Fig. 21) is rarely observed, because this type of injury (transitional fracture) occurs exclusively at an age when physiologic plate closure is mostly complete. If bridging occurs between the epiphysis and metaphysis with no radiologic evidence of primary injury, it may be assumed that a crushing injury has been sustained (Figs. 22 and 23). The bony bar inhibits growth in the area of the former injury.

It is hoped that our systematic treatment and theoretical discussion will serve as a useful introduction to the clinical contributions that follow.

Growth Disturbances after Injuries Outside the Epiphysis

K. H. Jungblut

The postnatal longitudinal growth of long bones is confined to the epiphyses and occurs almost entirely in the transitional region between the epiphyseal cartilage and the metaphysis.

Latitudinal (diametric) growth and remodeling of the long bones, on the other hand, are dependent on the osteoblastic and osteoclastic activities of the periosteal and endosteal systems.

With closure of the epiphyseal plates, the skeleton is mature and there is a cessation of endochondral ossification and longitudinal growth. However, functional adaptation through bone resorption and deposition, known also as "remodeling," continues largely as before in accordance with the transformation law postulated by Wolf [8] in 1982.

The following factors regulate the growth of the pediatric skeleton and have causal significance in growth disturbance:
1. stimulation of longitudinal growth,
2. inhibition of longitudinal growth,
3. unilateral acceleration of growth,
4. unilateral retardation of growth.

Stimulation of Longitudinal Growth

Ollier [5], in 1867, demonstrated clinically and experimentally the stimulation of longitudinal bone growth after periosteal injuries and especially after fractures. Since then a great many authors have confirmed and supplemented these observations. The phenomenon is equally common after the operative and conservative treatment of diaphyseal fractures. It is attributed to hyperemia and increased vascularization in the adjacent epiphyseal and metaphyseal tissues. The degree of growth stimulation depends on various factors, including the duration and extent of the increased blood flow. The implantation of internal fixation material, fracture nonunions, delayed unions, and infectious processes can perpetuate the hyperemic condition and provides a powerful stimulus for increased longitudinal growth.

Of 125 children with femoral shaft fractures treated by overhead traction or ordinary drill-wire traction between 1966 and 1972, 75 were available for follow-up more than 6 years after their injuries (Table 1). In one-third of the cases, roentgenographic measurements indicated a femoral length discrepancy in excess of 1.0 cm. Eighteen patients had 1.0 – 2.0 cm of leg lengthening, and 5 others had lengthening of 2.0 – 3.0 cm. Shortening was present in only two

Corrective Osteotomies of the Lower Extremity
Edited by G. Hierholzer, K. H. Müller

Table 1. Femoral shaft Fractures in Children: Length Discrepancies Measured on Roentgenograms. n = 25 ($33^1/_3$%)

cm	Lengthening	Shortening
1.1 – 1.5	8	1
1.6 – 2.0	10	1
2.1 – 2.5	4	
2.6 – 3.0	1	
	23	2

Table 2. Average Overgrowth after a Femoral Fracture (Weber)

Age less than 4 years	0.5 – 1.0 cm
Age 4 – 6 years	1.0 – 1.5 cm
Age 6 – 8 years	1.5 – 2.0 cm
Over 8 years	0.5 – 1.0 cm

Table 3. Frequency of Posttraumatic Leg Lengthening for Different Types of Femural Fracture

Transverse fractures	62%
Oblique fractures	41%
Spiral fractures	37%

patients. Increased longitudinal growth was mainly observed in children who had sustained their fractures between 4 and 8 years of age. Weber [7] confirms that the average overgrowth tends to be particularly high in this age range (Table 2). We observed a definite relationship between posttraumatic lengthening and fracture type. Lengthening was most common after transverse fractures, followed by oblique and spiral fractures (Table 3). No relationship was apparent between posttraumatic growth rate and the location of the fracture.

Compared with the femur, accelerated growth is far less pronounced after fractures of the tibia [7]. The average discrepancies range from 2 mm in transverse fractures to 5 – 6 mm in oblique fractures to a maximum of 10 – 13 mm following segmental and comminuted fractures. Discrepancies of this magnitude have relatively little impact on the statics of the limb.

Inhibition of Longitudinal Growth

Next to infectious lesions of the epiphysis, prolonged ischemia is the most frequent cause of the posttraumatic shortening of bone.

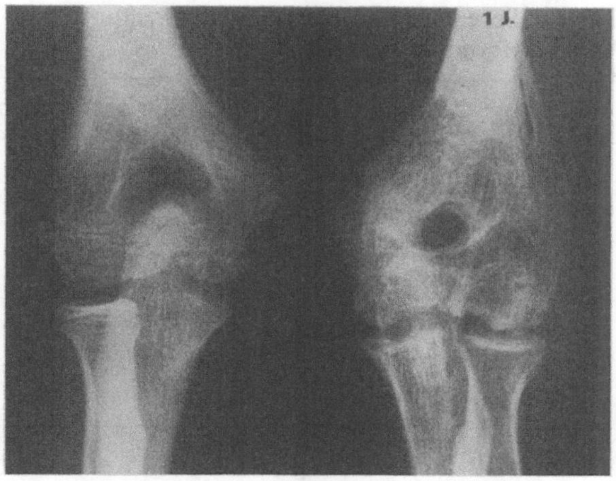

Fig. 1. This patient suffered a supracondylar fracture of the left humerus with injury of the brachial artery and prolonged ischemia, resulting in early closure of the epiphyses at the elbow

A supracondylar fracture of the humerus in an 11-year-old boy was accompanied by a laceration of the brachial artery. Primary repair of the artery was carried out. The repair was followed by secondary occlusion and protracted ischemia, resulting in significant soft-tissue contractures as well as premature growth plate closure at the elbow joint 1 year after injury. The humerus and forearm each showed 2 cm of shortening at the end of skeletal growth (Fig. 1).

Occasionally, spontaneous premature closure of the epiphyseal plate is described in the literature as a compensatory mechanism by which previously accelerated growth is corrected.

We have been unable to confirm this phenomenon, and we feel that, as a general rule, a spontaneous closure of this type cannot be relied upon.

Longitudinal growth can be temporarily or permanently arrested artificially by the Blount technique of epiphyseal stapling. The compressive forces exerted by the staples on the growth plate exceed the growth pressure of the tissue, and proliferation is halted.

Unilateral Acceleration of Growth

A localized, unilateral acceleration of bone growth occurs physiologically during skeletal maturation as the original varus position of the lower extremity is gradually converted to one of valgus.

This same mechanism can correct residual angular deformities after fractures. The younger the child, the greater the potential amount of spontaneous correction. This capacity for spontaneous correction shows a rapid and continuous decline after 10 years of age.

Among the 75 femoral shaft fractures that were followed, 12 varus deformities were noted at the conclusion of treatment (Table 4). At follow-up it was found that 10 of these deformities had corrected spontaneously. The remaining two patients showed minor degrees of improvement.

Table 4. Seventy-Five Femoral Shaft Fractures
Varus Deformities n = 12 (16%)

	End of treatment	Follow-up
Children under 5 years of age, n = 4	7°	–
	8°	–
	6°	6°
	10°	–
Children 10–15 years of age, n = 3	10°	–
	10°	–
	12°	–
Children 10–15 years of age, n = 5	8°	–
	10°	–
	14°	–
	14°	–
	22°	20°

Table 5. Seventy-Five Femoral Shaft Fractures
Valgus Deformities n = 21 (28%)

	End of treatment	Follow-up
Children under 5 years of age, n = 7	6°	–
	6°	–
	6°	–
	8°	–
	12°	–
	14°	–
	0°	6°
Children 5–10 years of age, n = 12	8°	8°
	5°	–
	6°	–
	8°	–
	8°	6°
	8°	7°
	10°	–
	10°	10°
	12°	–
	12°	–
	14°	–
	Unknown	6°
Children 10–15 years of age, n = 1	8°	–
Children over 15 years of age, n = 1	6°	10°

The valgus deformities, which were more prevalent, showed less favorable spontaneous outcomes (Table 5). In four cases spontaneous improvement was absent or minimal. In 1 patient over 15 years of age the valgus deformity increased slightly, and 2 children under 10 years of age who had no deformity when discharged subsequently developed a valgus deformity of 6–8° as a result of aberrant growth.

It is apparent that valgus deformities have less of a tendency to correct spontaneously than varus deformities.

It is also interesting to compare residual sagittal-plane deformities in this series. Residual forward displacement that was present at the end of treatment resolved completely in 14 cases and improved markedly in 1 case (Table 6). Among the 21 patients with backward displacement, 5 showed little or no improvement at follow-up (Table 7). In 1 patient over 15 years of age we found a marked progression of backward displacement from 6° to 19°.

It may be concluded that forward displacements secondary to pediatric femoral shaft fractures have a greater tendency to correct spontaneously than do backward displacements, and that the latter have a higher association with true growth disturbance.

The potential of various angular deformities of the tibia for spontaneous correction has been investigated by Weber [7]. Again, this potential is

Table 6. Seventy-Five Femoral Shaft Fractures
Forward Displacement n = 15 (20%)

	End of treatment	Follow-up
Children under 5 years of age, n = 8	6°	–
	6°	–
	8°	–
	8°	–
	8°	–
	8°	–
	10°	5°
	16°	–
Children 5–10 years of age, n = 3	6°	–
	10°	–
	16°	–
Children 10–15 years of age, n = 4	6°	–
	10°	–
	10°	–
	16°	–
Children over 15 years of age, n = 0	–	–

Seventy-Five Femoral Shaft Fractures
Rotational deformities exceeding 10°
n = 2 (2.6%) Internal rotation 17°
External rotation 21°

Table 7. Seventy-Five Femoral Shaft Fractures
Backward Displacement n=21 (28%)

	End of treatment	Follow-up
Children under 5 years of age, n=8	12°	–
	12°	–
	14°	–
	17°	–
	18°	12°
	20°	–
	24°	–
	24°	–
Children 5–8 years of age, n=11	12°	–
	12°	–
	12°	–
	12°	–
	12°	14°
	14°	–
	16°	–
	Unknown	16°
	18°	–
	20°	–
	40°	30°
Children 10–15 years of age, n=1	18°	18°
Children over 15 years of age, n=1	6°	19°

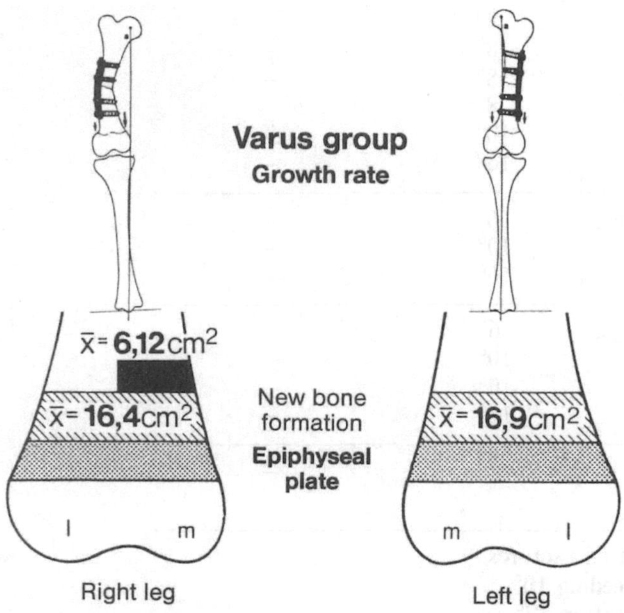

Fig. 2. Rate of asymmetric bone growth after osteotomy and varus angulation (20°) in experimental dogs

markedly higher for varus deformities than for valgus, and the capacity for corrections in the sagittal plane is minimal.

In the lower extremity, the epiphyseal plate has an excellent capacity for the correction of angular deformities under conditions of static loading. According to Pauwels [6] the plate corrects its alignment through eccentric growth until it is perpendicular to the resultant of the pressure forces created by muscular tension and body weight.

Together with Mommsen [4] and Dallek [1], we have been able to elucidate some biomechanical and anatomical principles that underlie the spontaneous correction of osseous deformities. Valgus angulation of the lower extremity exerts increased compressive forces on the fibular side, while varus angulation increases compression on the tibial side. Autoradiographic experiments were conducted in rats that had and induced varus or valgus deformity of the right hindlimb. Thymidine labeling revealed an increase of cellular proliferation on the side with the greater pressure load. This increased proliferation was evident on the fibular side of the epiphyseal plate in the valgus limb, and on the tibial side in the varus limb [4].

A similar experiment was performed in lambs in which both femora were osteotomized and plated after first manipulating the right femur into 20° of valgus or varus angulation. In each case fluorescent microscopy revealed an increase of bone deposition in the longitudinal direction in the pressure-load half of the epiphysis [4] (Figs. 2 and 3).

In another experiment we used polarized light to demonstrate the orientation of collagen fibrils in the epiphyseal plate [2]. In the columnar region of the plate, the fibrils are aligned in the direction of the prevailing

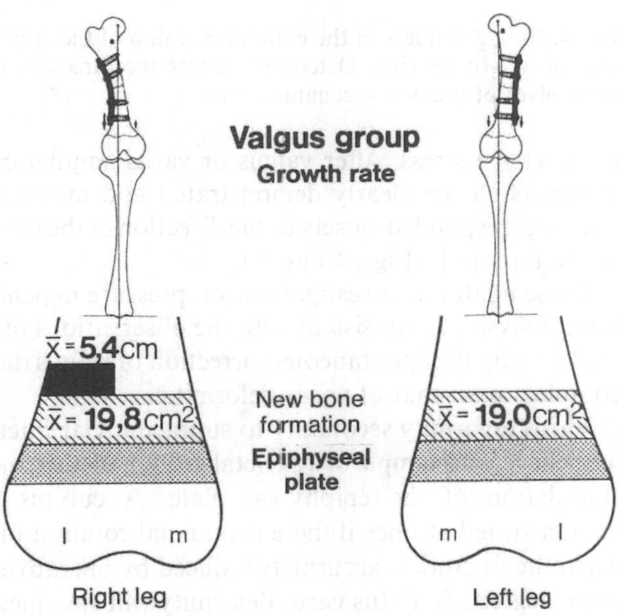

Fig. 3. Rate of asymmetric bone growth after osteotomy and valgus angulation (20°) in experimental dogs

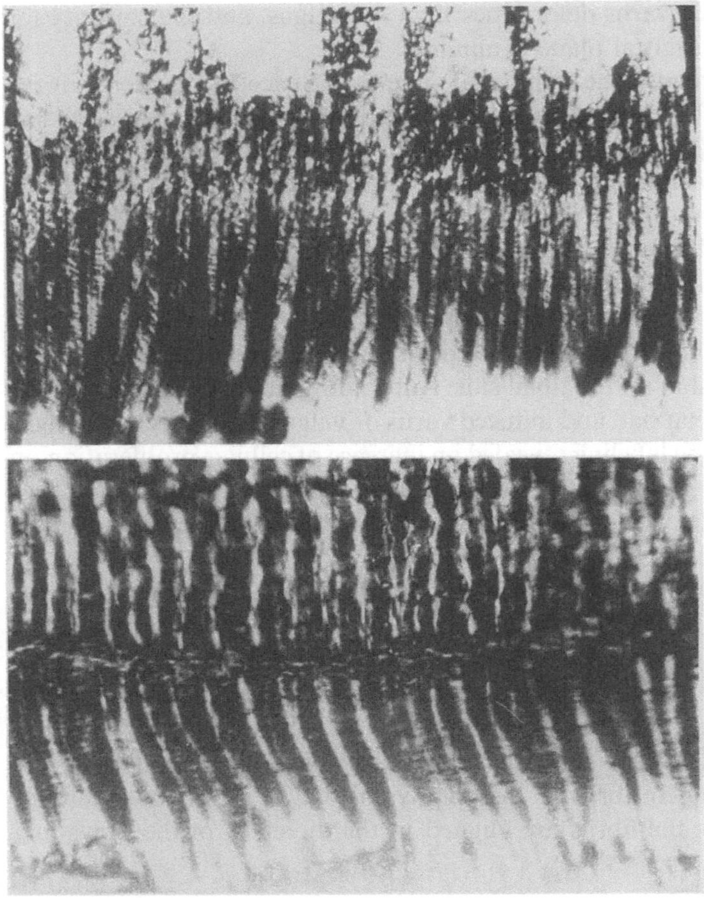

Fig. 4. Collagen fibers in the columnar region of the epiphysis are oriented along the axis of weight bearing. Osteotomy alters the direction of the fibers, which realign themselves of the new mechanical axis

compressive stress. After valgus or varus angulation, a reorientation of the system could be clearly demonstrated and measured. The direction of the fibrils corresponded closely to the direction of the new, altered mechanical axis of the limb [4] (Figs. 4 and 5).

These anatomic investigations on pressure-dependent growth processes in the epiphysis are consistent with the observations of Pauwels, but they fail to explain why the spontaneous correction of valgus deformities tends to be less complete than that of varus deformities.

Varus deformity secondary to supracondylar fractures of the humerus are, we believe, an example of a skeletal growth disturbance caused by asymmetric stimulation of the epiphyseal plate. A cubitus varus position can be demonstrated at once if there is minimal rotation of the fragments, but even when the fracture is accurately reduced by operative or nonoperative means, some degree of cubitus varus deformity will sbsequently develop in 20–40% of cases. Like other authors, we have found that the deformity shows no tendency toward progression once the fracture has united.

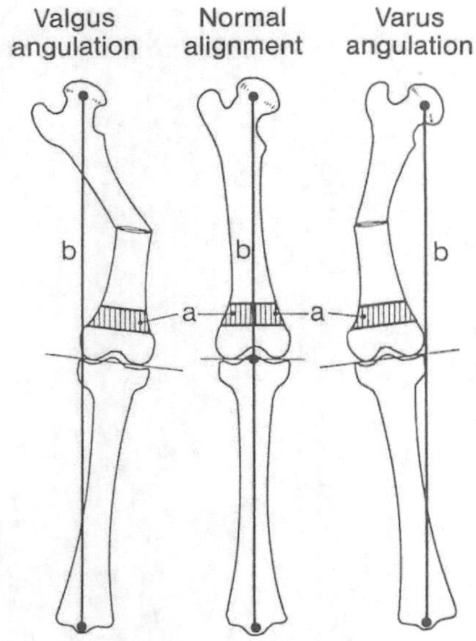

Fig. 5. Schematic representation of the change in collagen fiber orientation that occurs when the mechanical axis is altered by valgus or varus osteotomy

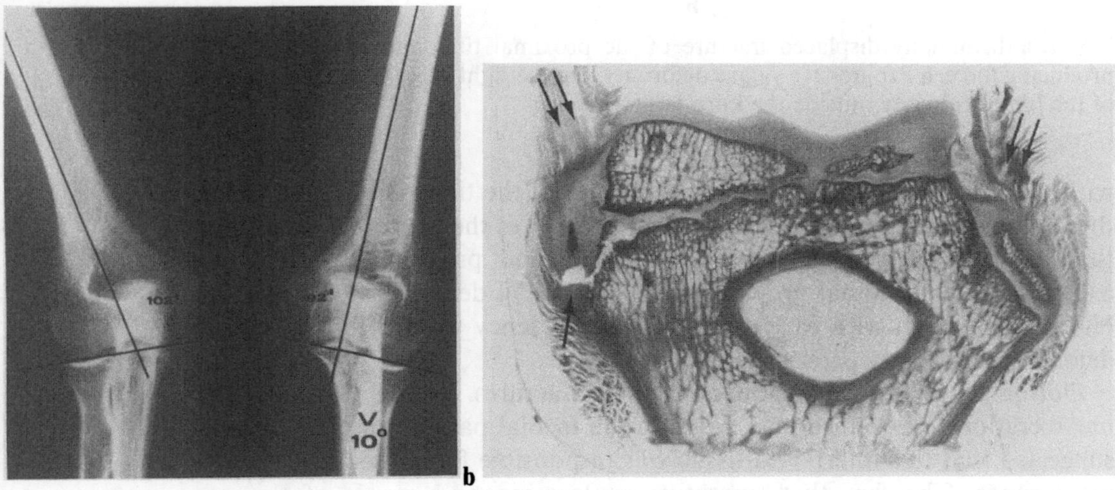

a b

Fig. 6. a This cubitus varus deformity followed on a perfectly reduced supracondylar fracture of the left humerus. **b** Asymmetric position of the ossification centers of the distal humerus. Hyperemia may account for the disproportionate growth on the radial side

One possible explanation for this pehenomenon may be an asymmetric anlage of the epiphyseal plate. Up to the age of about 11 years, only the radial part of the distal humeral epiphysis possesses an ossification center, while the trochlea on the ulnar side is still cartilaginous and lacks a true blood supply. As a result, the hyperemia that is induced by trauma and healing exerts a greater stimulative effect on the radial part of the epiphysis than on the ulnar trochlea (Fig. 6).

A special problem is posed by high tibial fractures caused by valgus-producing forces (Fig. 7 a). Fractures of this type have a very high association

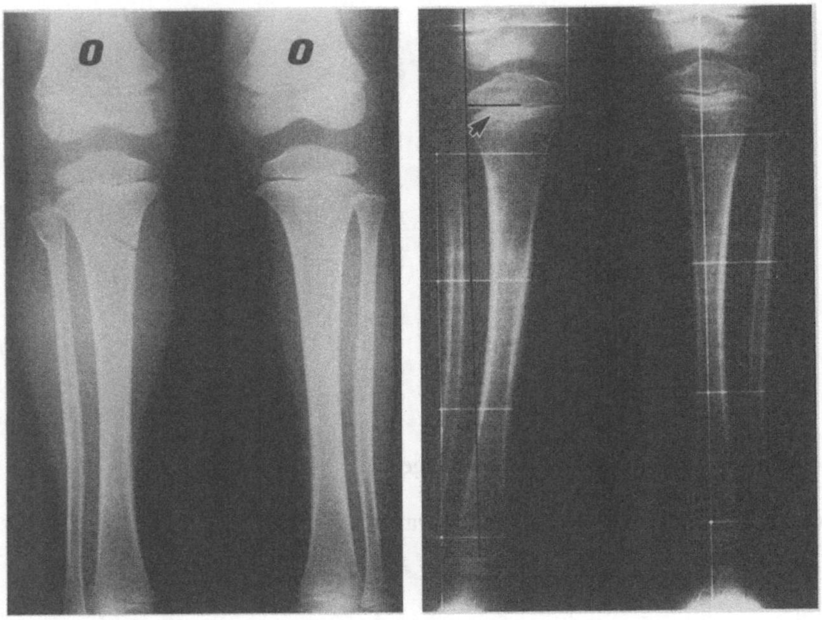

a b

Fig. 7. a Minimally displaced fracture of the proximal tibia caused by a valgus-producing force. **b** Progressive valgus deformity. On the right side the mechanical axis of the limb is already outside the knee joint (*arrow*)

with marked and refractory valgus deformity of the tibia (Fig. 7 b). Often there is an increase in cortical density at the level of the fracture. Distally the tibia becomes bowed as growth progresses, and proximally there is an asymmetric longitudinal growth which Weber [7] demonstrated using the Harris lines. Even with early osteotomy, a tendency toward further valgus deformity frequently persists.

During the operative treatment of these fractures, Weber [7] noted the incarceration of pes anserinus tissue in the medial part of the fracture and suggested that this interposed tissue was responsible for subsequent growth disturbance. The fact that operative exploration and repair of the pes anserinus prevented growth disturbance was accepted by Weber as proof of his theory.

Weber [7] as well as Klapp [3] see causal significance in the loss of the checkrein action of the pes anserinus on the periosteum. Klapp [3] suggests that the resultant loss of compression on the medial side of the epiphyseal plate serves as a stimulus for epiphyseal growth.

This concept is difficult to reconcile with clinical and experimental evidence that the epiphyseal plate responds to physiologic compression with increased growth.

Other pathophysiologic interpretations appear to be more plausible:

1. Injury to the periosteum in the region of the pes anserinus incites a local hyperemia in the medial portion of the tibial epiphysis, causing an asymmetric increase of longitudinal growth on the medial side.

2. There is a general stimulation of longitudinal growth in the proximal tibial epiphysis. But the powerful lateral checkrein effect about the knee from the combined action of the iliotibial tract and collateral ligament generates forces which exceed the physiologic, growth-stimulating amount. The result is an inhibition of growth on the lateral side.

Both explanations are supported by the fact that these progressive valgus deformities of the proximal tibia are associated with an overall increase in tibial length.

Summary

The tendency of deformities after metaphyseal and diaphyseal fractures to correct spontaneously in children depends on remaining growth potential, displacement and the primary degree of deformity at skeletal maturity. Because of these variables, spontaneous mechanisms do not always restore a normal skeletal configuration.

At the same time, the absence of some spontaneous improvement after epiphyseal and metaphyseal fractures is as rare as a true growth disturbance, i.e., a growth-related progression of the deformity.

Growth disturbances are known to relate to general or localized changes of epiphyseal blood flow due to trauma, with hyperemia being associated with growth stimulation and ischemia with growth inhibition. A special case is the greenstick abduction fracture of the proximal tibia. The pathophysiology of the valgus growth disturbance that consistently follows this injury has not been satisfactorily explained.

References

1. Dallek M, Jungbluth KH, Holstein AF (1983) Studies of the arrangement of the collagenous fibres in infant epiphyseal plates using polarized light and the scanning electron microscope. Arch Orthop Trauma Surg 101:239–245
2. Jungbluth KH, Dallek M, Mommsen U (1980) Die Bedeutung der Kollagenfasertextur der distalen Humerusepiphyse für die Verlaufsrichtung der Kondylenfrakturen. Hefte Unfallheilkd 148:424–427
3. Klapp F, Seiler H, Feth G (1982) Einfluß des Periosts auf das Längenwachstum von Röhrenknochen. Hefte Unfallheilkd 158:60–62
4. Mommsen U, Jungbluth KH, Dallek M (1981) Zur Korrektur von Achsenfehlstellungen langer Röhrenknochen am wachsenden Skelett – experimentelle Untersuchungen. Aktuel Probl Chir Orthop 20:69–72
5. Ollier L (1867) Traité experimental et clinique de la régénération des os de la production artificielle du tissu ossent, Vol 1. Masson, Paris
6. Pauwels F (1965) Gesammelte Abhandlungen zur funktionellen Anatomie des Bewegungsapparates. Springer, Berling Heidelberg New York
7. Weber BG, Brunner C, Freuler F (1978) Frakturbehandlung bei Kindern und Jugendlichen. Springer, Berlin Heidelberg New York
8. Wolf J (1892) Das Gesetz der Transformation der Knochen. Hirschwald, Berlin

Indications and Techniques of Osteotomies Near Joints

J. Müller-Färber and K. H. Müller

Introduction

Posttraumatic deformity in the growing patient differs from that in the adult in two contrasting respects: One is the potential for spontaneous correction of the deformity; the other is a tendency for the deformity to progress.

While osseous healing in the adult "fixes" a deformity that follows the closed or open treatment of a fracture, angular deformities after diaphyseal and metaphyseal fractures in children may correct spontaneously to some degree. This means that one must be cautious about the use of corrective surgery in this group. If an indication for surgery exists, a deformity of this type can be corrected by a single operation [11].

On the other hand, there are some types of posttraumatic growth disturbance which either increase during growth or become manifest only later in the course of longitudinal growth. These changes are the result of a disturbance in the function of the growth plate caused either by direct damage to the plate itself or indirectly, as by a fracture of the upper tibial metaphysis [3].

Depending on the nature and severity of the plate injury or dysfunction, the growth disturbance may increase causing serious deformities to develop as skeletal growth progresses. Accordingly, the age of the patient at the time of injury critically influences the amount of deformity that occurs after metaphyseal and diaphyseal fractures as well as fractures that affect the function of the epiphyseal plate.

Because the potential for spontaneous correction declines sharply after the age of 10 – 12 years, deformities after periarticular metaphyseal fractures cannot be expected to correct spontaneously after the age of 12, and operative treatment may be indicated. On the other hand, epiphyseal plate injuries during puberty, i.e., shortly before the end of skeletal growth (at which time 75% of growth plate injuries occur), cause minor growth disturbances that are not clinically significant and do not require operative intervention [3].

Before the age of 10 – 12 years, a growth disturbance based on an epiphyseal plate injury should still be corrected during the growth years because of the significant cartilage damage that can result from unphysiologic loading of the affected joints. Moreover, continuation of the aberrant growth will lead to major deformities that are much more difficult to correct later on. When surgery is elected in such cases, the likelihood of recurrences must be acknowledged. It may be necessary to repeat the operation one or more times

Corrective Osteotomies of the Lower Extremity
Edited by G. Hierholzer, K. H. Müller

until skeletal maturity is attained, and the parents should be informed of this possibility.

With all angular deformities, the affected limb is examined for the presence of concomitant lengthening or shortening. If a discrepancy in limb lengths is noted, the angulation must be corrected by means of a lengthening or shortening osteotomy.

A shortening osteotomy without angular correction should not be attempted until the patient is skeletally mature, at which time the true extent of posttraumatic lengthening can be appreciated. Corrective operations should always be preceded by a thorough clinical examination providing information on axial relationships, joint mobility, limb length, and possible fixed deformities of the spine resulting from the angulation [10].

Additional prerequisites are comparative roentgenograms of both lower extremities taken in identical projections to assess axial and articular relationships, and full-length standing roentgenograms to define the leg axes [7]. Drawings are made from the roentgenograms indicating the details of the proposed osteotomy and the result of the correction.

The Proximal Femur

Posttraumatic deformities of the proximal femur are most commonly observed after pertrochanteric and subtrochanteric fractures. Often there is significant varus deformity with backward displacement and retroversion of the femoral neck [11]. The associated limb shortening leads to a corresponding disturbance of statics.

Internal fixation of the proximal femur in children carries a significant risk of injury to the growth plates of the femoral neck or greater trochanter from a intramedullary nail or angled blade plate [12]. The typical result is a coxa valga deformity, whose severity depends on the age of the patient at the time of injury.

During the growth period, the function of the hip joint usually remains intact despite significant deformity of the proximal femur, although this should not be taken as justification for a wait-and-see approach. It is very likely that the effects of the altered statics on the abnormally positioned femoral head will lead to chondropathy and joint destruction. Furthermore, the proximal femur shows little potential for spontaneous correction, even in injuries that do not involve the growth plates [11]. If a relatively minor deformity develops in an older child, corrective osteotomy should be deferred until the cessation of skeletal growth. At that time the osteotomy is performed on the proximal femur according to standard principles followed in adults [6].

In corrective osteotomies of the proximal femur during growth, care must be taken that the implants do not injure the epiphyseal plates. Also, care is taken to use implants of appropriate size to minimize the destruction of osseous tissue. Corrective osteotomy for a femoral neck deformity should be done in the intertrochanteric region so that the position of the lesser trochanter will not be altered [12]. Numerous methods are available for the fixation of intertrochanteric osteotomies in children. The simplest according to Wagner is external fixation with Schanz screws, which are placed in accordance with the desired angle of correction.

For a varus osteotomy in hard bone, a medially based wedge is resected. In soft bone it is sufficient to align and impact the fragments without resecting a bone wedge [12]. The main advantage of the latter method is that it avoids extensive denudation of the bone surface. A disadvantage is the need for postoperative immobilization in plaster.

By contrast, internal fixation with a small angled-blade plate provides a stability that will allow early postoperative mobilization. Wagner [12] recommends that intertrochanteric osteotomies in children under 8 years of age be fixed with the modified hook plate of Becker, and in children over 8 years of age with the 90° angled blade plate of the ASIF (available as a "pediatric hip plate" for 8- to 12-year old children).

Valgus osteotomies of the femur tend to be difficult in the pediatric age group because the growth plate of the greater trochanter leaves little room for insertion of the seating chisel. In these cases the osteotomy can be fixed with Kirschner wires as described by Wagner for the treatment of congenital coxa vara. In this method two Kirschner wires are inserted into the femoral neck just distal to the growth plate of the greater trochanter and are clamped against the femoral shaft with a pair of one-third tubular plates. Another Kirschner wire is inserted obliquely across the osteotomy to prevent secondary migration of the fragments [12]. Corrective osteotomies after

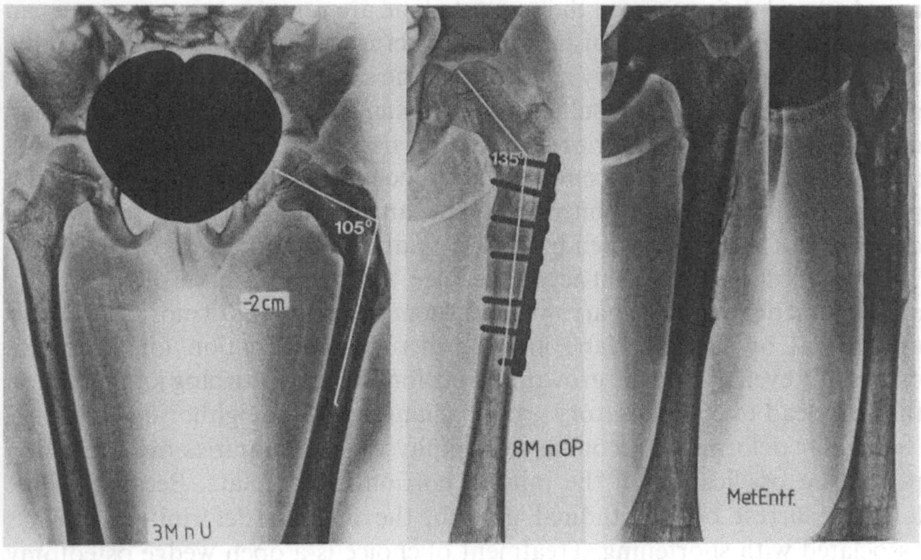

a b c

Fig. 1 a–c. a Seven-year-old girl (E.P.) 3 months after conservative treatment of subtrochanteric femoral fracture. Varus deformity with 105° CCD angle, backward displacement of femoral neck, and 2 cm of shortening. **b** Subtrochanteric wedge osteotomy stabilized with a narrow plate. **c** Anatomic axial relationships in frontal and sagittal planes after removal of fixation material

subtrochanteric fractures are less problematic, for the osteotomy and fixation are performed in the metaphysis and thus at a distance from the growth plates. The osteotomy can be fixed with a narrow plate (Fig. 1).

The Distal Femur

Growth disturbances secondary to epiphyseal plate injuries of the distal femur have serious effects on the position of the knee joint, and even minor disturbances can create an unequal load distribution that is damaging to articular cartilage. Angular deformities of 5–10° in the frontal or sagittal plane are considered to be an indication for corrective osteotomy [10].

Because growth changes in this region are usually associated with limb shortening, the open wedge osteotomy is preferred. Supracondylar osteotomies should not be fixed with angled blade plates before the growth plates have closed, and so Kirschner wires supplemented by plaster immobilization have to be employed.

The Proximal Tibia

We recognize two types of posttraumatic growth disturbance involving the proximal tibia: that caused by epiphyseal plate injuries, and genu valgum secondary to metaphyseal fractures.

The relatively rare epiphyseal plate injuries of the proximal tibia lead to progressive growth disturbance with an alteration of limb length and knee axis. Isolated deformities in the sagittal plane are rare. Genu recurvatum can occur as the indirect result of an evulsion fracture of the tibial tuberosity or the insertion of a intramedullary nail through the anterior part of the upper tibial growth plate [10]. The results are hyperextensibility of the knee joint and chronic stretching of posterior ligamentous tissues. Most angular deformities in the sagittal plane are accompanied by a coexisting deformity in the frontal plane. The sagittal component may be an antecurvatum or recurvatum deformity of the knee, depending on the nature of the injury.

Given the large loads that act on the knee, the tolerance limits of a deformity at that joint are relatively narrow. Thus, angular deviations of more than 10° in the frontal or sagittal plane are considered an indication for corrective osteotomy even during the growth period, for besides disturbing joint function they can lead to compensatory growth changes in the neighboring epiphysis.

Angular deformities secondary to epiphyseal plate injuries are caused by permature ossification of the injured portion of the plate. Because of the localized arrest of longitudinal growth, the angular deformity is always associated with shortening. Treatment of choice is a open wedge osteotomy which lengthens the limb while restoring angular alignment.

If the deformity exceeds 20° and there is preexisting scarring, it may be best to perform the correction in stages with the aid of an external frame to avoid undue trauma to soft tissues, nerves and blood vessels [3]. This is especially recommended for valgus deformities.

In the second type of growth disturbance, genu valgum after fractures of the proximal tibial metaphysis, there is an acceleration of epiphyseal plate growth on the medial side resulting in angulation and lengthening.

Various theories have been advanced as to the causes of asymmetric growth disturbances of the proximal tibia (cf. article by Jungbluth). While we cannot discuss these theories here, we can point to the general agreement that exists regarding the value of corrective osteotomies for certain angular deformities in growing patients. There is considerably less agreement regarding the optimum timing of surgical intervention.

Most authors believe that a corrective osteotomy should be done at the earliest possible opportunity, first because they place little reliance on spontaneous corrections in this region, and second because a compensatory varus angulation may develop leading to an S-shaped deformity that would require correction at two levels [3,8,13].

After corrective osteotomy the valgus deformity will commonly recur and necessitate reoperation, especially in younger patients [1,4,9].

A different approach is recommended by von Laer et al. [2], who state that corrective osteotomy should be deferred until 1–2 years after the injury. These authors believe that the growth disturbances are based on a combination of the primary deformity with a consequent disturbance of fracture healing, resulting in a partial nonunion that stimulates growth in the medial part of the plate. The authors further state recurrences after corrective osteotomy are most likely caused by the same mechanism responsible for the uneven distribution of interfragmental compression. An osteotomy performed too far proximally for a mild preexisting valgus deformity or a lack of compression will then reinitiate the cycle of impaired medial fracture healing and medial stimulation of the plate. Consequently, the authors recommend that a relatively distal osteotomy be performed at the junction of the metaphysis and diaphysis, which will coincide with the vertex of the deformity 1–2 years after the injury.

Because the angular deformity is accompanied by lengthening, a wedge-resection osteotomy is advised. Fixation of the osteotomy with Kirschner wires supplemented by plaster should be adequate, especially in younger children. In older children and with a more distal osteotomy plane, a plate or external frame may be needed, depending on the condition of the soft tissues (Fig. 2). When plating is used, it must be remembered that screws inserted into the medullary canal can create an additional stimulus for growth [10].

The Distal Tibia

The distal tibia is a more frequent site of epiphyseal plate injuries and associated growth changes than the proximal tibia. Besides the familiar fracture types classified by Aitken, particular attention should be given to the compression fracture of the distal tibial epiphysis, which often is not appreciated in x-rays and may initially be regarded as innocuous [5].

With a direct, crushing injury to the growth plate or damage to the epiphyseal blood supply creating a trophic disturbance, a localized epi-

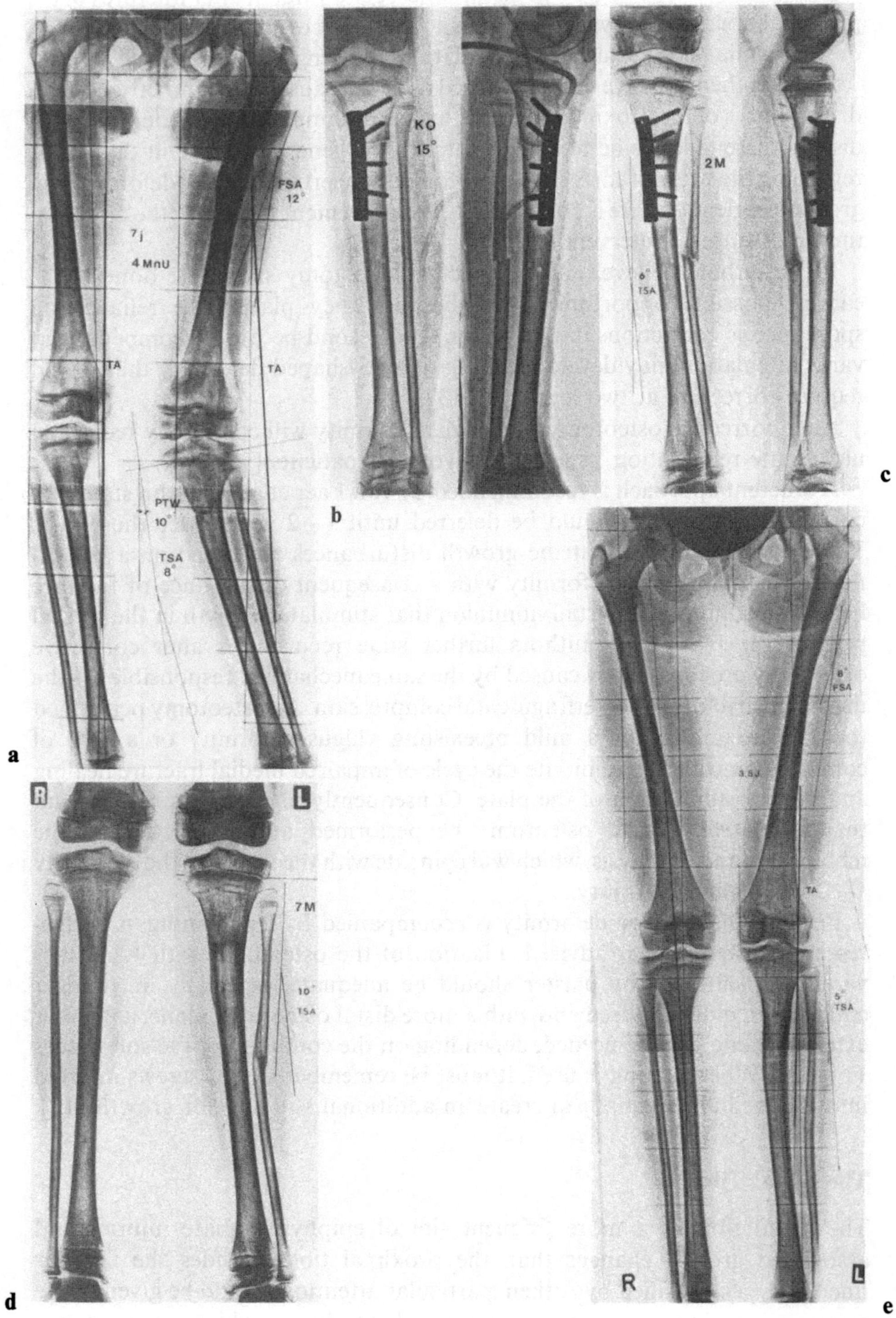
FSA
12°
4 MnU
TA
TA
PTW
10°
TSA
8°
a
KO
15°
b
2M
6°
TSA
c
R
L
7M
10
TSA
d
8°
FSA
TA
5°
TSA
R
L
e

physiodesis occurs that leads to asymmetric growth [3]. The result, depending on age at injury, is increasing angulation and shortening.

The surgical correction of this deformity should be undertaken during the growth period, both to spare the child years of functional disability and to prevent progression to more serious deformities that cannot be managed with a simple lengthening osteotomy [3].

According to Morscher and Jani [3], corrective osteotomy is indicated between 2 and 3 years after the primary injury. Longitudinal growth during this time is approximately 2–3 cm, enabling the angulation and shortening to be corrected with an open wedge osteotomy.

The osteotomy is performed in the metaphyseal region adjacent to the growth plate. We do not recommend a concurrent, permanent epiphysiodesis of the still-intact portions of the plate to prevent a recurrence, because considerable shortening can occur before cessation of growth. It is better to wait 2–3 years and perform another open wedge osteotomy as required. Of course, the operation may have to be repeated several times before the end of skeletal growth [3]. In almost all supramalleolar osteotomies it is necessary also to osteotomize the fibula to prevent undesired tension on the ankle mortise and tibiofibular syndesmosis [12].

When deformity is severe, it may not be possible to restore normal alignment right away, as this would place excessive tension on the soft tissues, nerves and vessels. In these cases the residual deformity can be corrected in a later operation [12].

If soft-tissue conditions are good, the narrow compression plate may be used to stabilize the osteotomy. Wedge-insertion osteotomies can be fixed with the buttress plate (spoon plate) of the ASIF.

If soft tissues are poor or the angle of correction is 20° or more, external skeletal fixation is preferred (Fig. 3). This will minimize the denudation of bone while avoiding the tension on soft tissues that would result from an internal fixation device.

◀

Fig. 2 a–e. a Girl (G. S.) 7 years of age with complex valgus deformity after conservative treatment of fractures of the left femoral shaft and proximal tibia. The mechanical axis (**TA**) lies outside the knee joint. The left leg is 1.5 cm longer than the right leg, which shows posttraumatic genu varum. The deformity of the left leg consists of a 12° valgus deformity of the femoral shaft (**FSA** femoral shaft axis) and an 18° combined valgus deformity of the proximal tibia, is composed of a valgus deformity at joint level (**PTW** proximal tibial angle) and at the junction of the metaphysis and diaphysis (**TSA** tibial shaft axis). **b** Shortening varus osteotomy with wedge resection at the junction of the tibial metaphysis and diaphysis. **c** Two months after osteotomy the **TSA** shows 6° of recurrent valgus angulation, whose vertex is at the distal end of the plate. Cause: growth stimulation by the implanted material. **d** Progression of angulation to 10°. Implants are removed at 4 months after osteotomy. **e** Result at 3.5 years after osteotomy (age 10.5 years). Spontaneous correction of the diaphyseal deformities is apparent but is inadequate; length discrepancy is 2.5 cm. Plan of treatment: Allow another 2 years for spontaneous recovery; at that time assess the need for a shortening varus osteotomy of the femur

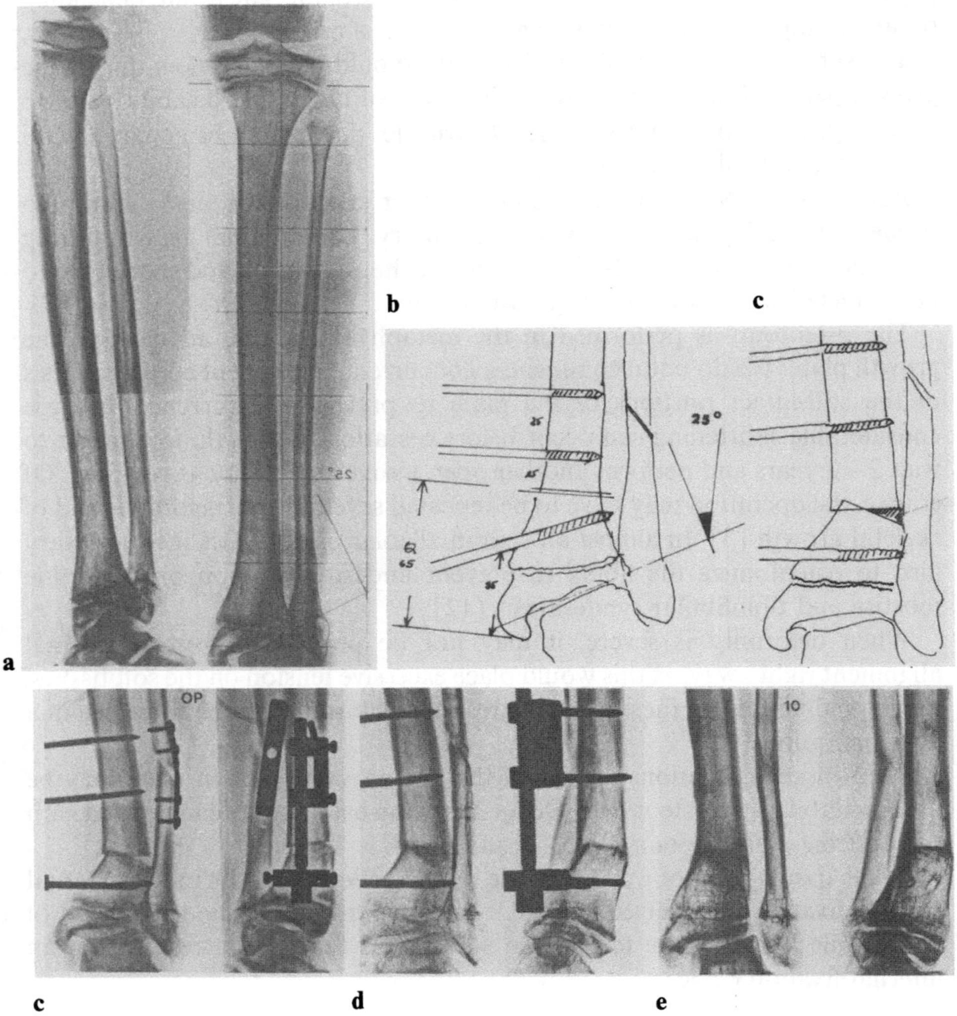

Fig. 3 a – e. Boy (Z. C.) 13 years of age who suffered an untreated ankle sprain about 2 years previously. Medical attention was sought for increasing "deformity" of the ankle mortise and pain in the area of the medial malleolus. **a** 25° Valgus deformity secondary to injury of the lateral part of the distal tibial growth plate and possibly of the lateral malleolus. Preoperative drawings **b** and operative result **c** of the supramalleolar varus osteotomy. The two Schanz screws flanking the osteotomy site define the angle of correction. The medial cortex of the distal fragment is impacted into the proximal fragment, and the lateral defect is filled with cancellous bone. Fibula is lengthened by oblique osteotomy. The tibial osteotomy is stabilized with the small threaded-rod external fixator of Müller, and the fibular osteotomy is fixed with a one-third tubular plate. **d,e** Roentgenograms taken at 3 and 10 months after corrective osteotomy. Additional angular correction and fibular lengthening may be necessary after the cessation of growth

References

1. Jackson DW, Cozen L (1971) Genu valgum as complication of proximal tibial metaphyseal fractures in children. J Bone Joint Surg [Am] 53:1571
2. Laer L von, Jani L, Cuny C, Jenny P (1982) Die proximale Unterschenkelfraktur im Wachstumsalter. Unfallheilkunde 85:215
3. Morscher E, Jani L (1977) Korrekturosteotomien bei posttraumatischen Wachstumsstörungen. Orthopäde 6:113
4. Müller KH, Biebrach M (1977) Korrekturosteotomien und ihre Ergebnisse bei Kniegelenknahen posttraumatischen Fehlstellungen. Unfallheilkunde 80:359
5. Müller ME, Ganz R (1974) Luxationen und Frakturen: Untere Gliedmaßen und Becken. In Rehn J (Hrsg) Unfallheilkunde bei Kindern. Springer, Berlin Heidelberg New York
6. Müller ME, Allgöwer M, Schneider R, Willenegger H (1977) Manual der Osteosynthese. Springer, Berlin Heidelberg New York
7. Oest O, Sieberg HJ (1971) Die Röntgenganzaufnahme der unteren Extremitäten. Z Orthop 109:54
8. Parsch K, Manner G, Dippe K (1977) Genu valgum nach proximaler Tibiafraktur beim Kind. Arch Orthop Unfallchir 90:289
9. Rettig H, Oest O (1971) Das Genu recurvatum als Folge der proximalen Tibiaapophysen-verletzung und die resultierende Valgusfehlstellung nach Fraktur im proximalen Tibiabereich. Arch Orthop Unfallchir 71:339
10. Rüter A, Burri C, Kreuzer U (1978) Korrektureingriffe nach Epiphysenverletzungen im Bereich des Kniegelenks. Unfallheilkunde 81:649
11. Tscherne H, Gotzen L (1978) Fehlstellungen im Wachstumsalter. In: Zenker R, Deucher F, Schink W (Hrsg) Chirurgie der Gegenwart, Bd 4 a, Beitrag 52. Urban & Schwarzenberg, München Wien Baltimore
12. Wagner H (1977) Prinzipien der Korrekturosteotomie am Bein. Orthopäde 6:145
13. Weber BG (1979) Die proximale metaphysäre Tibiafraktur. In: Weber BG, Brunner C, Freuler (Hrsg) Die Frakturenbehandlungen bei Kindern und Jugendlichen. Springer, Berlin Heidelberg New York D

Indications and Techniques of Diaphyseal Corrective Osteotomies after Trauma

K. P. Schmit-Neuerburg, J. Hanke and H. W. Hölter

Introduction

The main objective of fracture treatment in growing patients, as in adults, is to restore axial alignment in all three planes with equality of limb lengths. This applies equally to the femur and tibia. The reputed ability of the growing skeleton to correct even gross deformities prior to cessation of growth is true only to a limited degree and is influenced by three main factors [2,16,21,24]:

Age of the Child

Within limits, time and growth potential are able to correct even severe angular deformities in children under 10 years of age. The potential for spontaneous correction is minimal following the second growth spurt around age 10 (Fig. 1).

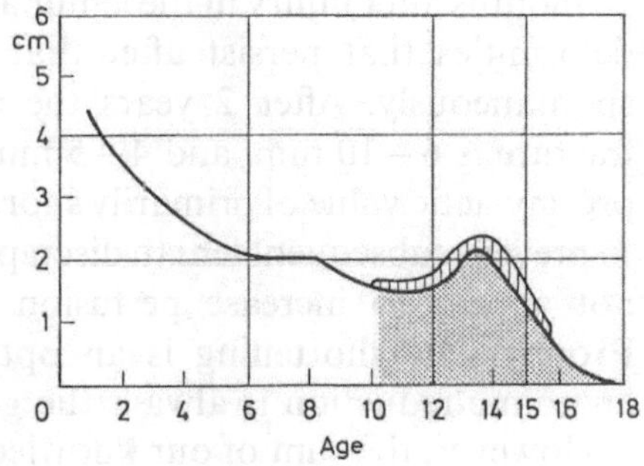

Fig. 1. Mean longitudinal growth of the femur and tibia [14]

Location of the Fracture

Seventy percent of femoral shaft fractures are located in the middle third. Most are unstable transverse and oblique fractures with varus and backward displacement. The potential for correction by compensatory epiphyseal growth is smallest in the midshaft area, and a complete correction is possible only in small children.

Type of Deformity

Valgus, anterior and posterior angulations show little if any tendency toward spontaneous correction. Rotational deformities can be compensated to some degree by the two derotation spurts that occur at 5 – 7 and 11 – 13 years of age [8]. However, this derotation affects only the uninjured side, producing a decrease of femoral neck anteversion in the healthy leg which more closely matches that of the injured side [1,5,8,17].

Corrective Osteotomies of the Lower Extremity
Edited by G. Hierholzer, K. H. Müller

Angular and rotational deformities: Persistent angular deformities of the femoral diaphysis at skeletal maturity are still reported in 10–15% of cases, and rotational deformities in 40% of cases, although functional disturbances and painful unphysiologic loading of the joints are uncommon [1,7,8,18,19,21].

Length discrepancies: Inequality of leg lengths, a more serious complication, is present in 70% of healed femoral shaft fractures and averages 10–15 mm [8]. But discrepancies as small as 5 mm can cause painful disturbances of spinal statics in patients who do not wear a corrective shoe. Increased longitudinal growth is related in a complex way to fracture type, instability, angular deformity, and repeated reductions. It can also relate to the use of intramedullary implants (medullary nail, Ender nails, Rush pins, medullary wires), which, by disrupting the intramedullary blood supply, promote the development of a collateral circulation that is the true stimulus to epiphyseal growth. Thus, medullary fixation tends to greatly accelerate the growth of the injured bone within a short period of time (Fig. 2). By contrast, the stable plating of a bone without periosteal stripping is associated with only about 10–15 mm of lengthening.

According to the studies of Reynolds [14], the posttraumatic acceleration of bone growth reaches a maximum of 6 months after injury in the femur, and at 3 months in the tibia (Table 1). Thereafter, with regression of the collateral blood supply, the growth rate progressively declines and returns to normal at 24 months after injury in the femur and at 18 months in the tibia [14]. Angular deformities that persist after that time are extremely unlikely to correct spontaneously. After 2 years the average length increase after a femoral fracture is 6–10 mm, and 4–5 mm after a tibial fracture [2,3,8,10,16]. The prophylactic value of primarily shortening a femoral shaft fracture by 1–2 cm to prevent subsequent length discrepancy is controversial; in any case this does not appear to increase perfusion of the distal epiphysis [2,3,8,10,16,21]. Prophylactic shortening is an option only in the femur; in the tibia, an anatomic reduction is always the goal.

However, the sum of our knowledge and experience suggests that the best strategy for achieving normal limb axes without significant length discrepancy after femoral or tibial shaft fractures is to tolerate angular and length

Table 1. Duration of Posttraumatic Longitudinal Growth of the Femur and Tibia: Statistical Averages for 125 Clinical Cases of Reynolds, 1981 [14]

126 Cases treated conservatively	Maximum months	Minimum months	Normal months	Total (maximum) mm
Femur	6	18	24	8 (17)
Tibia	3	12	18	4 (11)
Independent of:	age, sex, location			
Dependent on:	primary shortening			

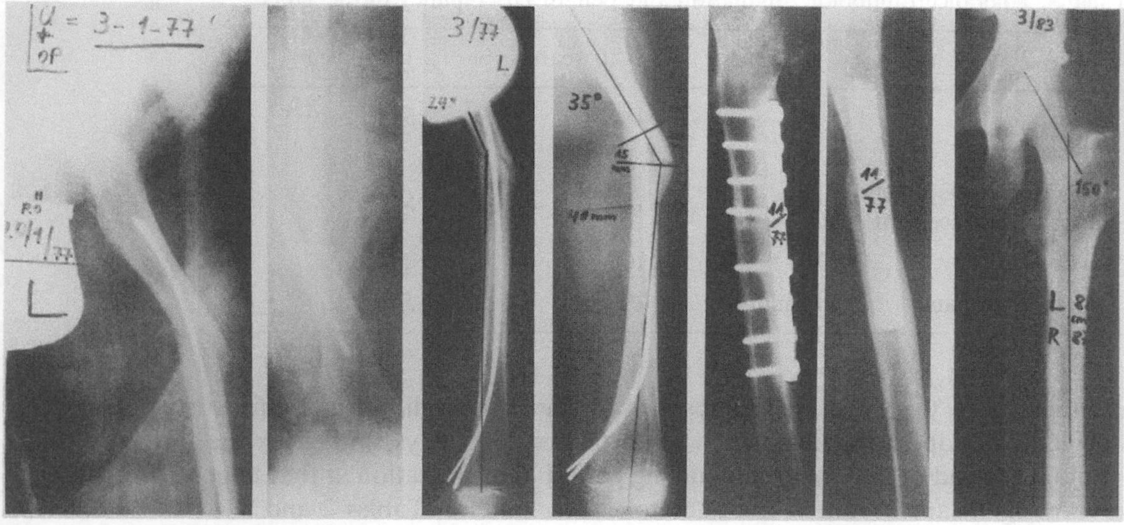

a b c d e f

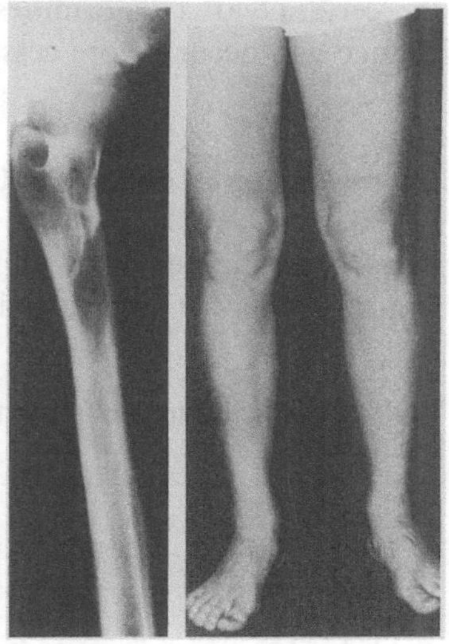

g h

Fig. 2 a – h. Compound fracture of the left femur with vascular injury sustained in a fall from a sled. **a – c** Immediately the main fragments were stablized with Ender nails, and a plaster cast was applied. **d** The cast was removed at 3 months, revealing a gross 35° angular midshaft deformity. Even so, the injured leg was already longer than the uninvolved leg. **e** At corrective operations the nails were removed, and a generous bone wedge was resected to correct angulation and shorten the femoral shaft by 40 mm. **f – h** Roentgenologic and clinical result: The left leg is still almost 1 cm longer than the right despite its good alignment. The patient has no complaints and wears a slightly elevated right shoe

Table 2. Tolerance Limit for Angulation and Length Discrepancy in the Femur

Deformity	1–5 years	5–10 years	10–15 years
Varus Valgus	20°	15°	10°
Backward displacement Forward displacement	20°	15°	10°
External rotation Internal discrepancy	15° 10°	10°	10°
Length discrepancy	15 mm	10 mm	5 mm

Table 3. Tolerance Limits for Angulation and Length Discrepancy in the Tibia

Deformity	1–5 years	5–10 years	10–15 years
Varus	20°	10°	5°
Valgus	10°		
Backward displacement Forward displacement	10°	10°	5°
Torsion	±10°	10°	10°
Length discrepancy	15 mm	10 mm	5 mm

discrepancy in the three age groups only within narrow limits, administer definitive, nonoperative treatment within the first 5–7 days, and check the result at the end of the 2-year remodeling period. If examination at that time reveals significant deviation from the tolerance limits in Tables 2 and 3, a corrective operation should be seriously considered, it being unlikely (except for certain varus deformities of the femur) that significant spontaneous change will occur before cessation of growth [2,16,24].

Internal Fixation during the Growth Period

Reports on the frequency of primary and secondary internal fixations of the femur or tibia for various indications range between 8 and 44% (Table 4).

Table 4. Indications for Internal Fixation in the Growth Period (Diaphyseal Fracture)

Author	Year	Rate of internal fixation, %	Site
Daum [4]	1969	43.7	Femur
Rehbein [13]	1963	22	Femur
von Oelsnitz [11]	1972	19	Femur
Weber [21]	1978	14	Femur, tibia
Schmit-Neuerburg	1983	15	Femur, Tibia
Müller [9]	1967	10	Diaphysis
Weller [22]	1972	8	Absolute indication

Extramedullary Implants (Plates, Pins and Frame)

The primary use of these devices within the first 2–3 weeks after injury do not stimulate increased bone growth, and so shortening of the bone is not required.

Intramedullary Implants (medullary Nail, Rush Pin, Ender Nail)

These devices stimulate growth by 2–4 cm [11,16]. A stable fixation is essential, for unstable implants provoke considerable growth stimulation through callus formation and increased collateral blood flow.

Corrective Osteotomies

Plates are best for the stabilization of diaphyseal osteotomies. Preoperative drawings based on clinical findings and scale roentgenograms are used to plan the correction in all three cardinal planes. Computed tomograms also may be obtained for accurate evaluation of rotational deformities. The planes of resection are marked with Kirschner wires. To avoid thermal necrosis these wires should not be drilled directly into the bone, but inserted into 2-mm predrilled holes (Fig. 3). In younger children 10 mm of shortening is desirable and should be allowed for when the bone wedge is resected. Orkan [12] has

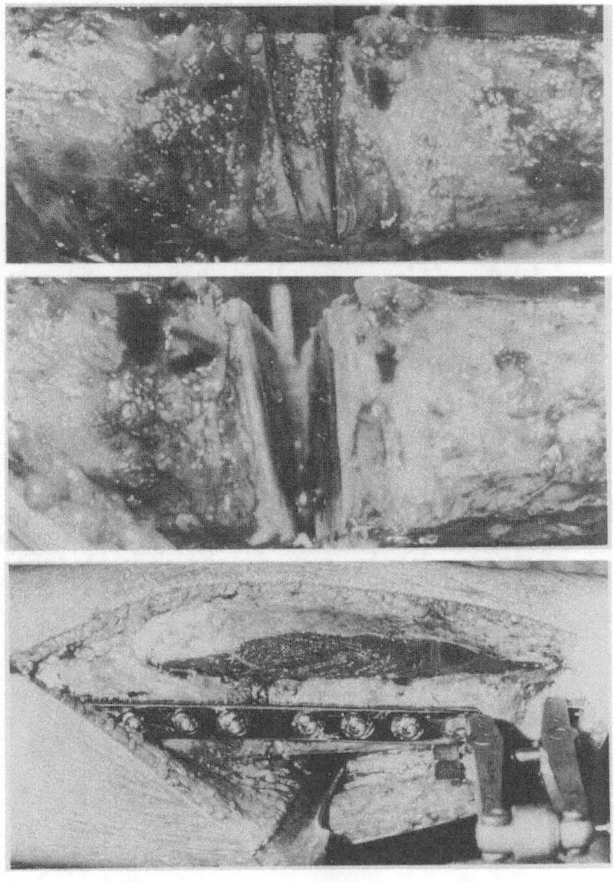

a
b
c

Fig. 3 a–c. Corrective osteotomy of the tibial diaphysis in the growing patient. **a** Without stripping the periosteum, the planes of section are marked with Kirschner wires introduced into predrilled holes. **b** The bone wedge is resected, and roentgenograms are taken to check for accuracy of correction. **c** The osteotomy is stabilized under compression (tension device) with a narrow dynamic compression plate

Table 5. Trigonometric Table for Determining the Height b of the Resected Bone Wedge for a known Correction Angle α and Bone Diameter *a*, after Orkan [12]

a

α	10,0	12,5	15,0	17,5	20,0	22,5	25,0	27,5	30,0	32,5	35,0	37,5	40,0	42,5	45,0	47,5	50,0	mm
5°	0,8	1,0	1,2	1,4	1,6	1,8	2,0	2,2	2,4	2,6	2,8	3,0	3,2	3,4	3,6	3,8	4,0	
10°	1,7	2,2	2,6	3,0	3,5	4,0	4,4	4,8	5,3	5,7	6,1	6,6	7,0	7,5	7,9	8,4	8,8	
15°	2,6	3,3	4,0	4,7	5,3	6,0	6,7	7,4	8,0	8,7	9,4	10.0	10,7	11,4	12,0	12,7	13,4	
20°	3,6	4,5	5,5	6,4	7,3	8,2	9,1	10,0	10,9	11,8	12,7	13,6	14,5	15,5	16,4	17,3	18,2	b
25°	4,6	5,8	7,0	8,1	9,3	10,5	11,6	12,8	14,0	15,1	16,3	17,5	18,6	19,8	20,9	22,1	23,3	
30°	5,7	7,2	8,6	10,0	11,5	13,0	14,4	15,8	17,3	18,8	20,2	21,6	23,0	24,5	26,0	27,4	28,8	
35°	7,0	9,0	10,5	12,0	14,0	16.0	17,5	19,0	21,0	23,0	24,5	26,0	28,0	30,0	31,5	33,0	35,0	
40°	8,5	10,5	12,5	14,5	17,0	19,0	21,0	23,0	25,0	27,5	29,5	31,5	33,5	35,5	38,0	40,0	42,0	
45°	10,0	12,5	15,0	17,5	20,0	22,5	25,0	27,5	30,0	32,5	35,0	37,5	40,0	42,5	45,0	47,5	50,0	mm

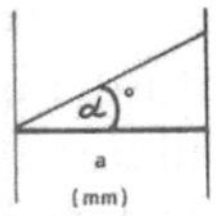

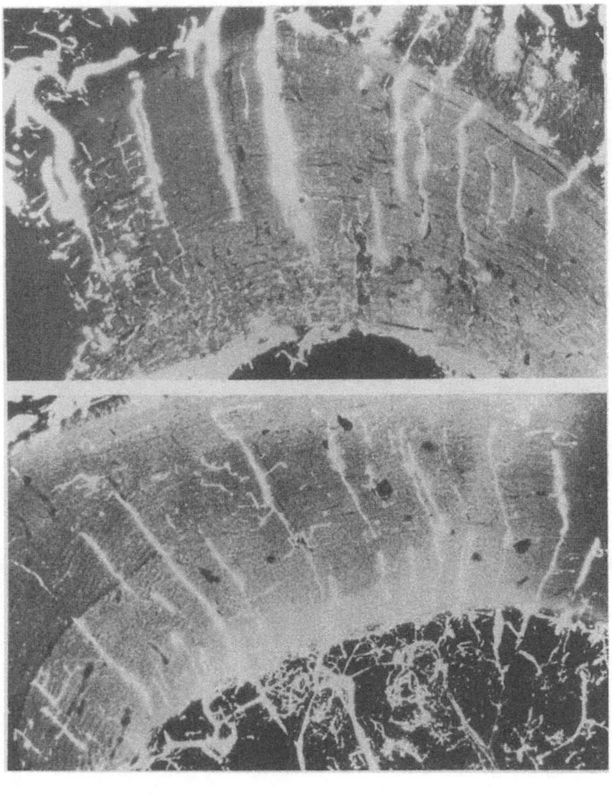

Fig. 4 a,b. Comparison of the vascular supply of the tibia in the midshaft area (300-μm decalcified sections, vessels perfused with Micropaque). **a** In the juvenile bone of a 6-month-old sheep, 4/5 of the compact substance is supplied by the periosteal vessels. **b** The mature bone of a 4-year-old female sheep is supplied by the medullary vascular system

published a trigonometric table from which the height of the resected wedge can be directly read when the angle of correction and bone diameter are known (Table 5). This obviates the need for check roentgenograms or angle measurements during the operation.

Management of the periosteum: During exposure, osteotomy and plating of the bone, the surgeon should be careful to leave the periosteum intact, and he should apply the plate over the periosteal sleeve. This recommendation is based on the peculiar blood supply of juvenile bone, four-fifths of which is derived from the periosteal vessels, in contradistinction to the medullary blood supply of the long bones in adults (Fig. 4). Elevation of the periosteum for subperiosteal plating inevitably leads to devitalization of the diapyseal compact bone, whereas epiperiosteal plating leaves the nutrient vessels intact (Fig. 5). Although the compact bone will eventually be revascularized via medullary system, the devitalization poses an increased risk, especially since the compact bone under the plate distal to the fracture and osteotomy is *also* cut off initially from the medullary supply (Fig. 6). Plating over the periosteum would preserve osseous nutrition via the natural periosteal supply.

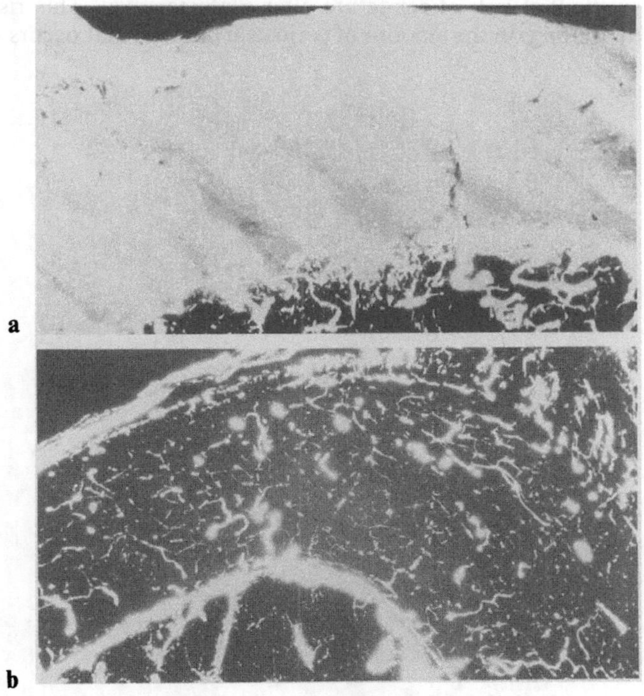

Fig. 5 a,b. Blood supply of the compact bone of the juvenile tibial shaft after osteotomy and plating. **a** Six weeks after osteotomy and subperiosteal plating the bone under the plate is still completely devitalized; there is evidence of early invasion by medullary vessels, but these will revascularize only about 1/3 the cross-section of the bone. **b** A similar plate was applied over the periosteum on the contralateral tibia of the same animal. The periosteum under the plate does not become necrotic and remains well perfused. The cross-section shown here is proximal to the osteotomy, and so the medullary blood supply is still intact

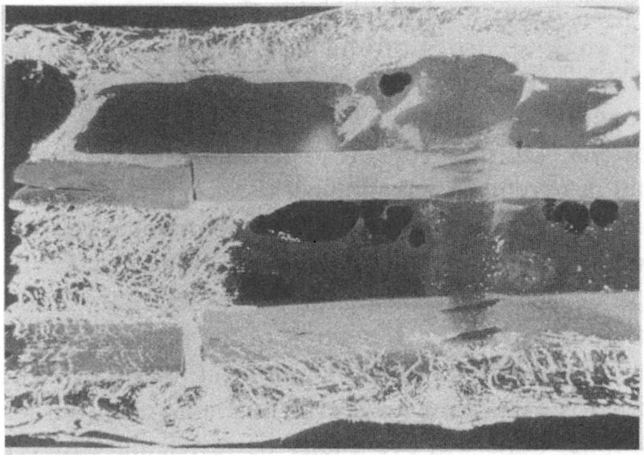

Fig. 6. Longitudinal section through the juvenile tibial shaft 6 weeks after subperiosteal plating of the osteotomy visible in the *left* part of the picture. Note that the elevated periosteum overlay the plate and could not reach the plated portion of the bone. The compact bone proximal to the osteotomy still appears avascular but is already being revascularized by the medullary system and by capillary ingrowth from the outside. The bone distal to the osteotomy is still completely devitalized. After about 3 months this bone would have been revascularized but greatly thinned by resorption, posing a substantial risk of refracture after plate removal. This risk also exists in children, depending on the amount of periosteal damage that occurs when the plate is attached

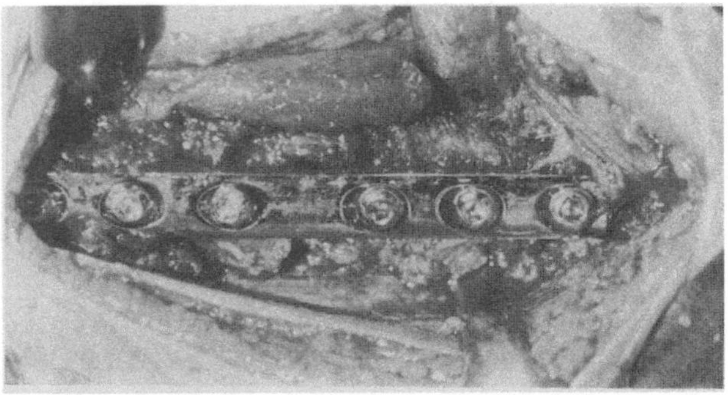

a

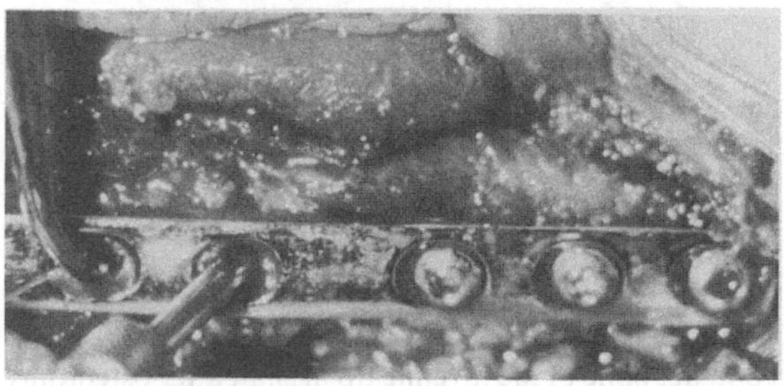

b

Fig. 7 a,b. Plate fixation of a femoral shaft fracture in a 5-year-old boy. **a** After osteotomy and wedge removal, the fragments are reduced and secured with a plate attached over the periosteum. **b** Before the screw on the *right* side of the picture was inserted, the position of the plate was defined by twisting the drill sleeve into the predrilled gliding hole. After stressing the plate with the tension device and inserting the distal screw, the thread hole was drilled through the far cortex and a lag screw inserted. This increases the rotational stability of the fixation by 30–50%

Table 6. Internal Fixations and Corrective Osteotomies of Diaphyseal Fractures in the Growth Period (Essen University Clinic, 1974–1983)

310	142	Femoral fractures – 29 internal fixations (20%)
	168	Tibial fractures – 17 internal fixations (10%)
	46	Internal fixations and corrective osteotomies 15%

These peculiarities of the blood supply of immature bone, which have been demonstrated experimentally in sheep and dogs [23], apply without restriction to human bone.

Another technical detail in the plating of juvenile bone concerns the *lag screw*, which we use even in transverse osteotomies that are compressed with the ASIF tension device. The use of a lag screw in these cases increase stability by 30–50%. Accurate placement of the lag screw is made easier by first drilling an oblique gliding hole under vision that is directed toward the center of the osteotomy surface. After the fragments are reduced, the plate is fixed with a drill sleeve through the gliding hole, whereupon the plate is stressed and the screws inserted in the usual manner. Then the thread hole is cut through the drill sleeve, the hole is tapped, and the lag screw is inserted (Fig. 7).

Removal of the plate is done at 6 months in preschool children and at 8–12 months in school-age children. After the last stage of growth (the "adolescent spurt") at about 14 years of age, the same guidelines are applied to plating, intramedullary nailing, and the removal of implants as in adults.

During the past 10 years at the Department of Trauma Surgery of Essen University Clinic, we have performed internal fixations and corrective osteotomies in 29 of 142 femoral fractures (20%) and in 17 of 168 tibial fractures (10%) in pediatric patients (Table 6). Overall, this corresponds to a 15% rate of internal fixations, which is considered a reasonable rate of selection for procedures of this type.

Indications for Diaphyseal Corrective Osteotomies of the Femur and Tibia

In the classification of Brunner [3] these indications are:

- *Primary angular and rotational deformities* that develop during the course of fracture healing.
- *Secondary angular deformities* based on a disturbance of epiphyseal growth.
- *"Functional" growth disturbance* unaccompanied by traumatic damage to the growth cartilage.
- *Length discrepancies* resulting from accelerated or inhibited growth.

Early Correction of Primary Angular and Rotational Deformities

Primary angular and rotational deformities that are present during or within four weeks after fracture healing most commonly occur at the junction of the proximal and middle thirds of the femoral shaft. Muscular rotation, flexion and abduction of the short proximal fragment tends to produce varus angulation with malrotation and shortening. In a 5-year-old chid with a grotesque malunion of the femoralshaft coexisting with craniocerebral trauma

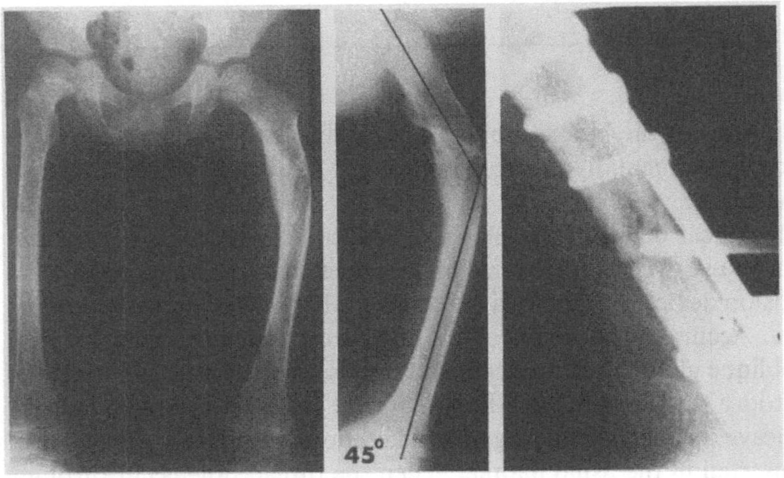

a b c

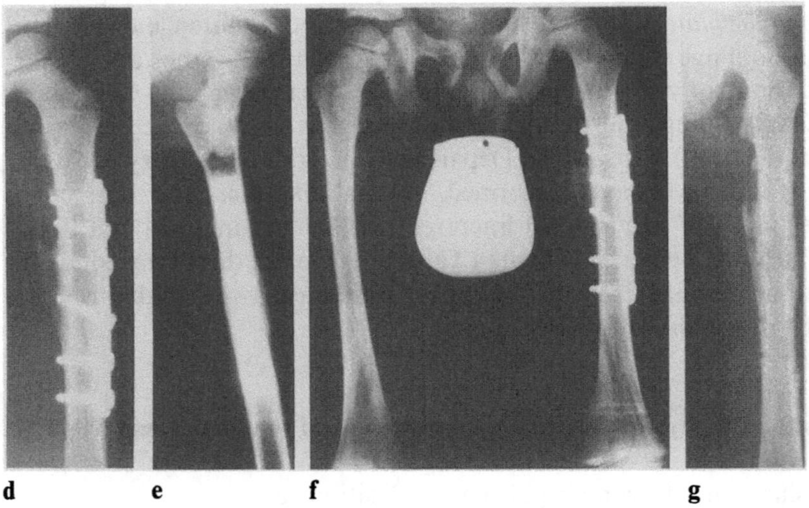

d e f g

Fig. 8. a,b Grotesque malunion of the femoral shaft in 5-year-old boy with 40° varus, 45° backward displacement and external malrotation following hospitalization for neurosurgical treatment. **c,d** Wedge-resection osteotomy was performed and stabilized with an epiperiosteal plate and lag screw. **c** Image intensification shows the drill sleeve in the gliding hole of the plate. **d,e** This mode of fixation is so stable that the narrow 6-hole plate on the femur is sufficient to permit full weight bearing. **f** Primary limb shortening of 7 mm. **g** Plate removal after 6 months. At follow-up 1 year after osteotomy the femoral shaft has healed in excellent alignment with only 5 mm of residual length discrepancy

(Fig. 8), it is still advisable to perform a corrective osteotomy fixed with an epiperiosteal plate in order to facilitate rehabilitation of the neurologic injury. At follow-up 1 year later (6 months after removal of the plate), the femoral shaft had healed in good alignment with 5 mm of residual length discrepancy.

The early correction of primary angular and rotational deformities is also important in older children between 10 and 12 years of age, as these patients

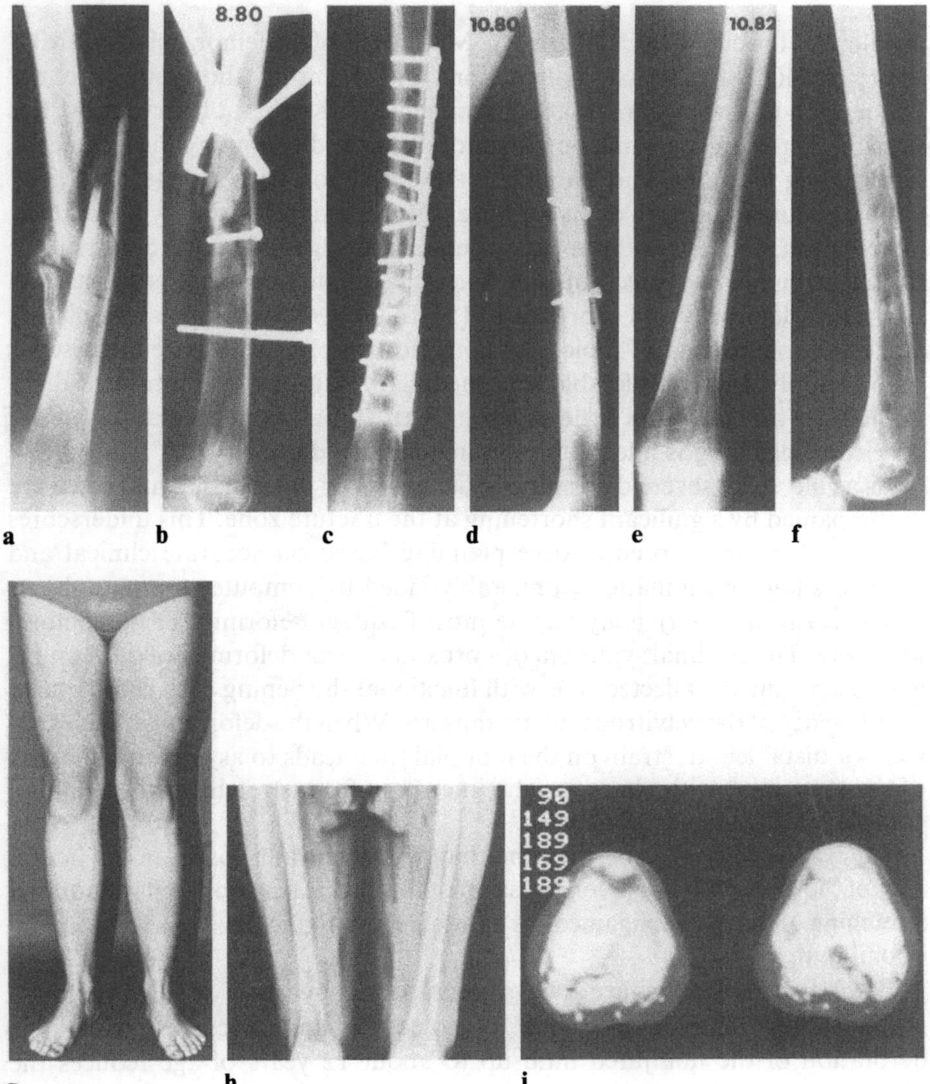

Fig. 9. a Ten-year-old girl who was referred to us 4 weeks after a femoral shaft fracture healed with varus, external rotation, and shortening. **b** We performed an osteotomy through the freshly healed fracture and applied the Müller distractor, which enables the gradual correction of limb alignment in 3 planes as the distraction is carried out. **c,d** Subsequent plate fixation; plate was removed 1 year later. **e–h** Follow-up at 2 years (skeletal maturity) shows equal limb lengths with no angular deformity. **i** Results is verified with CT scans, which are also useful preoperatively for evaluating rotational alignment

Table 7. Femoral Diaphysis

Varus:	Leg shortening, strain on iliotibial tract, asymmetric loading of knee ("medial meniscus")
Valgus:	Overcompression of lateral femoropatellar joint, asymmetric loading of knee, stretching of medial ligament

are close to the end of skeletal growth. Malunions of the femoral shaft with 30° of varus, 40° of external malrotation, and 4 cm of shortening are not uncommon following conservative treatment. With prompt intervention, it is possible to restore a normal limb by mobilizing and realigning the fragments, lengthening the bone, and stabilizing the correction with a plate (Fig. 9).

As absolute indication exists for the early correction of primary angulation, malrotation, and length discrepancy between the ages of 5 and 15 years if the degree of deformity is well outside tolerance limits and there is substantial rotational deformity and shortening [15]. In these cases compression plating is the fixation method of choice. An epiperiosteal plate will spare the osseous blood supply and is preferable to a medullary nail or other intramedullary implant in that it causes little or no growth stimulation, so that 10 mm of surgical shortening is adequate even in small children.

As a rule, these severe deformities exist in two or three planes and often are accompanied by significant shortening at the fracture zone. This underscores the need for careful preoperative planning based on accurate clinical and roentgenologic examinations, preferably aided by computer tomography.

The *varus deformity* is by far the most frequent deformity of the femoral diaphysis. The cardinal symptom of a proximal varus deformity of the femur is a limp favoring the affected side, with functional shortening of the limb due to insufficiency of the pelvitrochanteric muscles. When the deformity involves the shaft or distal femur, strain on the iliotibial tract leads to asymmetric loading of the knee joint with characteristic knee pain from stretching of the lateral capsule and ligaments (Table 7).

The *valgus deformity*, on the other hand, concentrates loads on the lateral part of the knee with hypercompression of the lateral femoropatellar joint and stretching of the medial ligament. A painful genu valgum develops very rapidly in children.

Rotational deformities are always accompanied by varus or valgus deformity, but they rarely exceed the 10° tolerance limit because physiologic derotation of the uninjured limb up to about 12 years of age reduces the difference between the anteversion angles of the two femora.

Secondary Angular Deformities of the Diaphysis

Most deformities of this type result from a disturbance of epiphyseal growth. Three-fourths present as a genu valgum and/or genu recurvatum deformity. A frequent cause is a proximal avulsion fracture of the lateral collateral ligament across the epiphyseal plate, followed by collateral epiphysiodesis after

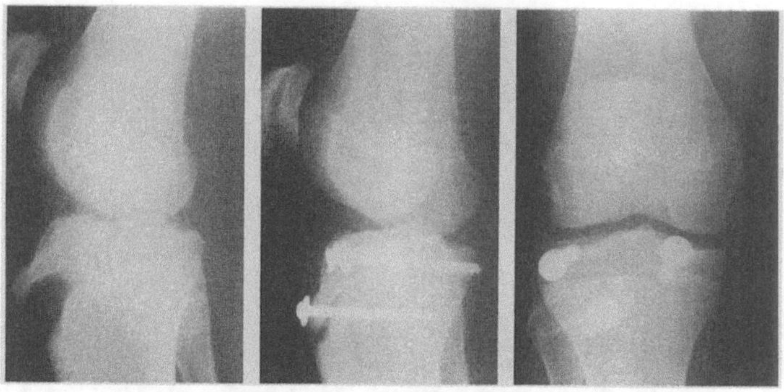

Fig. 10 a–c. a Avulsion of the tibial tuberosity and fracture of the epiphyseal plate. **b,c** Emergency reduction and screw fixation, which is permissible in adolescents close to the end of skeletal growth. In younger children it is necessary to use drill wires, possibly combined with a tension band. An incomplete reduction can lead to growth disturbance with consequent genu recurvatum and genu valgum

reattachment of the ligament. The result is a severe, recurring genu valgum that can be corrected *only* by repeated supracondylar osteotomies of the distal femur until skeletal growth ceases.

Fracture-separations of the proximal tibial epiphysis and especially avulsions of the tibial tuberosity with associated epiphyseal fractures cause growth disturbance leading to genu recurvatum unless accurate reduction and fixation are carried out. Screw fixation of the tibial tuberosity is appropriate only in adolescent patients (Fig. 10).

The high, transverse fracture of the tibial metaphysis can cause a partial epiphysiodesis due to its proximity to the growth plate, and this can also produce a genu recurvatum or genu valgum pattern of deformity.

An unusual variant of the tibial metaphyseal fracture is its combination with a fracture of the ipsilateral femoral metaphysis. Open, grade III fractures of this type with associated vascular damage occurred in an 8-year-old boy who sustained a severe crushing injury in an accident with a forklift truck. During primary treatment in 1976, the femur was fixed with a medullary nail, and the upper tibia was plated. Neither fracture united, however, and both went on to atrophic nonunion (Fig. 11). The femoral nonunion finally consolidated after two revisionary platings and cancellous bone grafting. Meanwhile, distal migration of the necrotic tibial nonunion resulted in a valgus deformity which was due not to nonunion but rather to epiphyseal damage occasioned by the crushing injury. Because the tibial plate had previously been removed, a refracture occurred that was initially treated conservatively. But now a growth arrest developed distal to the nonunion, necessitating a radical necrectomy with extensive decortication and cancellous grafting, correction of the valgus deformity, and the application of a long plate. Although the plate did not loosen, a 10° valgus deformity nevertheless recurred and was corrected by a high tibial osteotomy fixed with Kirschner wires. One year later the long plate was removed and replaced with a shorter one applied over the periosteum, allowing progressive revitalization of the compact bone until final plate

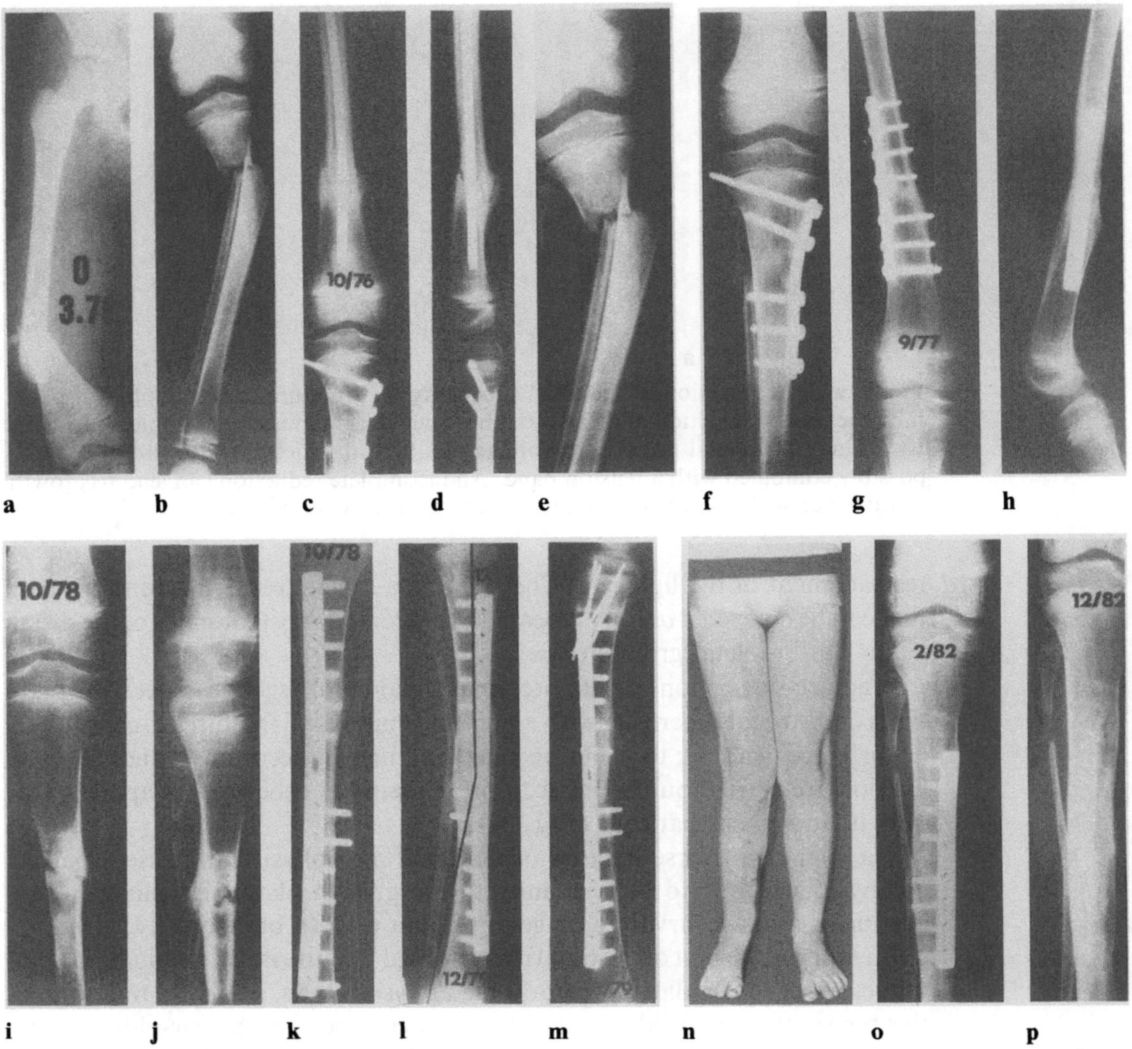

Fig. 11 a – p. An 8-year-old boy was injured in 1976 by a forklift truck, sustaining a high tibial metaphyseal fracture and an open grade III femoral fracture of the right leg with a ruptured artery and vein. **a, b** Preoperative roentgenograms. **c – f** In primary treatment elsewhere vascular lesions were repaired with interposed vein grafts, a thin intramedullary nail was inserted into the femur, and the tibia was plated. Soft tissues healed uneventfully, and normal perfusion was reestablished in the right leg. **g, h** About 1 year later an avascular nonunion developed in the distal femur, which was successfully treated by removing the intramedullary nail and plating the femur. The tibial plate was also removed, leaving behind a necrotic zone in the tibial diaphysis which migrated distally with growth. **i, j** Refracture and casting failed to accomplish union. **k** In October, 1978, a long plate was applied to the tibia, necrectomy and decortication were carried out at the site of the nonunion, and the defect was filled with autologous cancellous bone. A secondary valgus deformity was corrected at the same time. **l – n** The plate did not loosen, but a progressive, clinically apparent valgus deformity developed that was treated by metaphyseal wedge osteotomy and Kirschner wire fixation. **o, p** One year later the long plate was removed because of a plate bed fistula and was replaced with a shorter plate attached over the periosteum. This was followed by a rapid revascularization of the bone that continued until fall of 1982, when the plate was removed. During that period the accelerated bone growth induced by the growth arrest below the nonunion was able to correct the length discrepancy

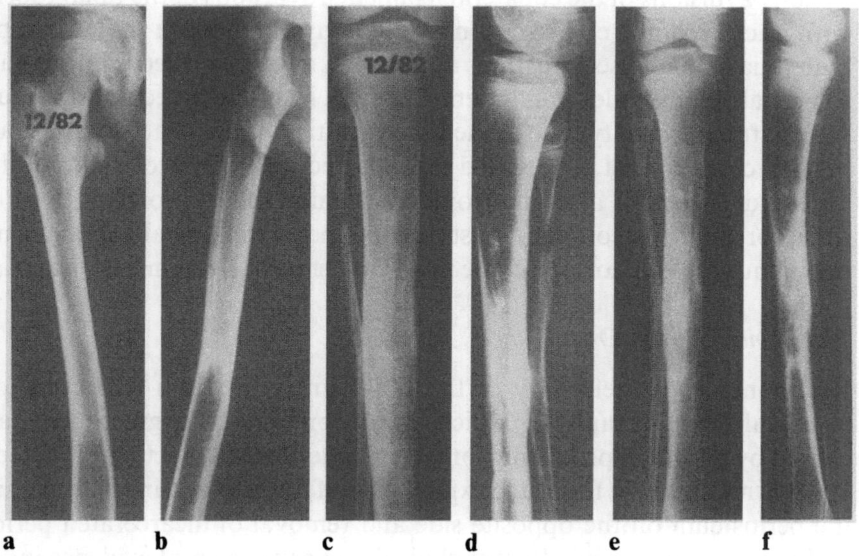

a b c d e f

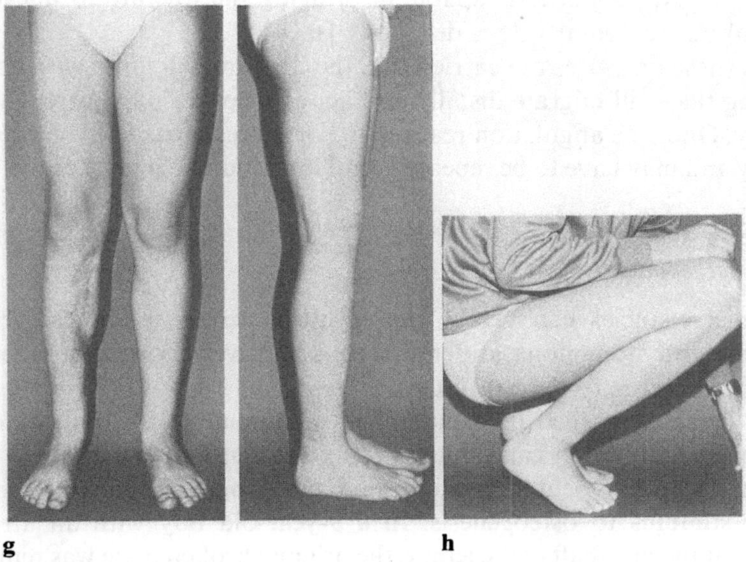

g h

Fig. 12 a–h. Same case as in Fig. 11 seen at follow-up 6 years after injury. **a,b** Roentgenologic result in the femur. **c–f** Roentgenologic result in the tibia. **g,h** Clinical appearance and functional result: Almost equal leg lengths with 5 mm lengthening on the right side, normal leg axes with 7° of residual valgus. The patient does not limp and bears weight normally

removal in August, 1982. Growth of the bone, while initially inhibited, was so stimulated by the multiple operations that the operated limb was 5 mm longer than the uninjured limb at 6 years after injury. The tibial nonunion was solid with a residual valgus of 7°. Now that the patient is skeletally mature, it is hoped that the correction will be permanent and no additional operations will be required (Fig. 12).

Bony avulsions of the collateral ligaments, avulsions of the tibial tuberosity with fracture of the epiphysis, and the epiphyseal damage that accompanies high tibial metaphyseal fractures are rare but often neglected injuries that lead to partial epiphysiodesis of the femur or tibia resulting in recurrent valgus and recurvatum deformity. The limited therapeutic options that are still available in such cases consist of repeated axial corrections when tolerance limits are exceeded. If there is also an atrophic nonunion of the proximal third of the tibia, corrective osteotomies must be combined with radical debridement and cancellous grafting to correct the problem before skeletal maturity is reached.

Functional Growth Disturbance

Recurrent valgus deformity of the tibia can result from a fracture of the proximal tibial metaphysis, which always presents as a greenstick fracture caused by a torsion-producing force. A simple closed reduction is inadequate. What is required is a thorough exploration of the fracture line with division of the periosteum on the opposite side and removal of incarcerated periosteal and pes anserinus tissue. Recent clinical and experimental evidence indicates that this procedure alone is capable of bringing the fracture to uneventful union without recurrent valgus deformity [6,18].

Unless these measures are carried out, the fracture will unite with cortical thickening that will migrate distally and act as a source of recurrent valgus deformity. Once the angulation reaches 10° or more, corrective osteotomy is necessary and may have to be repeated until longitudinal growth ceases (Fig. 13).

Length Discrepancies

Length discrepancies can result from disturbance of epiphyseal growth, malunions, and nonunions and must be operatively corrected when the discrepancy reaches or exceeds 2 cm.

In the femur shortened by a malunited or nonunited fracture, thorough decortication followed by cancellous grafting and distraction with the Wagner apparatus is an excellent procedure, and the progressive distraction is a powerful stimulus to osteogenesis. In a 9-year-old boy with an atrophic nonunion at the midshaft of the femur, the original broken plate was removed, and decortication, grafting and distraction were carried out. This procedure not only corrected the growth arrest but also stimulated an increase of growth which equalized the leg lengths. At 3 months a strong, well-structured callus was present that allowed removal of the Wagner device (Fig. 14) [20].

If the femur has to be lengthened by 2.5 cm or less and there is coexisting rotational deformity that requires correction, we can also recommend the following procedure that was used in a young girl whose subcapital nonunion had been managed by repositioning osteotomy and electrical stimulation. After the nonunion healed, there remained 2.0 cm of limb shortening and 20° of external malrotation of the distal fragment (demonstrated by CT). To maintain a strong medial buttress with a good blood supply, we first resected a 10-cm-long medial fragment equal to almost half the diameter of the shaft,

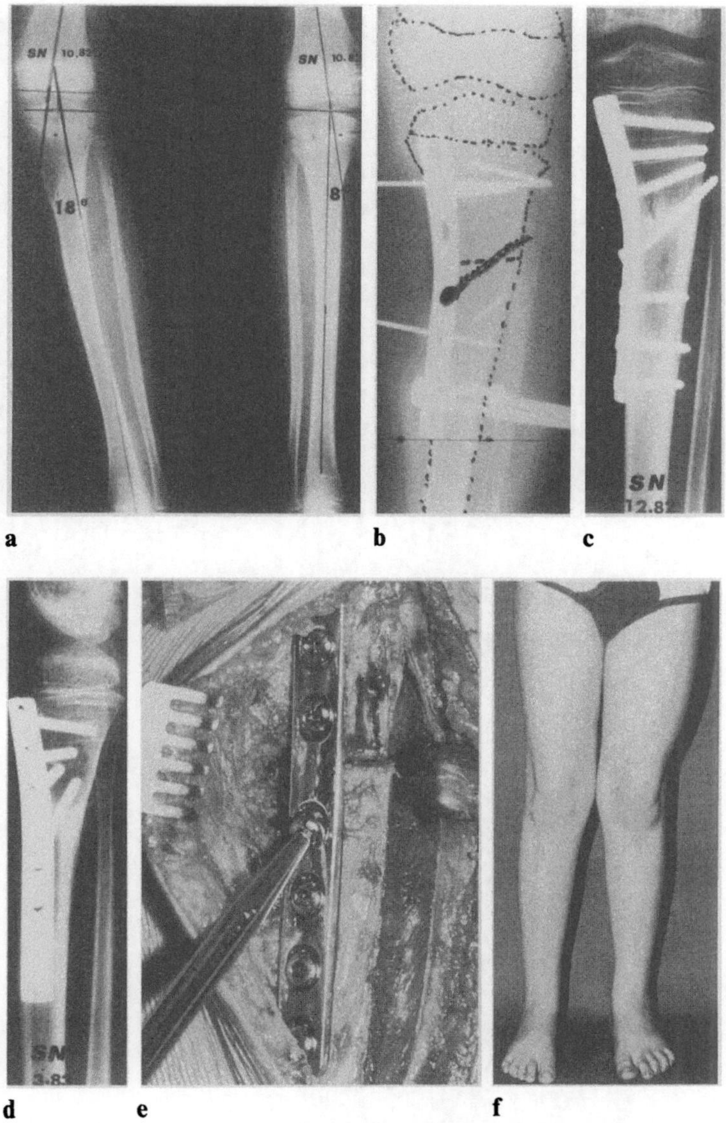

Fig. 13 a–f. Recurrent functional growth disturbance in the right tibia after a metaphyseal greenstick fracture that was set and immobilized in plaster. **a** The 8-year-old boy is undergoing his 2nd corrective operation after the valgus deformity again exceeded the 10° limit. **b** Intraoperative roentgenogram. **c, d** Postoperative roentgenograms show normal axial alignment. **e** Epiperiosteal plate with a lag screw across the osteotomy. **f** Clinical result

freed it proximally and distally together with adherent soft tissues, and retracted it medially. We then sectioned the remainder of the shaft and gently lengthened the gap with the Müller distractor while correcting rotational alignment [9]. A 2-cm-long block of homologous bone was interposed between the bone ends, whereupon the medial fragment was reapposed to the shaft and secured with 4 screws inserted in lag-screw fashion through the new lateral plate (Fig. 15).

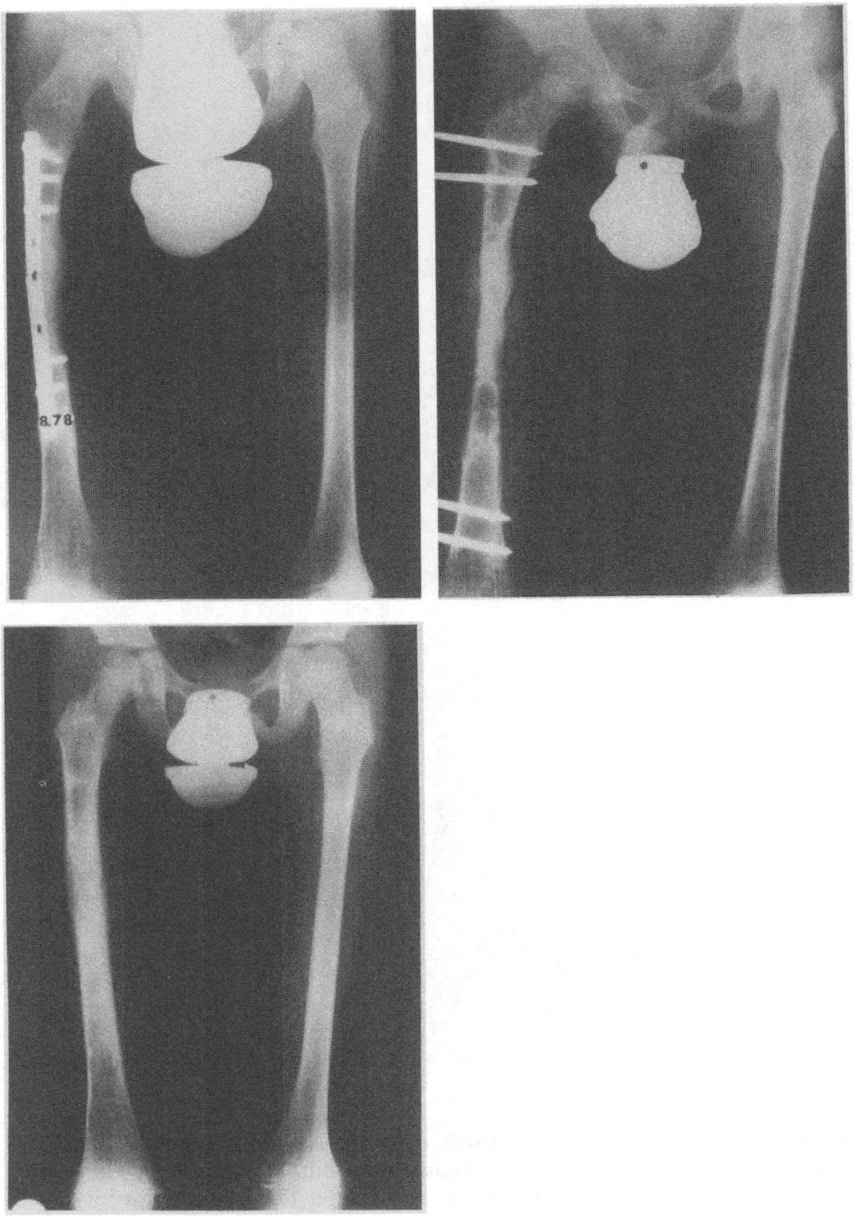

a b c

Fig. 14. a Boy 9 years of age with atrophic nonunion after primary subperiosteal plating of the femoral shaft. Plate fracture has occurred. **b** The old plate is removed, the Wagner distractor is applied, and decortication and cancellous grafting are carried out. **c** At 3 months the bone is solid and exhibits normal length owing to the growth-stimulating effect of the Wagner device

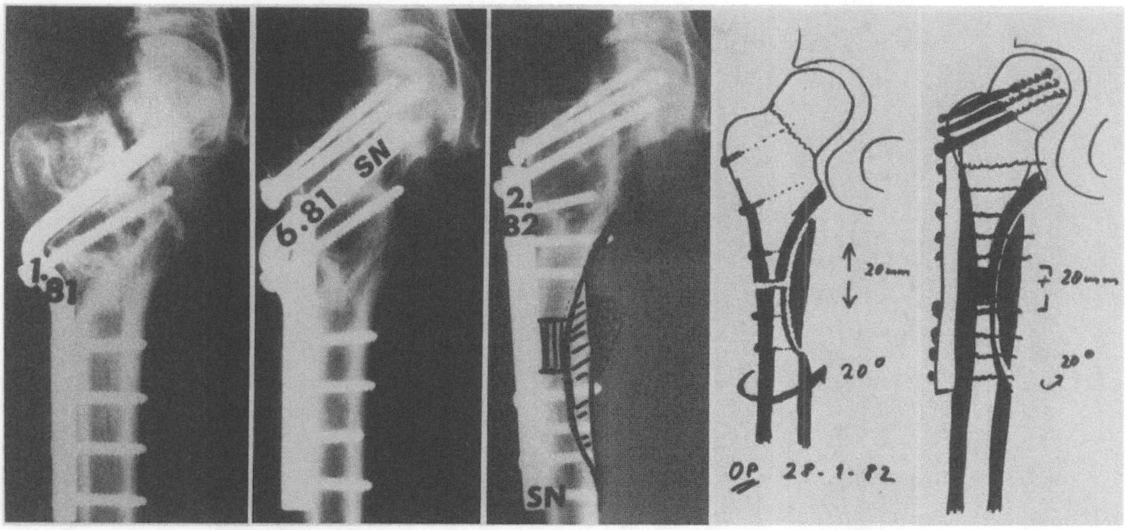

a b d c

Fig. 15 a–d. Nonunion of the femoral neck. **a** Even a repositioning osteotomy failed to accomplish union. **b** At 1st reoperation the plate was replaced with one having a shorter blade, and an electromagnetically induced current was applied through 2 lag-type electrode screws to stimulate healing. At 5 months the nonunion is consolidated. **c** Preoperative planning for the 2nd reoperation in which the femur is to be lengthened and derotated 20° (according to CT measurements). The steps involved are: plate removal, resection of a long, medial bone fragment encompassing about half the femoral shaft diameter, medial retraction of the fragment and soft tissues, transverse osteotomy of the rest of the shaft, derotation of the shaft, insertion of a homologous bone block to lengthen the femur 2 cm, and reattachment of the resected fragment with a Wagner plate to provide a secure medial buttress. The advantage of this procedure is that the well-perfused autologous graft makes a superior medial buttress; an interposed full-diameter homologous block would first have to be invested by a callus cuff. **d** Status at 1 month after surgery, with osseous remodeling

Primary angular deformities of the tibia are uncommon since most tibial fractures heal in satisfactory alignment. An exception occurred in the case of a 10-year-old girl with 4 cm of tibial shortening that resulted from the union of a short oblique fracture with overriding. This case was managed by osteotomy and distraction with the Wagner device: In addition to osteotomizing the tibia and fibula, it was necessary to screw the distal end of the fibula to the tibia to prevent subluxation and deformity at the ankle. As always, the Wagner device was applied to the medial side of the extremity, and distraction was effected at a rate of 2–3 mm per day; this increment was removed immediately at the first sign of paresthesia or diminution of the pedal pulses. When slightly more than the desired amount of distraction had been obtained, the defect was filled with autologous cancellous bone and stabilized with a lateral bridge plate. At that time there was still 5 mm of residual shortening on the operated side, which was left alone so that further growth before skeletal maturity would not cause excessive lengthening (Fig. 16). At follow-up two years after plate removal leg lengths are equal, and there is no angular deformity or limitation of motion

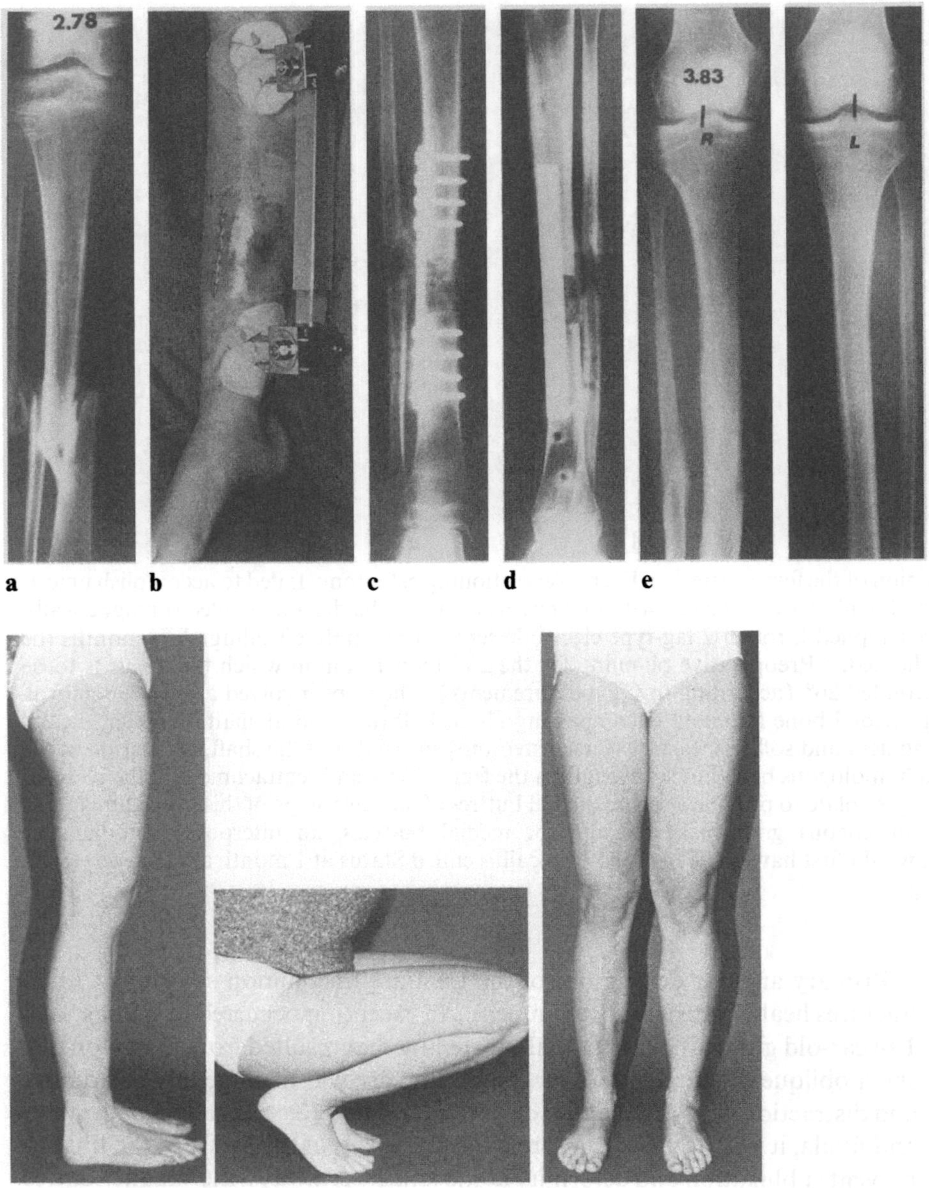

Fig. 16 a–h. J. L., who was hospitalized at 11 years of age for treatment of a tibial fracture. **a** Roentgenogram on admission shows a malunited fracture with 3.5 cm of shortening and lateral displacement. **b–d** Six months later the tibia and fibula are osteotomized, and the distal end of the fibula is screwed to the tibia. The Wagner device is applied medially, and distraction is carried out in millimeter increments for 2 months until 4 cm lengthening is achieved. A Wagner plate is applied laterally, and the defect is filled with autologous, compressed cancellous bone; metal is removed at 1 year postoperatively. **e** Roentgenologic status at follow-up 3.5 years after plate removal. **f–h** Clinical and functional status at follow-up: equal leg lengths, no complaints, normal recreational ability

Summary

Indications for Corrective Osteotomy

Osteotomies of the femoral and tibial diaphyses are performed mainly for primary angular deformities that are noted during or shortly after fracture healing and are stabilized by plating after alignment is restored. An epiperiosteal compression plate will not damage the blood supply to the bone and will permit up to 10 – 15 mm of limb lengthening. Osteotomy is indicated in the presence of severe angular deformity, or if there is deformity well outside tolerance limits after the cessation of posttraumatic bone remodeling two years later.

Secondary Angular Deformities

These most commonly affect the tibia and result from a medial or lateral epiphysiodesis caused by high tibial metaphyseal fracture with crushing of the epiphysis or by unrecognized fracture-separations, avulsions of the tibial tuberosity, or bony avulsions of the collateral ligaments.

Functional Growth Disturbance

This likewise creates a specific valgus deformity of the tibia. In this case the medial incarceration of periosteal and pes anserinus tissue in a high metaphyseal greenstick fracture causes a recurrent valgus deformity which must be corrected if it exceeds 10°.

Length Discrepancies

Length discrepancies are corrected in the shafts of the femur and tibia with the Wagner or Müller apparatus when shortening reaches or exceeds 2 cm.

Published Data on Diaphyseal Corrective Osteotomies

The reported frequency of these operations in the growing skeleton is between 10 and 20%. Of the 310 femoral and tibial fractures that were treated at the Trauma Surgery Department of the Essen University Clinic from 1974 to 1983, an internal fixation or corrective osteotomy of the diaphysis was performed in 45 children and adolescents (15%). It is apparent that stricter criteria should be applied to the reduction and fixation of pediatric diaphyseal fractures of the lower extremity due to the high percentage of valgus, antecurvatum and recurvatum deformities and malrotations that go uncorrected in these patients. When primary reduction and traction was carried out on the Weber traction table, femoral shaft fractures as well as tibial fractures can be reduced to within 10° of physiologic alignment. This would limit the indications for internal fixation in pediatric patients basically to fresh open fractures, multiply injured and unconscious patients, and fractures that have united with deformity.

References

1. Best PNB, Verhage CC, Molenaar IC (1972) Torsion deviations after conservative treatment of femoral fractures. Z Kinderchir [Suppl] 11:814–821
2. Blount WP (1955) Fractures in children. Williams & Wilkins, Baltimore
3. Brunner C (1974) Spätfolgen kindlicher Frakturen. In: Rehn J (Hrsg) Unfallverletzungen bei Kindern. Springer, Berlin Heidelberg New York
4. Daum R, Metzger G (1969) Analyse und Spätergebnisse kindlicher Femurschaftfrakturen. Arch Orthop Unfallchir 66:18
5. Dunn JM (1952) Anteversion of the neck of the femur. J Bone Joint Surg [Br] 34:181–186
6. Houghton GR, Rooker GD (1979) The role of the periosteum in the growth of long bones. J Bone Joint Surg [Br] 61:218–220
7. Klapp F (1981) Diaphysäre und metaphysäre Verletzungen im Wachstumsalter. Hefte Unfallheilkd 152
8. Laer L von (1977) Beinlängendifferenzen und Rotationsfehler nach Oberschenkelschaftfraktur im Kindesalter. Arch Orthop Unfallchir 89:121–137
9. Müller ME (1967) Posttraumatische Achsenfehlstellungen an der unteren Extremität. Huber, Bern Stuttgart
10. Neurath F, Van Lessen H (1972) Die unter Verkürzung geheilte kindliche Oberschenkelfraktur. Z Kinderchir [Suppl] 11:791–802
11. Oelsnitz G von der (1972) Marknagelung kindlicher Oberschenkelschaftfrakturen. Z Kinderchir [Suppl] 11:803–814
12. Orkan E, Roth VG, Rousso M, Harness D (1977) A new method of achieving accuracy in osteotomy of any long bone. Arch Orthop Unfallchir 89:157–162
13. Rehbein F, Hofmann S (1963) Knochenverletzungen im Kindesalter. Langenbecks Arch Klin Chir 304–539
14. Reynolds DA (1981) Growth changes in fractured long bones. J Bone Joint Surg [Br] 63:83–87
15. Rippstein J (1955) Zur Bestimmung der Antetorsion des Schenkelhalses mittels 2 Jahre Röntgenaufnahmen. Z Orthop 86:345–360
16. Saxer U (1974) Die Behandlung kindlicher Femurfrakturen mit der Vertikal-Extension nach Weber. Helv Chir Acta 41:271
17. Staheli LT, Clawson DK, Hubbard DD (1980) Medial femoral torsion: Experience with operative treatment. Clin Orthop 146:222–225
18. Tachdjian MO (1972) Pediatric orthopedics. Saunders, Philadelphia London Toronto
19. Vontobel V, Genton N, Schmied R (1961) Die Spätergebnisse der kindlichen dislozierten Femurschaftfraktur. Helv Chir Acta 28:655
20. Wagner H (1972) Technik und Indikation der operativen Verkürzung und Verlängerung von Ober- und Unterschenkel. Orthopäde 1:59–74
21. Weber BG, Brunner C, Freuler F (1978) Die Frakturenbehandlung bei Kindern und Jugendlichen. Springer, Berlin Heidelberg New York
22. Weller S (1972) Spezielle Gesichtspunkte bei der Behandlung kindlicher Frakturen. Z Kinderchir [Suppl] 11:655–659
23. Wilde CD, Stürmer KM, Weiss H (1977) Veränderung der Knochenstruktur durch Plattenosteosynthese am Röhrenknochen bei Versuchstieren im Wachstumsalter. Langenbecks Arch Chir [Suppl]:85–89
24. Witt AN, Walcher K (1972) Korrektur-Operation nach kindlichen Verletzungen. Z Kinderchir [Suppl] 11:841–861

Summary: Posttraumatic Deformity of the Growing Skeleton

J. D. Wolf

The differentiated morphologic growth processes that occur in the epiphyses of the pediatric skeleton respond sensitively and at times unpredictably to traumatic insult.

Bone growth may be stimulated or inhibited in response to traumatic and pathologic influences, producing a result that is difficult to assess until the patient approaches skeletal maturity.

The clinical significance of posttraumatic deformity is most apparent in the lower extremity, where deformities directly affect the statics of the spine, hip, knee, and foot.

Recent studies have shown that besides the known ability of anteroposterior and varus/valgus deformities to correct spontaneously, small amounts of *rotational deformity* also have a capacity for spontaneous correction.

Complete stimulative growth disturbances (disturbances that increase overall growth in the epiphyseal plate) can be favorably influenced only by indirect means when there is minimal primary deformity, i.e., by conservative management, by shortening the duration of remodeling, by avoiding delayed reduction maneuvers, and by simplifying any operative measures that are required.

Partial growth disturbances (those affecting a portion of the epiphyseal plate) exacerbate posttraumatic deformity according to the age and sex of the patient and the location and primary displacement of the fracture. The potential for spontaneous recovery during growth may obviate the need for corrective intervention on the one hand, but it can also make treatment more difficult by aiding the progression of deformity. Conflicting hypotheses on posttraumatic corrective mechanisms have been proposed in an effort to explain the spontaneous correction of deformities.

After 12 years of age the potential for spontaneous correction declines sharply, and the presence of unacceptable deformities at this stage is an indication for corrective surgery. Even in patients younger than 12, severe deformities secondary to epiphyseal injuries should be corrected at the earliest possible opportunity, even if additional operations may become necessary in the future. Every corrective operation should be preceded by careful planning based on a thorough clinical evaluation aided by comparative roentgenograms of both extremities and drawings documenting the correction.

Even if clinical function of the extremity appears to be good owing to the unphysiologic position of abnormally loaded joints, the physician is cautioned against taking a wait-and-see approach toward operative intervention.

Corrective Osteotomies of the Lower Extremity
Edited by G. Hierholzer, K. H. Müller

If the result of the correction cannot be adequately stabilized by conservative means, the surgeon should use only a minimum of internal fixation material in the growing skeleton. The implant of choice is the Kirschner wire, which causes negligible growth disturbance even when inserted across epiphyseal plates. Corrective operations on the upper extremity in the region of the wrist and elbow generally will heal well when fixed with Kirschner wires supported by an external plaster dressing. For corrective osteotomies about the hip and knee that are performed close to epihyses, use of the specially designed pediatric hip plate (90° ASIF) may be advised. Particular attention should be given to compression injuries of the distal tibial epiphysis, which often are dismissed as innocuous. Progressive growth disturbances from this injury may necessitate multiple corrective operations on the tibia as well as the fibula to prevent damage to the ankle joint. In this region, which is a "problem area" where soft tissues are concerned, external skeletal fixation may be the most appropriate means of stabilizing the osteotomized bone.

In all corrective operations and especially in operations for length discrepancy, particular concern should be given to the condition of the soft tissues, and established tolerance limits should not be exceeded. Limb lengthenings in excess of 2 cm should be carried out in staged fashion using the Wagner or Müller distraction device. Diaphyseal lengthenings of 10 – 15 mm can be obtained in one stage using compression plates applied over the periosteum.

Posttraumatic deformities of the growing skeleton place very great demands on the treating physician in every respect.

Critical observation and regular follow-up examinations are very helpful in determining the best time for corrective surgery. Thorough clinical examinations and preoperative planning will establish the necessary amount of the correction and the most suitable mode of fixation. The details of the treatment program, which can be quite lengthy, should be thoroughly explained to the parents. This, combined with proper guidance of the juvenile patient, are absolutely essential to a successful outcome. Under no circumstances should deformity be accepted as an inevitable consequence of trauma. If the potential for spontaneous correction in the growing skeleton does not produce an acceptable result, a number of effective operative and conservative procedures are available for treatments of the deformity.

VII. Epilogue

Changing Attitudes toward the Disabled

H. Schadewaldt

There is little of an authoritative nature that a medical historian can say on the subject of Corrective Osteotomies of the Lower Extremity after Trauma, especially when surgery and orthopedics are not his areas of expertise. This fact has prompted me to examine the related issue of changing attitudes toward the physically disabled over the course of history. On the one hand, this frees me from having to deal with complex questions of differential diagnosis in individual cases. On the other, it gives me the opportunity to bring art into the discussion, a subject that has been a lifelong interest and formed the basis of a recent book on surgery in art that was introduced at the 100th meeting of the German Society for Surgery in Berlin in 1983. In my introduction to that book I noted that art and medicine appear at first glance to be contrasting disciplines. An artwork is unique, nonreproducible, individual, and subjective. Aesthetic comparisons, psychoanalytic interpretations, and historical observations can never penetrate to the inner core of the deeply personal process of artistic creation. Always, the value of an artwork is determined by the *percussio*, or impact, that it has upon the observer. Medicine is quite different. Its standards appear to be the objectifiability of its research results, which must be weighable, measurable, comparable and reproducible if they are to be accepted as scientific. Thus, all the qualities that distinguish a work of art – the unique, the individual, the subjective – count for little in medicine and are even regarded with suspicion. Objectivity, general validity, and reproducibility are its postulates.

But a quite different picture emerges when we look at medicine from the standpoint of the patient. For him, disease is a highly individual, nonreproducible and subjective phenomenon. He cares little about subtle diagnostic distinctions and etiologic explanations. His main concern is to be successfully treated, the most spectacular form of this treatment being the surgical operation, which the patient indeed experiences as a unique occurrence. And because artists generally are on the side of the patient or at least the potential patient, they have attempted throughout history to take the patient's point of view, be it in a realistic, caricaturizing, heroizing, or even sarcastic manner. Apparently artists appreciated the social component of disease much earlier than the physicians themselves, sensing the isolation of the sick in society and the difficulty that society has in dealing with persons who are conspicuously ill.

These persons are particularly well exemplified by "the crippled," or physically disabled. Understandably, the very word "cripple" is taken by many as a slur, and it has been largely erased from our vocabulary as "homes for the crippled" have been renamed "orthopedic institutes." This evolution of

Corrective Osteotomies of the Lower Extremity
Edited by G. Hierholzer, K. H. Müller

attitudes and nomenclature is similar to that which has taken place in psychiatry. In both cases society has faced the need to overcome antiquated predjudices toward persons with a conspicuous illness. An important source of the equation of sickness with inferiority was the idealistic philosophers of ancient Greece. None less than Plato charcterized the sick person as a *kakos*, or "defective," especially if he suffers from a chronic illness or permanent disfigurement; for to Plato, complete physical and spiritual health meant unity with the cosmos, a harmony of the body and soul according to the prized concept of *kalokagathia*, meaning the union of beauty with health. Consequently, it was believed that sickness was a negative attribute, and the sick person, especially when lame or disfigured, was viewed with suspicion or contempt because of his persumably unsound character. Plato was even more explicit in his *Republic*, where he states that Asclepius created the art of healing only for the curably and "innocently" sick. The incurably or constitutionally ill, writes Plato, are better left untreated, for treatment would only promote a lengthy invalidism, and neither the sick nor their offspring would be of any use to the state. Rather, the medical art should be reserved for those who can be restored to complete health. It is better for the seriously or chronically ill to work until they die, says Plato, than to lie idly in bed and be a burden to their families, and the physician is advised to "withhold treatment from bodies that are diseased inwardly and throughout."

Plato was not alone in cautioning against treatment of the chronicaly sick. The *Corpus Hippocraticum* contains numerous passages that offer similar counsel. While the guiding principle of *Corpus Hippocraticum* was the "complete elimination of the sufferings of the sick and alleviation of the severity of suffering," the physician is nevertheless advised to "keep away from those who are already overcome by disease."

This attitude persisted until the rise of Christianity, which viewed all men as fellow creatures of God and stressed the virtue of "misericordia" (compassion) toward all, especially the sick and infirm. Indeed, there was a tendency to venerate the suffering and tend meticulously to their needs, giving particular consideration to the lame, who for the Greeks had been an object of contempt.

We can appreciate this change of outlook when we compare Greek mythologic concepts with the essentially human concept of the deity that prevails in Christianity. All peoples have developed concepts of their deities and of the demons who serve or combat them. If animal or plant symbols were originally identified with these powers, the deities tended to assume zooanthrophmorphic forms, as exemplified by the half-human, half-animal gods of ancient Egypt. The early Greek sculptors also represented their gods in animal form, such as the serpentine Zeus Meilichios, the forerunner of Asclepius. Other examples are the harpies and sirens, the spirits who served the gods and who, incidentally, have phocomelic features that somewhat resemble the unfortunate victims of the thalidomide catastrophy. This group might also include Babylonian depictions of unclean spirits, which apparently inspired Christian concepts of the Devil, and whose most conspicuous features where their cloven hooves, which relate directly to our theme. Other artistic representations of disease are known from ancient Egypt. A famous example is the depiction of the "Queen of Punt," who once a year accompanied a procession from the Abyssinian highlands to Egypt to pay tribute to the Pharoah. On an Egyptian relief dating from the Eighteenth Dynasty, roughly between 1500 and 1480 B.C., the Queen Ati is shown following her husband Parihu, who is presenting the Pharoah's emissary with gifts. Ati is pictured quite differently from her husband and their attendants. Large rolls of fat hang from her arms, legs and buttocks, and the lordotic curve of her lumbar spine is greatly exaggerated. Experts have suggested a variety of diagnoses for this curious condition, ranging from rickets and chondrodystrophy to progressive muscular dystrophy and bilateral dislocation of the hips. It is certain, however, that these early representations are pertinent to our consideration of the changing status of the disabled. A similar problem of diagnosis is presented by a sacrificial monument to the goddess Ishtar at he Ny-Carlsberg Museum of Sculpture in Copenhagen, which probably dates from the same period. This stone pillar shows the priest Ruma with an apparent atrophy, shortening and pes equinovarus deformity of the right leg and walking with the aid of a staff, while his wife and son appear completely normal. Suggested diagnoses range from poliomyelitis and infantile paralysis to infantile coxities, making this relief one of the best known depictions of illness from the Egyptian world.

In this context we should also mention Hephaestus, the limping metal-founder of the gods, who has a Germanic counterpart in the legend of Wieland the Blacksmith. Hephaestus, who also practiced surgery as a sideline, was the son of Zeus and Hera. For various offenses he was cast out from Olympus and, in the fall to earth, sustained severe foot injuries which crippled him for life. In another account Hephaestus was born lame, and because his two sons, the club-wielding Perphetes and Palaemon, were also lame, it is suggested that a clubfoot may have been the model for this legend. Because of his deformity, which rendered him unfit for other services, Hephaestus devoted himself to the art of metal forging under the earth and became the god of smithery and fire. The respected Austrian medical historian, Edwin Rosner, suggests that Hephaestus actually was a victim of lead and arsenic poisoning, which once was a fairly common ailment among mineworkers and often is accompanied by symptoms of paralysis in the lower extremities.

It is often speculated that the god of medicine, Asclepius, was himself a cripple, for he is always shown holding the staff of Aesculapius, which he lays aside only when sitting. This would be consistent with the selection of Asclepius as the heavenly patron of the sick and those seeking a cure. A marked difference in godly attributes becomes apparent when we consider the wand of his colleague Hermes, a heroldic staff with two entwined snakes, which unfortunately was adopted as the insignia of the U. S. Army Medical Corps, even though Hermes/Mercury was not only the god of merchants and thieves but also the guide to Hades for departed souls – not the most fortunate symbol for a physician!

I mentioned earlier that the rise of Christianity brought with it a new attitude toward mankind, especially with regard to the chronically sick. In fairness, however, it should be noted that stoic philosophers had already postulated a new ideal of humanity some time before. Seneca, who was not a Christian but lived in the 1st century A.D., stressed that *homo res sacra homini*, or "man is sacred to man." Earlier, in the 2nd century B.C., the physician Serapion described his ideal colleague as follows: "The physician must first heal his own son and help himself; then, like a god, he will equally be savior of poor man and slave, of rich man and ruler, and will to all be a brother." Scribonius Largus, who was a Christian, stated in the 1st century A.D. that "The physician must have a heart full of compassion and love of mankind" (*plenus miserecordia et humanitatis animus*), for "the healing art takes no notice of the person, but promises help equally to all those who seek it." This placed those previously regarded as incurable into the category of those worthy of treatment.

The motto of Seneca, *non deformiate corporis foedari animum, se pulchritudinae animi corpus ornari* ("ugliness of the body does not harm the soul, but a beautiful soul ennobles the body"), also became the guiding principle of the new Christian anthropology. Particular concern was given to the aged, sick and infirm, a typical example being the veneration that was enjoyed by Hermanus Contractus the Lame, from the island of Reichenau, both during his life and for many centuries thereafter. Born in 1013, Hermanus was severely crippled from childhood. His pupil Berthold wrote:

By the cruelty of nature, he was so crippled and disfigured in all his limbs that he was unable to move from the place where he was set down. Any activity was done only with the greatest effort... Yet this miserable body was tenanted by a matchless spirit and a will of strength that was beyond all measure.

Hermanus Contractus was a Benedictine monk at the cloister of Reichenau, where he worked both as a scholar and as a great composer of hymns until the age of 42, when death freed him from his physical suffering. His antiphons "Slave regina" and "Alma redemptoris mater" are still sung in cloisters and Catholoic churches.

But while many disabled persons enjoyed an increase in social prestige, others did not. Many had to continue their existence as wandering, mendicant cripples, and artists throughout the centuries have called attention to their catastrophic social situation while appealing to the benevolence and Christian charity of their unafflicted environment. A book by Hans Wurtz, published in 1932 and titled *Throw Away Your Crutches. The Plight of the Crippled, the Stepchildren of all Ages and Peoples, in Words and Pictures*, makes reference to 2502 artworks and 779 literary works and remains unsurpassed in its broad depiction of the historical plight of the handicapped. Wurtz also compared the two Biblical concepts of the Redeemer – one envisioning Him as sick and afflicted, and the other as an idealized image of the coming Messiah. While Isaiah 53:3 tells us:

He was despised and rejected by men; a man full of pain and sickness; and as one from whom men hide their faces he was despised, and we esteemed him not.

we read in Isaiah 63:1:

...he that is glorious in his apparel, marching in the greatness of his strength.

The artistic representations of the crippled are far removed from this second apotheosis, and even if we direct our attention to the rendering of diagnoses, we cannot help but pity the misery of those who are afflicted in this way. Today as before, the largest numbers of cripples become so because of accidents or war wounds, and these have attracted the greatest attention of artists. A wealth of drawings and paintings depict persons who have suffered leg amputations or have been otherwise maimed such that they must rely on more or less makeshift crutches for locomotion. An especially poignant image is that of the cripple hobbling along on a cane, which was widely regarded as a social indictment of their merciless environment. For artists of all periods, mendicant cripples and especially disabled war veterans have served as a symbol of the ingratitude of their fellow men, who sent these victims of senseless conflicts into battle with cheers and brass bands, but turned their backs on them when they returned home as crippled veterans. The 19th-Century Italian artist Preciosi gave us masterly portrayals of the war-injured veteran, though even he observed that the hordes of those truly deserving of sympathy included a number of malingerers who feigned war injuries in an attempt to arouse the pity of passersby. Of course congenital malformations, such as clubfoot, have also been widely represented in art, as have certain acquired infectious diseases such as tuberculosis and tuberculous arthritis, rheumatoid arthritis, which once was a common source of grotesque deformity, and tabes, which produced paralytic symptoms such as hemiplegia. Rickets and beriberi also were a common source of lameness before they were recognized as being vitamin deficiency diseases. And we must not forget a paralytic disease that today is all but extinct in North America and Europe, leprosy. By destroying nerve pathways, the form known as tuberculoid leprosy often led to bizarre contractures which rendered the patient unable to walk and relegated him to the status of beggar or prompted his isolation in a leprosarium.

Regardless of whether the reaction elicited by the depictions of these illnesses was contemptuous or charitable, medical treatment prior to the 1800's was limited to the production of more or less customized canes and cruthches that gave the disabled at least a passable form of locomotion. It was not until the 19th Century, with the advent of orthopedic surgery (though still without benefit of anesthesia and antisepsis) that significant advances were made in the management of these cases. German surgeons in particular, most notably Dieffenbach, Karl Ferdinand von Graefe, and the true founder of German orthopedics, Jakob von Heine, were instrumental in breaking new ground and greatly improving the prognoses of these patients. As mentioned previously, it was the change from the "cripple" mentality to modern operative treatment methods and the turning away from conservative prosthetics that brought significant improvements in patient care and gave this discipline the status of a full-fledged surgical specialization. Fifty years later the slogan of Hans Wurtz, "Throw away your crutches," has become a reality. Many persons who, even since World War II, have had to live as unfortunate victims of war wounds or traffic accidents have been able to discard their rutches after successful surgery and take their place in society as normal, i.e. unobtrusive citizens. But even for patients who still must rely on orthopedic aids in their daily lives, far better options are available today than begging on street corners. Through social activism on behalf of the handicapped, public awareness has been directed to the necessity of special access ramps, lavatories, telephones and other facilities which, though grudgingly accepted by some, have nevertheless greatly improved the quality of life for this segment of our population.

This symposium, dedicated to corrective osteotomies of the traumatized lower extremity, attests to the significant progress that medicine and presumably humanity as well have made in this area. And while the historian is reluctant to use the word "progress" because he knows that much that was touted as progress in the past subsequently failed to enrich medical science, I believe that this word is well considered and justified when used in reference to the life's work of Jörg Rehn. Under his direction, the Bergmannsheil Clinic in Bochum has become one of the leading trauma centers in Europe, and it is due largely to the initiative of Prof. Rehn that spectacular operations have been performed there and cases that appeared hopeless have gone on to recovery. For this, Prof. Rehn, you have earned not only the thanks of this assembly, which is in any case assured, but also the recognition of the many patients whom you have treated and cared for in the course of your academic career.

Subject Index

FSC
www.fsc.org
MIX
Papier aus verantwortungsvollen Quellen
Paper from responsible sources
FSC® C105338

If you have any concerns about our products,
you can contact us on
ProductSafety@springernature.com

In case Publisher is established outside the EU,
the EU authorized representative is:
Springer Nature Customer Service Center GmbH
Europaplatz 3, 69115 Heidelberg, Germany

Printed by Libri Plureos GmbH
in Hamburg, Germany